DENISE AUSTIN

A FIRESIDE BOOK

Published

by

Simon

&

Schuster

J U   P S   T

JUMPSTART

THE 21 DAY PLAN

to Lose Weight,
Get Fit,
and
Increase
Your Energy
and
Enthusiasm
for Life

FIRESIDE
Rockefeller Center
1230 Avenue of the Americas
New York, NY 10020

Copyright © 1996 by Denise Austin
All rights reserved, including the right of reproduction
in whole or in part in any form.

First Fireside Edition 1998

FIRESIDE and colophon are registered trademarks of Simon & Schuster Inc.

DESIGNED BY BARBARA MARKS

Photos pages 182–248 by Mary Noble Ours; photo page 8 by Bernard Boudreau;
photos pages 18, 93, and 302–17 by Diane Walker; photo page 63 by David West;
photo page 101 by Rafael Fuchs.
All other photos property of Denise Austin or used by permission.

Manufactured in the United States of America

1 3 5 7 9 10 8 6 4 2

The Library of Congress has cataloged the Simon & Schuster edition as follows:

Austin, Denise.
    Jumpstart : the 21-day plan to lose weight, get fit, and increase your
energy and enthusiasm for life / Denise Austin.
        p.   cm.
    1. Weight loss.   2. Physical fitness.   3. Health.   I. Title.
RM222.A97   1996
613.2'5—dc20   95-43279   CIP

ISBN 0-684-80220-1
ISBN 0-684-82698-4 (Pbk)

To Jeff,
Kelly, and Katie,
who jumpstart my life
every day
with their love.

ACKNOWLEDGMENTS

I am so grateful to my mom, whose love and endless dedication to us kids made my childhood so happy and filled with such life. And to my dad, for teaching me that the harder you work, the luckier you get. And to my wonderful grandmother, who gave me the gift of faith that will always be with me and will continue through my family.

To all my sisters and my brother, who are my best supporters and are always so proud.

Without my husband, Jeff, I would not have the true freedom to live this dream. As my grandmother used to say to me, "Your marriage is made in heaven." I've always believed it. Thank you, Jeff, for so much, especially our two precious girls, and your constant support, great humor, and real love and respect. Most people don't get this much happiness in a lifetime! I love you and I'm so grateful.

I want to thank Bob Asahina of Simon & Schuster, who made it all happen. And thanks to Jan Miller, my literary agent, for believing in me. Also, thanks to Sarah Pinckney, my editor at Simon & Schuster, who was a joy to work with.

Special thanks to Steve Kostorowski, who helped "shape" this book. And to Moira McGinty Klos, who "organized" so much. And to Cal Pozo, my ultimate "sounding board." Also, thanks to Laurin Morgan, who spent countless hours on the computer.

Thank you, Colleen Pierre, registered dietician, for your help with planning nutritious meals. And many thanks to all who contributed recipes, especially Rita Calvert, Carmen Lewis Goddin, and my dear friend Betsy Volkert.

There have been so many people who have helped "form" my career. Thanks to my close friend Marijane Levee for her P. R. intellect. Many thanks to all my friends at ESPN for giving me ten great years on TV (and hopefully more). And there's a special place in my heart for Paul Fireman, who believed in me from the start! I also want to thank everyone at P.P.I., my video company, especially Donald Kasen and Shelly Rudin. And thanks to all my friends at Spalding.

I have so many good friends professionally and socially that have truly helped me in some way that I know I have left out. But you know who you are . . . and thank you.

CONTENTS

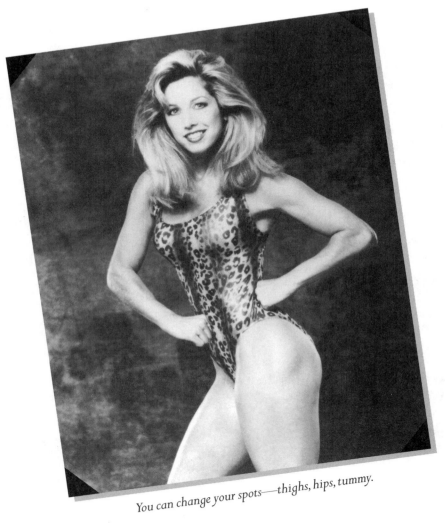

You can change your spots—thighs, hips, tummy.

Dear Denise,

I am thirty-six years old and I weigh 187 pounds. I've been fat my whole life. I just had my third child and my stomach and hips have never looked this bad. Sometimes I don't want to get up in the morning because I hate the way I look. I'm so depressed. Can you help me?

——Joyce, Little Rock, Arkansas

Dear Denise,

I can't stand the way I look. I've gained so much weight and have gotten so loose that I close my eyes while getting into the shower so I don't have to see myself in the mirror. You probably want to know why I don't do something about it if I'm so disgusted, right? You've probably heard this before, but I don't have time for a workout. My drive to work is an hour and a half each way. To avoid traffic I go in early and stay late. Moving isn't an option right now because of my husband's job. When the weekend comes, I'm too tired to move, and, anyway, I know two days isn't enough to do any good. I've tried every diet in the world but nothing has worked. My husband says I'm beautiful but I know he doesn't mean it. He can't! On the rare occasions that I've been home during the week I've seen you on ESPN. You seemed so nice that I decided to write for help. I'm really feeling down. Any suggestions?

——Rosa, San Bernadino, California

i, I'm Denise Austin! Do you recognize yourself in these letters? Then, honey, *keep on reading!!*

9

I receive more than 600 letters every week from people all over the country asking me for advice. People not only want to share their weight concerns with me, but also wonder how they can find and harness the energy missing from their lives. They ask me what I eat, how I have so much energy, how I always stay "up," how I flattened my tummy after a baby, how to get rid of cellulite in the thighs, and, of course, how old I am. Now I have the chance to offer my best advice in this one complete book: *JumpStart!*

I want your body, your mind, your heart and soul for 21 consecutive days. Let me show you how to jump-start into a new you. I want to change your body. I want to empower your mind with positive energy. I want to improve the quality of your life. I will provide you with all you need to lose weight, all you need for a healthier, more energetic life, in 21 days!

Please don't misinterpret the name *JumpStart*. Yes, it is set up so that you'll see results quickly. But in reality we are redesigning your lifestyle, how you eat, and how you feel both physically and mentally. This is a process, a way of life, and a new way of thinking that never ends. This is not a diet. Yes, you will lose weight. But it is a way of living. As a matter of fact, did you know that the word *diet* comes from the Greek *diaita* and means "a manner of living"? Living, that's it! Not starving, not suffering, not denying. That's why I believe in *eating.* Eating is essential to keep your metabolism and energy up. I never miss a meal, and neither should you. And it is what you eat in those meals that's important. I eat healthily 80 percent of the time and absolutely crummy junk food 20 percent of the time. And I don't feel guilty. I love food. It is for both health and enjoyment. Everything in moderation!

As a fitness professional for over 17 years, I have learned that you don't have to exercise that much to enjoy tremendous health benefits. All you need is five minutes here and there in a day to accumulate 30 minutes of activity. It could be 10 minutes of walking, 10 minutes of toning—like squats while you're blow-drying your hair—and 10 minutes of stretching. I am here to tell you that I only exercise 30 minutes a day. You too will learn that exercise speeds up your metabolism, making you feel more energetic, and I will make exercise just as easy a part of your day as brushing your teeth!

The number one excuse I hear is "I don't have the time to exercise." Well, you'll learn in this book that you'll never have to use that excuse again. I will give you several different exercise routines that range from 5 minutes to 30 minutes. I will give you exercises you can do in a hurry. I will even show you exercises like a tummy tightener that you can do while stuck in traffic and a buttocks firmer while in line at the grocery store. You will see that you don't need to have a block of time, a lavish home gym, or belong to an expensive club, in order to get fit. You can do it right there in the privacy of your own home.

Exercising regularly is one of the most positive habits you can develop. It can and will change your entire life! I have listened to thousands of people and to their weight-loss stories, especially their successful ones. (You will read about them in this book.) And one thing that has been proven to me, over and over, is that the real problem is not just food, not just lack of time, not just lack of know-how, not just lack of family support, and not just lack of energy and will. The real problem lies in *bad habits* that block, time and time again, any resolution you make to improve your body.

The underlying element, the key ingredient, behind every successful weight loss story is the ability to abandon old eating and exercise habits and replace them with new *positive habits.*

All the success, good health, energy, happiness, and peace of mind I have enjoyed are directly related to *positive habits.* These are nothing more than simple changes we make in our daily choices. When a positive change in your life becomes routine and pleasurable, then a new habit is born. *Positive habits* will improve the quality of your life because they funnel down into your relationships, your energy level and self-confidence, and your ability to succeed in getting what you want out of life. The basis of my philosophy of *positive habits* is that there are major areas in our lives that we can control and master. They are your *attitude,* your *eating habits,* and your *exercise habits.*

I will teach you the formula with which to govern each day with successful small changes that will eventually grow into new *positive habits.* Let me help you replace bad habits with healthy new ones. These *positive habits* are the principles, or laws, that you should follow to create lifelong changes. *Positive habits* don't happen overnight.

Behavioral scientists now agree with a theory originally introduced by Benjamin Franklin, who believed that it took 21 days of concentrated repetition of an activity for it to become a permanent habit in your life. Studies have proven that just three weeks of constant practice can alter your current behavior. You can, and will, change the way you eat, the way you feel about exercise, and the way you see yourself by changing personal habits, negative ones, that have gotten you to where you are right now: probably not too happy with the way you look and feel about yourself.

The 21 Day JumpStart Plan is designed to be the framework for eating well, exercising regularly, and thinking positively:

Week 1—Your body adjusts to the initial change (detoxifies).

Week 2—The body begins to respond and function better.

Week 3—The results are noticeable.

"Sure, Denise," some of you might now be saying. "Change a lifetime of eating and exercise habits in twenty-one days? Are you crazy? That's impossible!"

No, I'm not crazy, nor is it impossible. We are all creatures of habit, and I also know that no one is going to do away with a lifetime of habits in twenty-one days. What I am saying is that in twenty-one days I will give you, day by day, all my secrets and easy tips for how you, too, can transform your current bad habits into positive ones. I will give you the blueprint to a healthier way of life.

Fitness Is Not a Fad.

It's a Lifestyle!

My 21 Day JumpStart Plan is just that: a jump start. It's a way for you to fire up. Get you going on the right track. Psych you up. A road paved with positive tools and techniques that will help you glide to success. You know down deep inside that the best way to set yourself up for success is to follow a plan, a blueprint. A blueprint provides all of the detailed information a builder requires before beginning construction. It literally eliminates all guesswork. Everyone needs a plan—a fresh start; something to ignite them, something in front of them that gives all the information they need. That's just what I'm giving you: all the essentials that have led to successful changes in the way people ate, exercised, and conducted their lives.

I can say that this book is the culmination of all my seventeen years of experience in the fitness business. It contains all the tools, techniques, and ideas I have learned and shared throughout my career. It contains all the information you need to lose weight in twenty-one days and beyond.

This book is divided into three parts. Part I, "Getting Started;" Part II, "The 21 Day JumpStart Plan," which includes "Healthy Recipes"; and Part III, "Keeping It Off."

Part I, "Getting Started," is just that: It gets you on the right track to begin your 21 day plan. These chapters target your attitude, your physical activity and your eating habits. While I've always said that exercise is the key to a lean, firm body, maintaining a regular exercise schedule is hard without a positive mental attitude. I will teach you ways to improve your self-esteem, increase your self-worth, and improve the way you feel about yourself.

Part II contains the 21 Day JumpStart Plan. Years of professional experience helping and motivating people to exercise regularly and eat healthily have gone into the 21 Day JumpStart Plan. Everything thousands of women have told me in their letters about weight-loss success has been considered and included in designing this plan. I've left nothing out: What you need to do to get yourself to think positively, your body to be fit and firm, and your taste buds to feel satisfied, never deprived. The JumpStart

Plan comes complete with detailed daily menus featuring tasty low-fat recipes that will take 15 minutes or less to prepare. I have even supplied you with a grocery shopping list so you can start each week with everything you need for healthy eating.

Increasing your physical activity level is an important part of the 21 Day JumpStart Plan. I have designed two different workouts for each day with photographs and detailed instructions. There's Denise's Daily Dose, a five-minute routine designed to start your day, to stretch and tone your body from head to toe. It's your minimum daily requirement workout. The Activity Menu includes aerobic and muscle toning exercises on alternating days that start with just a few minutes each day and, over the days, build up to 30 minutes of aerobic and 20 minutes of toning exercises.

And, of course, there's my Daily Deniseology. People always ask me, "Denise, where do you get all that energy?" "How can I stay up all the time?" "What's the secret to your success and your positive outlook on everything?" The answers to these and many other questions regarding positive attitude and self-esteem are found in "Deniseology," personal stories that will give you insights into my theories on positive attitudes. Each story is filled with positive messages that will inspire and motivate you to think "I can do it," "I am worth it."

Also included are Healthy Recipes, featuring the recipes found in your daily menus. You might be surprised to find some family favorites that I have been able to include by decreasing fat content, like French toast, pizza, tacos, and even a turkey burger! I have counted the calories and fat grams, and each recipe will take no more than 15 minutes to prepare. The appendix includes In-a-Hurry Recipes, ones you can count on for quick and healthy dinners, plus a list of healthy sandwiches for lunch. A section entitled Food Lists contains many low-fat choices for snacks, breads, dairy products, condiments, and so on, and even desserts!

Part III, "Keeping It Off," is your reference guide. The information in its chapters will further help you to continue on your way to improve your body, your mind, and your eating habits. You didn't think I was going to leave you hanging after twenty-one days, did you? In Part III, I have included everything you ever wanted to know about sex—not really!—fitness. It covers everything from what to order at restaurants to tips on walking, to special back exercises to working out with weights. I'll tell you how to give added time and concentration to those troublesome spots: tummy, hips, thighs, and buttocks, and twenty In-a-Hurry exercises you can do anywhere, even in the office. In Chapter 14, "Babies, Business, and Biceps," I will share with you my personal philosophy as to how to balance your family and career and squeeze in a little time to take care of yourself. Part III is all about maintaining your healthy habits. You've got to keep it

Optimism gets people in motion and gives them a JumpStart. Optimism is the magical way to be healthy.

13

going to be fit for life. And remember, knowledge is positive power, and in Part III you will find a wealth of additional positive reinforcement and motivation.

This is not another diet book. What distinguishes this program from others you may have tried in the past is that it can be followed not only for the three weeks it takes to start looking and feeling better, *but for the rest of your life.*

This is a book about attitude. *Your attitude* about your life, your body, and *who you are.* It is a book about total fitness: heart, body, and mind. And it is about taking care of you, first and foremost, so that you have the energy and self-confidence to handle all that life demands as the wife, the mother, the housekeeper, the cook, the chauffeur, the daughter, the employee, the friend . . . the multitalented, multifaceted, unique and beautiful woman that is *the one and only you.*

I know that each and every one of us has the potential to reach beyond our current boundaries and to achieve new goals. I believe strongly that every "body" can do it. *You deserve to look and feel great and live better,* and this book is your way to achieve those goals.

Over the next 21 days and beyond, you and I are going to develop a great, close relationship. From the minute you wake up in the morning to the time you go to bed, I'll be with you. I will be your own personal trainer, your motivator, and your coach. I have taken all the hassles out of the way so that you can concentrate on the most important person in the world. *You.*

JumpStart is working for thousands of people. They are losing weight, losing inches and, most of all, they are feeling better about themselves. Now you can do it too!

> *I can't believe the difference in only three weeks. I am so proud of myself. I lost ten pounds and thirteen inches.*
>
> —*Vicky, Cincinnati, Ohio*

> *I'm ecstatic. I lost three inches in my waistline in only three weeks. And I ate more food than I was used to. Thanks, Denise.*
>
> —*Diane, Fort Worth, Texas*

> *"You have only one life to live. This is not a dress rehearsal. It's the real thing."*
>
> —DENISE AUSTIN

PART I

GETTING STARTED

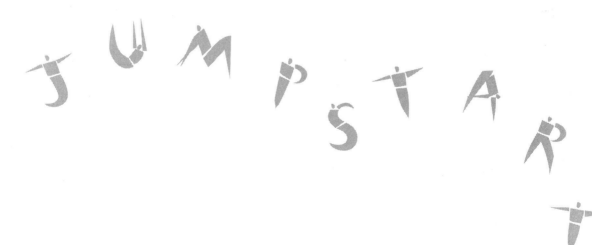

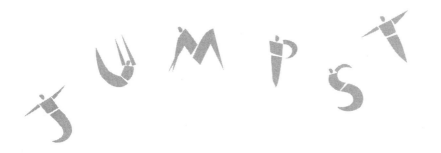

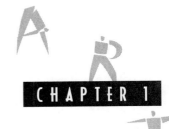

CHAPTER 1

FULL ESTEEM AHEAD!

Dear Denise,

I was diagnosed with multiple sclerosis ten years ago. I found your exercise program on ESPN two years ago and I am so thankful. You are so encouraging! "Just do the best you can do," saved me from becoming a chubby, immobile person. I've gone from a size 14 to a size 9 and I have more energy than I ever thought possible. I'm forty-seven years old and I feel like a new person. I've gone from 5 minutes of exercise a few times a week to 30 minutes every day. Thank you for such an encouraging, informative, sensible and sensitive program that really works. God bless you and keep up the great programs! —*Margot, Fontana, California*

Dear Denise,

I don't know how to express my appreciation for what you have done for me. Through your motivation, I've lost 43 pounds and have never felt better. I never thought I could do it, but somehow you knew, even when I doubted myself. Although I'm thirty years old, in some ways I feel like my life is just beginning. Yesterday I went to the beach and actually played in the water, wearing a bathing suit for the first time since I was a little girl. It was so much fun! The truth is everything seems to be fun these days—even exercise and low-fat eating! Thank you for all your help. I'm a real fan. —*Kathleen, Ocean City, New Jersey*

Most of you know me from my daily TV show on ESPN, *Getting Fit,* which aired for ten years (now I can be seen weekdays on Lifetime TV's *Denise Austin's Daily Workout*); my exercise videos; or my appearances at QVC or from seeing me on NBC's *Today Show;* or in magazines and newspaper articles. I have been a fitness professional for over seventeen years. In addition, I have proudly served as a consultant to the President's Council on Physical Fitness and Sports for twelve years, but of greater importance is the fact that I'm just like you.

I am not a health nut, a fitness addict, or the fat police. I work hard to have a fulfilling career; be an attentive, loving wife; raise two beautiful children; maintain a home that at least passes for clean; attempt some semblance of a social life; support my community and church; and carve out at least a couple of minutes for me. And yes, you are reading it here first, sometimes I am too lazy to exercise and eat like a pig!! There are days when I say "to heck with it" and collapse on the couch with a bag of chips! But those occasions do not last too long, since ultimately I know how much better I feel and how much more energy I have when I include regular exercise and healthy foods into my daily routine. To be honest, being fit is the only way I can keep up with the hectic pace of life!

I am the wife of Jeff Austin, a sports attorney representing professional athletes. He is the most wonderful, supportive husband in the whole world. I am the mother of two beautiful, healthy, energetic little girls (Kelly Angela, five, and Katherine Reed—we call her Katie—two). I am also a housekeeper, car pool driver, sister, daughter, and friend.

I grew up Denise Katnich in southern California in a big Catholic family, the middle child of four sisters and one brother. I do come from an athletic family. My dad played professional baseball (St. Louis Browns Organization, '46–'47) and my mom was a jump-rope champion (high school), but out of five kids I was the only one who made a career out of it. I have been active since I was a kid. When I was five, I couldn't wait to do cartwheels across the dance floor after a ballet class. At eleven, I was trampolining away at the local Y. At twelve, I took gymnastics classes after school. At fourteen, I was enthusiastically putting in five hours a day, five days a week with a gymnastics team. I won lots of awards competing both nationally and internationally, and was offered twenty-one college athletic scholarships. I chose the University of Arizona, then transferred to California State University, Long Beach, from which I graduated with a bachelor of arts degree. My area of study was exercise physiology in the physical education department.

After graduation, in 1979, I started my own company in Los Angeles, setting up fitness programs at corporations and health clubs. I trained twenty-five instructors who then taught for me at the different places I set up. It was about this time that a new buzz word was floating around—aerobics. Very few people actually knew what aerobics was. Since I had just graduated from college, I was at the forefront of fitness and knew all about it. I was there, in Los Angeles, right where it all began! Here I was, a specialist in the field, with a background in gymnastics from childhood. I went at aerobics with gusto. I worked day and night to become the best in my field, but I loved every minute of it! Then, in 1981, Jack LaLanne gave me my first start in television: I became the co-host of his TV show with his wife, Elaine LaLanne.

From that point on I became a fitness expert, demonstrating and lecturing all over the country, and appearing on national talk shows like *Merv Griffin* and *Hour Magazine*. In 1982, I got my own show on KABC in Los Angeles, *DayBreak LA,* which aired five days a week at five thirty every morning. It was then that I started to receive letters from viewers telling me that I was really making a difference in their lives. My grandmother had been right. She always told me that God had given me the gift of being able to touch people, that my exuberance was contagious. I knew I could put a smile on people's faces. The truth is, I really believe in people and that they have the power to change their lives. But it was through the TV show that I first knew I was motivating and inspiring people to get off the couch and exercise with me right there in the privacy and convenience of their own homes.

In 1982, I met Jeff Austin while I was setting up an aerobics studio at a tennis club where he and his sister Tracy Austin were practicing. A year later, we were married. Right after the wedding, Jeff accepted a position as a sports attorney for a

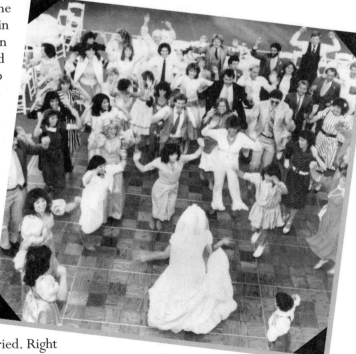

Leading aerobics, even on my wedding day, in a gown and all . . .

Washington, D.C.-based sports-management firm. It was a great opportunity for him so I encouraged the move, even though it meant I would have to give up my TV show and everything I had worked for.

You would have thought I would have wallowed in self-pity. And yes, I did for a few days. But not for long. I turned it around and made it a challenge. I knew my goal: a national TV show. After hundreds of phone calls, resumes, letters (you name it!), persistence paid off. I finally got hold of NBC's *Today Show*'s executive producer, and I pitched my idea to him. At that time no one had ever done a regular fitness segment on television. He said he would give me one chance. In 1984, I appeared for the first time on the show. Within a week, I received over ten thousand letters. I got a four-year contract! I succeeded because I truly believed in myself.

In 1987, I finally got my own national show, *Getting Fit with Denise Austin*, shown daily on ESPN. I had always dreamed of having a trim-and-travel show, one in which people could exercise with me in some of the most beautiful places in the world. After ten years, it is viewed in eighty-two countries. Imagine, in America alone, over a million people exercise with me every day on Lifetime TV's *Denise Austin's Daily Workout*. In addition to filming my show, I was able to produce and choreograph two videos a year. Today, I have over twenty different videos ranging from step aerobics to TrimWalk to workouts for pregnant women to my latest Hit the Spot series. Through relentless energy and hard work, I am proud to say I have sold over five million copies. From all my fan letters and knowing more people wanted to work out in their homes, I took the initiative to develop my signature line of home exercise equipment. I take great pride in placing my name on this, since it all evolved from your letters. I'm constantly developing new products to help you on the road to fitness.

As you can see, my story is one of persistence and determination. It all came from within. My parents were always encouraging me but never pushing me. My mom was way too busy raising five young kids on her own (my parents divorced when I was eight). Nothing was handed to me. I worked to succeed. Failing many times. Bouncing back. Succeeding. And ultimately, believing in myself. I am here to tell you not that I did it, but that if I can do it, *you can, too.* Of course, I have bad days. There are days I look in the mirror and I see huge thighs and in more recent years the changes in my body due to childbearing, or lines around my eyes that weren't there in my twenties.

And whenever the least bit of self-pity or dissatisfaction creeps in, I will teach you how to reflect on your blessings, how to keep on track with motivation, and I will give you positive "self talk." A positive attitude reflects how you feel about yourself and how you perceive the way you look. I will teach you how to adopt a healthier lifestyle by making changes in the way you think and therefore act regarding yourself, exercise, and food.

JumpStart focuses on three areas of life: These areas are *mental attitude, positive eating habits,* and *positive exercise habits.* These three elements, no matter if you're trying to lose weight, improve your sex life, or just want to feel better, are key to jump-starting your quality of life. We all need a place to start. Here's your chance to begin today with a clean slate, a fresh start. . . . Plus we all need a plan, some type of structured blueprint, to be successful.

Developing a Positive Mental Attitude

For each of the 21 days you will begin your day with a Deniseology, which is a daily positive reinforcement tool. These tips, thoughts, and motivational techniques lead toward a healthy mind as well as a healthy body. Each of the 21 days will have its own theme so you can focus on a particular aspect in your life. Some examples of topics I talk to you about in my Deniseologies are how to have a positive attitude, how to gain enthusiasm, how to improve your confidence level, and how to lift your spirits. All these optimistic viewpoints are components of my formula for creating happiness and joy in all facets of your life.

Without positive reinforcement, changes in habits and attitudes are difficult, if not impossible, to make. I'll be there for you every day for twenty-one days, talking to you and urging you to keep going, so that you will look ahead toward a new, happier you. Every morning before breakfast, you'll start with a Deniseology story and positive reinforcement thought that will be your thought of the day. You know life is so busy and hectic and we often don't take the time to "nourish" our souls. So each day we will reflect on selected thoughts to enjoy with a little happiness and encouragement as you go along. Take the clutter out of your head and I'll fill it with new inspiration and put a positive attitude into your spirit. Repetition is one of the greatest tools in making habitual changes. Believe me, you may say to yourself "I can't do it," a negative reinforcement that will get you nowhere, but you can as easily keep telling yourself "I can do it," a positive reinforcement that will get you where you want to go every time, all the time. You are going to learn how to increase your self-worth, improve your self-esteem, and wake up each day to a new vitality and zest for life. You are going to discover the energy inside you. . . . Believe me, it will come out! Think of Deniseology as my way to keep you motivated and on track . . . like your own personal motivator.

You have to change old bad habits into positive new habits. I know of no better way to motivate you to make those changes than by first letting you meet, through their letters and pictures, some of the many people who have already changed their bodies and their lives with my 21 Day JumpStart Plan.

Developing Positive Eating Habits

While Deniseology will feed your brain with positive reinforcement, my twenty-one day meal plan will feed your body with fabulous food. I have created a program that teaches you techniques to not only help you lose weight but also keep it off for life. *Food is fabulous. Eating is essential.* You will eat three meals a day, plus snacks and even dessert, and still lose weight. Yes, I eat. As a matter of fact, I never miss a meal and neither should you. No more yo-yo dieting. No more starving.

The JumpStart eating plan is designed to make it easy for you to eat well, with low-fat recipes that are plentiful, tasty and so easy to prepare they take 15 minutes or less. Fully planned menus, including breakfast, lunch, dinner, and snacks are provided for each day. I have counted all the calories and calculated all the fat grams. Each day your calories will come from three meals and two snacks, totalling between 1,350 and 1,500 calories, with 30 grams of fat (that is, 20 percent of calories from fat). All these recipes are healthy, quick, and simple to make.

My JumpStart eating plan will never dip below 1300 calories per day, so your metabolism stays high. Go ahead. I know you're dying to look at them. Check out the menus and you'll see that you are eating real food, that you are not on a fad diet. I'm giving you new liberty to eat! Enjoy!

Developing Positive Exercise Habits

Think of yourself as the *architect* of your body. By the way you sit, by the way you stand, you design the overall framework of your body. Let me explain: Muscles are like modeling clay, and their shape is determined by the way you form them. If you're sitting there right now, slumped over, your tummy has nowhere else to go but out. But if you sit up nice and tall, your tummy has a place to stay—tucked in.

Here is a pop question: Which do you think would be more effective to flatten your stomach: pulling in your tummy throughout the day, or doing 500 sit-ups? The answer is pulling in your tummy throughout the day, and here's why. Imagine there are sixteen waking hours of the day that you can train your abdominal muscles, versus five minutes of sit-ups. Don't get me wrong, sit-ups are effective. But think of how much faster you'll get that flat stomach when you become *aware* of those muscles constantly during every waking hour. The first step toward becoming your own architect—and getting a rock-hard tummy!—is to think about good posture. Good posture is critical to how you feel and how you look. Sitting up straight (the average person sits for over seven-and-a-half hours a day!)

opens up the chest and gives you maximum potential to bring in fresh oxygen, which in return gives you *more energy*. Now look at yourself. How are you sitting right this minute? *Sit up straight.* There. In two seconds you have tremendously improved your appearance. You look more confident and I'll bet you look 10 pounds thinner.

A rock-hard tummy has been my trademark for years. I have had more people than I can count feel my tummy—everyone from Bryant Gumbel to Phil Donahue to Regis and Kathie Lee, Dustin Hoffman to Martina Navratilova to David Robinson to Colin Powell to CEOs all over the world, even the then-President of the United States, George Bush. It is through a combination of good posture and sit-ups—being my own architect—that I have been able to maintain my rock-hard tummy—even after having two kids!

Remember, *you* completely control the outward appearance of your body. The general features and inherent chemistry are genetic. Your bony framework and your skeleton you cannot change. Your parents gave you that. But yes, you *can* change your muscles. You have over 640 muscles in your body that you can reshape and tone, and as these muscles adapt to your new positive exercise habits, they will become strong and firm. So how you sit, stand, and move are completely up to you.

How you carry yourself, your posture, your mannerisms, and the way you speak and respond to others: All of this communicates *your attitude!* According to *Webster's Dictionary,* an architect is "one who plans and achieves an objective." That is what we are doing here: planning to achieve the objective of living life to the maximum with a healthy body and a healthy mind every day!

The two biggest barriers that keep people from exercise are time and a negative feeling about themselves. You might feel that it's hard to picture yourself out there exercising and you might have this image of how you will look and how you will fit in. For instance, you're not comfortable with your present appearance and/or size. You're embarrassed by your level of physical condition—you huff and puff climbing up a flight of stairs. And maybe, you think you're too old (you're never too old to start exercising). But, I'm here to let you know you need to break down these barriers. Forget about any stereotyping, because that perception is what is holding you back from feeling the best you can! I'm going to get you to move past that self-protective and incompetent feeling. I can offer you a chance to improve your self-esteem and I hope I can give you the assurance to become fit and happy within yourself. Remember that every person in my book who has lost from 10 to 180 pounds first lost one pound. *You can do it now!*

You know that with every hour that passes throughout the day, a woman's time gets gobbled up by other commitments. Unless you absolutely can't function in the early morning (you'll never know unless you give it a try), I suggest taking the half-hour before your day usually begins and make it your own. If the word *exercise* doesn't sit well quite yet, think of it as taking a walk to organize your thoughts. Or better yet, get a friend or two and turn it into a fast-paced gab session! Remember, the half-hour is going to pass anyway. You can either be done with it or think about it for the rest of the day.

I personally work out Monday through Friday because it fits into an already structured schedule. Everything is regimented during the work-week anyhow. All I do is get up 30 minutes earlier (before my children get up), because as the day progresses I find more excuses not to exercise. Since you're already set in a routine, the perfect solution for finding time to exercise would be to give it a permanent place in this regular schedule. When you were a kid, Monday through Friday were structured school days. Now as an adult, it's still a routine. For instance, I do aerobic fitness three days a week and do two days a week of toning. Saturday is my free day to do a fun activity with the family like go for a bike ride. For you, like me, it could be a free day or it could be a make-up day—in case during the week there was one day where you couldn't do it (always do the 5-minute DDD—your minimum daily requirement). Use Saturday as your substitute day. And for those who would like to add another aerobic activity, add it on a Saturday. Actually, in a perfect world you should do your cardiovascular workout (aerobic activity) four days a week—that would be great!

There are three main components to a well-balanced fitness program:

1. Aerobics: Cardiovascular exercise to burn fat and condition the heart and lungs.
2. Toning/Resistance Training: Strengthening exercises for firming muscles and toning, body sculpting, and reshaping your muscles.
3. Flexibility: Stretching exercises to improve joint flexibility and to reduce muscular stress and tension.

Sounds like a lot? It isn't. The JumpStart exercise plan starts with just 20 minutes of aerobic exercise only three days a week; 25 minutes in the second week; and 30 minutes in the third week. The muscle conditioning exercises will be done twice a week: 10 minutes in the first week; 15 minutes in the second week, and 20 minutes in the third week.

Exercise is the key ingredient in losing weight—and in keeping it off. I want to get you moving! Get off that couch—get out of that desk chair! Get your blood pumping and your blood flowing. You need to ignite that metabolism. You need to create stronger, leaner, muscles that will eat fat, fat, and more fat.

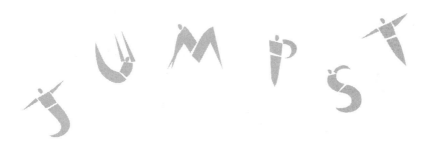

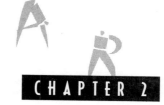

PRACTICE MAKES PERFECT

Dear Denise,

21 Day JumpStart has given me the opportunity to lose those awful last 10 pounds—and more. I had been getting a little lazy. But you got me back on track again. Thanks.

—Joyce, Watauga, Texas

Dear Denise,

I loved the JumpStart Plan. I lost 13 pounds and 14 inches from all over! Your planned menus were great. Thank you, Denise. I feel so much better about myself!

—Dianna, Luverene, Alabama

A habit becomes easy to perform through practice. When an act becomes easy through constant repetition it becomes a pleasure. If it is a pleasure, it becomes second nature, and you will do it often. When a habit is a part of your subconscious, it becomes a natural part of you, and then a new *positive habit* is born.

We have all heard the old saying "Practice makes perfect." Well, it's true! I consider creating *positive habits* to be the most important tool I will share with you in this book. I want these *positive habits* to be at the center of your life. They will improve your eating habits, your activity level, your energy, and your attitude. I will teach you the formula to govern each day with successful small changes that will eventually grow to become new *positive habits* in your life. Let me help you replace bad habits with healthy new ones. These *positive habits* are the principles or laws that you should follow to create lifelong changes.

I have based my entire career on being *positive*! I will never tell you that you are wrong not to exercise. I just keep reinforcing how much I believe in you and all that you would accomplish with a fit body and mind! (And, as you will see later on, I offer you ways of sneaking exercises into your daily activity so that you won't even know you are exercising.) I will never tell you to give up the foods you love. I believe all foods are good foods! I teach that good health, fitness, and yes, even weight loss are all about making choices and staying active, not deprivation. And I will absolutely never ever tell you to be fit in order to conform to others' standards of attractiveness! I want you to be totally fit so you have tons of energy, feel strong and confident, and live life to the fullest every day.

The two most important *positive habits* that will lead to a healthy, trim, energetic body that will remain with you for the rest of your life are a *positive attitude* (big surprise, huh?), and *moderation in everything*. Incorporate these two basic principles into your daily existence and you cannot go wrong. As easy as this sounds, however, it really requires a great deal of work. In modern society, the media bombards us with unrealistic images of who and what we need to find happiness. When we have not achieved the prosperity levels of *Dallas* or *Dynasty,* we become negative about all that we do have. Without money, power, a mansion, a personal Lear jet, and the perfect body, how could one possibly be happy? What a lot of malarkey!

I'm here to tell you I don't have all those things and I am extremely happy! I have good health, a very supportive husband, two beautiful children, close family ties, a close relationship with God, and a career that allows me to help others. These things are the source of my true happiness.

"Yeah, yeah. That is all well and good, but I want to lose weight! Counting my blessings will not stop me from eating french fries and a Big Mac at McDonald's!" (I can just hear you thinking to yourself.) Well, I think that it can! A *positive attitude* reflects how you feel about yourself and how you perceive you look.

Right now you might *feel* bad about yourself, and you *perceive* that you are a failure, fat, and unattractive. How could you possibly maintain a positive attitude with all that baggage! I have a girlfriend who has lost over 30 pounds in the last two years. You would think she would be proud and confident. But it seems that no matter how thin and toned she gets, she continues to see her old image. She has a *negative attitude* about her body and that negativity is clouding her judgment. She still perceives herself as fat and unattractive. In her mind she remains a failure! Her body has changed, her mental attitude has not. I can talk to her until I am blue in the face, and she simply refuses to believe me. *Please do not let this happen to you!* That is why it is *so important* that you work on your mind perhaps even more diligently than you work on your body. The principles of weight loss are really fairly basic and easy to apply. True success is found inside your head!

You will learn that it is not willpower that you lack—it is all in your *attitude!* I can train you to become more positive in life. There are simple techniques that will help you achieve happiness. This is your opportunity to wake up every day with a smile on your face (which goes a long way!) and say to yourself, "Life is short—make it the best!"

I want you to feel my presence and literally hear my positive reinforcement every day! Each day, Deniseology will provide a bit of inspiration based on my personal experiences for you to think about and suggest a focus for the day. Don't be surprised if the topics are not diet issues—remember, our goal is to change how you process information about your food, your body and your life. You will learn how to:

- Feel better about yourself
- Improve your self-esteem
- Believe in your abilities
- Take action and control your destiny

One of the purposes in writing this book is to encourage women to feel good about themselves. I want to share my feelings with you as a mother, wife, and career woman. I feel passionately that everyone deserves to feel good and embrace life. We all have so much to live for! I hope this will open a door to your future, and help you live out your dreams to the fullest.

Moderation Is Not Deprivation

You should know up front that I *love to eat!* Food is not only half my energy source, but meals are a time for bonding with my family and socializing with my friends. In spite of how easy it is these days to be frightened by all the conflicting reports we hear and read about, I happen to believe that food is still fabulous! I even find a place—in moderation—for treats like ice cream, hamburgers, and french fries. Eating foods like that more than just occasionally, however, doesn't make me feel as good as eating foods low in fat. Low-fat cooking has come a long way in a short time. Many times it's impossible to taste the difference between the kind of meals you think you love and the kind of meals that love you! I'm going to give you all sorts of tips on buying and preparing food to fit your particular needs and taste—tips designed to make your time spent in the kitchen short and sweet.

Eat in Moderation. Stop for a moment and consider how you care for

Enjoy Life and Feel Like a Million Bucks!

the most important vehicle you own: your body. Do you realize that the average person pays more attention to how she takes care of her car than her body? That's crazy! Our cars are replaceable items, our bodies are not! We should give at least as much attention to the quality and quantity of food we put into our bodies for optimum performance as we do the gas we buy. Too much of a good thing is just as bad as too little.

Starving yourself and skipping meals actually becomes counterproductive even though you are ingesting fewer calories. Our bodies are pretty smart. They will constantly fight—even you—to survive in all circumstances. In spite of all the marvelous developments with computers, robotics, and the like, *nothing* surpasses your body in the ability to automatically assess a situation and adapt to keep itself alive.

When you skip meals, the body registers "starvation." It does not know whether you are stranded on a mountaintop with perhaps days to face before rescue, or whether you chose to skip breakfast and did not have time for lunch! It will automatically slow down your metabolism in order to reserve energy. It will not burn fat, *it will save fat for its final reserves!*

By the same token, overeating causes lethargy and sleepiness. Being too full can make it difficult to move properly, and sometimes causes abdominal discomfort. When you overeat, the body will *take only what it needs.* It will store or excrete the rest. You know what that means . . . WEIGHT GAIN! Bear in mind that calories do count, even low-fat calories. Too much of a good thing is just as damaging as too little. Combine intermittent starvation with binges and you have got a body that is extremely bewildered and struggling to keep up!

A little consistency and a few simple changes can make all the difference! Did you know that by eliminating just 1 tablespoon of oil from your diet each day, over the course of a year you would lose 4 pounds? Just 1 tablespoon! Anyone can do that! We are talking about adjusting here and there over the course of a lifetime, not major self-denial.

My husband, Jeff, loves to tell stories about the first time someone eats a meal with me. I guess because of my occupation, people are often too intimidated to have what they really want. Inevitably, when the waiter approaches, the table will fall silent and everyone will look at me expectantly. I try to pop up and take the initiative of ordering first. Jeff says he loves to see their faces when I ask for a juicy hamburger with all the fixings! Boy, are they surprised! Well, I am not about to live my life on plain lettuce leaves, and neither should you. I love a good hamburger! On occasion, I do not think twice about ordering one because I know that on a day-to-day basis my diet is quite low in fat, moderate in calories, and very healthy.

Life is to be lived and food is central to our lives. Food should be our

DID YOU KNOW?

After puberty, fat cells remain constant. They will never disappear but you can shrink them by sticking to a low-fat diet and exercising . . . so let's "downsize" those fat cells!

28

sustenance, not our enemy! Truly, all food is good food (yes, even chocolate ice cream!). We just need to make better decisions—one meal at a
time. I contend that if we can succeed in revamping your attitude toward
food, exercise, your body image, and your life, while you adapt to a healthier routine over the next 21 days, the changes to your body will be long-
lasting.

Weight loss is a simple matter of calories in and calories out. If you eat
more calories than you burn, your body will store the excess as fat and you
will gain weight. If you burn more calories than you eat, your body will be
forced to utilize your stored fat and you will lose weight. The more active
you are, the more calories you burn. That is why you must move, move,
move throughout the day.

21 Day JumpStart Eating Plan

My 21 Day JumpStart Eating Plan comes complete with planned
menus for each day (including breakfast, lunch, and dinner), shopping lists, and great low-fat recipes. The calories and fat content have been
tabulated and listed for you so you don't have to guess about anything. And
if you're the least bit concerned about the taste of the meals on my plan—
don't be! I would never suggest you commit to 21 days of eating anything
that wasn't absolutely delicious. In fact, I wouldn't expect you to eat tasteless meals for even *one* day! The food in this plan is food I eat, feed my family, and serve to guests in my home. The recipes are my personal favorites
that ensure great taste, nutritional value, and ease of preparation (no more
than 15 minutes).

Even though I call it my 21 Day JumpStart Plan, you'll probably be
using these menus for the rest of your life. They are that good! If I gave you
recipes for food you'd only want to eat temporarily, the effects would only
last temporarily. And, let's face it, temporary weight loss you've had. I
want you to be in the habit of eating great tasting food that will, in turn,
leave you feeling great!

Enjoy every meal. Even if you do not consider yourself talented in the
kitchen, I want you to relax. Despite how good this food tastes, I promise
it is easy and uncomplicated to prepare. (That was a top priority because,
like you, I am always on the go!) Nearly all of the recipes do not require
more than 15 minutes of preparation, though some might need additional
baking, broiling, or simmering thereafter. Use the cooking time to visit
with your husband and children. Meals should be relaxing, guilt free, and
satisfying.

Of course, I am fully aware that there are always days when there is no
time to prepare anything! Why else would companies be making billions
selling fast food? Sometimes it is nice to go out and let someone serve you!

Don't worry! You will be prepared for these occasions. I have devoted an entire section of this book to such situations in Chapter 8, "Eating Out." You can replace any of the scheduled meals with a multitude of healthy alternatives. I have included in the appendix more "In a Hurry" recipes for more variety. It is perfectly all right to modify a recipe slightly, mix and match, or substitute one meal for another, although I hope you will be brave enough to try them all at least once.

Remember, this is not a diet with a beginning and an end. The purpose of this program is for you to learn a new way of eating. Whatever your culinary proficiency, I hope you will approach this new way of cooking as a positive adventure. Enjoy your food. Eating should be fun!

Energy, the Ultimate Commodity

Believe it or not, oxygen is a great source of *increased energy* and a component of *reducing stress!* No, I am not kidding! And, yes, I am going to talk about good posture again. You already know that when you sit and stand correctly you look and feel better. Why? One simple reason. When you stand with your shoulders back and your chest wide, your lungs can expand to their full capacity, taking in maximum quantities of air. Your heart then pumps the oxygen-rich blood to the furthest reaches of your body: the brain, the hands, and the legs (some pretty important places)! When oxygen supplies are limited, your body has to work twice as hard to get all that it needs. Hence, you feel tired.

Do you know why you get drowsy late in the afternoon? It is not because you are truly sleepy, but because your posture (whether seated or standing) has limited the supply of fresh air your lungs take in. To see what I mean, try this: Sit down and allow your shoulders to slump, let your spine curve out, and try to take the biggest breath you can. Now do the same exercise sitting straight. See how much more air your lungs can hold. Bad posture actually robs you of the energy you need by causing shallow breathing. To avoid this take three deep breaths. After the third, if you are a bit dizzy, then you really needed that fresh air and to exhale all the carbon dioxide out of your body. So . . . from today on, instead of caving in to a sugary sweet craving at 3 P.M., get up out of that chair (whether you are at work or at home), stand up straight, and take deep breaths. Better yet, go for a 5-minute brisk walk and really get that oxygen flowing. It's a great energy boost. No more afternoon doldrums! Take an exercise and water break instead of a coffee break (water is another great source of energy). For those of you who have a desk job, try to take breathing breaks and walk around the office every two hours. That way you will end the day with more energy.

This practice is also a great stress reliever. Stress causes our muscles to tense. Just as our built-in defense mechanisms react to food, when the body detects stress it prepares to defend itself. Like when you skip a meal, your body does not know if you have a big presentation at the end of the week, or if you are preparing to run should a wild animal jump out at you in the forest. Stress puts our muscles on high alert! Tense muscles equal constricted muscles. And constricted muscles cannot handle a great deal of blood flow. After a while, muscles adapt to that constricted state. That begins to hurt. The only way to eliminate the tension is to bring blood back into the area by stretching and moving the muscles. That is why doctors recommend exercise programs to their patients who work in high stress environments. Yes, once again, get up, get moving! Stretch your arms, roll your head, and raise and lower your shoulders as you walk. Take a moment and give those hard-working hands and fingers a little massage. *Get that blood flowing!* Not only will you feel more energetic and less tense, I bet that you will find it easier to concentrate, too!

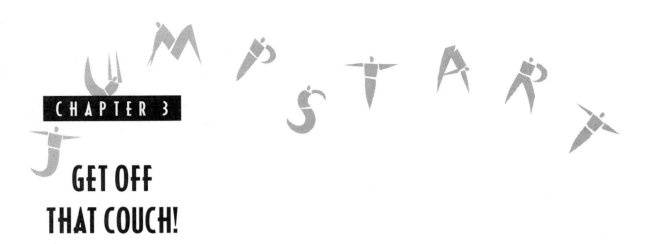

CHAPTER 3

GET OFF
THAT COUCH!

Dear Denise,

After giving birth to three boys and being a stay-at-home mom, I was up to 194 pounds. I relied on your exercise, diet tips, and encouragement to realize my goal. It took almost one year to drop 70 pounds. Your cheerful enthusiam helped me to reach my goal of 124 pounds. Thanks to you, Denise.

—Marilyn, Birmingham, Michigan

For seventeen years, I've been saying that the key to weight loss is exercise. Increase your activity level so that you burn more calories and speed up your metabolism, and you will lose weight and keep it off. Now, new research findings being published prove what I've been saying for years. Exercise regularly and you will control your weight for life.

One study, conducted in 1995 at Rockefeller University in New York, and reported in the *New York Times*, found that to keep weight off you have to eat less, but also exercise more—permanently. That's right, it has to be a lifetime commitment.

Too many people reach their ideal weight and think that's it, they have done it. Now they can go right back to the pints of ice cream, the bags of french fries, and the couch. And what happens? Their weight goes right back to what it was before—and then some. No, the moment you reach your ideal weight is not the end. The process of keeping excess weight off is a lifetime process. It does not have an end.

Another study conducted by researchers at the Universities of Pittsburgh and of Colorado, involving a national registry of people who lost 30 pounds and kept it off for over a year, stated that 94 percent of the successful losers "increased their activity level to accomplish their weight loss."

Exercise, again, is the key. And input versus output is the solution. Unfortunately, a lot of people get confused with the input/output theory. Over the past few years fat has become the popular word in health and fitness, and a lot of people think that if they just watch their fat content they don't have to worry about gaining weight. As a result, reports are that weight gain, even among those who watch their fat content, is at an all-time high. Why? Because many are watching their fat gram content but not watching their total calorie intake. Don't get me wrong: Low-fat eating is important, but calories are still calories. If the calories you consume on a daily basis are greater than the total calories you burn through physical activity—exercise—you will add pounds and inches.

There is no other way out. Exercise is the key ingredient. If you've tried to get in shape before and it didn't work, *don't worry about it.* I don't want you to dwell on past disappointments. Don't let the memory of old failures stop you from trying again. You've moved on from failures since early in your life, so many that you probably can't remember half of them. Don't stop moving on now; the best time of your life is just around the corner.

How can exercise become a daily habit you enjoy and not one you dread? One way is to concentrate on the proven mental and physical results you get from exercise: the vitality, increased energy, alertness, increased self-esteem, rejuvenation of facial and body lines, youthful posture and carriage, the way your clothes feel and look—I could go on and on.

Many people get an impulse to start exercising from seeing bodies of models in magazines and on television. Admiring thin, beautiful models is fine if it doesn't set up images and expectations that are unrealistic and therefore start to diminish how you feel about yourself. Unfortunately, in our society we equate happiness with slim bodies and fat bank accounts: "You can never be too thin or too rich." Ridiculous! We should not use fat, finances, or occupation as our barrier to happiness. Why would we want to give something with no power, power over us? Why should our weight, height, or any other aspect of our appearance or life circumstances affect how we feel inside? Not only do we allow such things to rule our emotions, we permit them to debilitate us and our best exercise and eating intentions. I will teach you how to love yourself for what and who you are, physically and mentally. You will still find yourself admiring those models. Why not? They are beautiful. But you will not need that type of motivation to continue with your positive exercise plans. Your own beauty, the power within yourself, will do that.

Some people use important events as motivation to exercise and get in shape: an anniversary, a wedding, a high school or college reunion. *You are the most important event in your life.* Your mind, your body, your health are on display all the time—to yourself. After the special party is over, after beach weather has come and gone, you are still as important. Exercise for the marvelous, unique, beautiful person you are. *You are beautiful.* Remember that, always.

21 Day JumpStart calls for you to exercise regularly. 21 Day JumpStart is a completely balanced, 21 day fitness program. It has all the *essentials.* If you want to lose inches and reshape your body, you must follow *both* the exercise and the eating plan.

Variety Is the Spice of Life

Especially when it comes to exercise! Just as training yourself to make the right food choices is easier when you realize you have plenty of foods to choose from, getting yourself on a regular exercise schedule is easier to do when you have lots of ways of exercising to choose from. And while exercise is only one part of the 21 Day JumpStart Plan, it is a very important one.

Knowing that the more exercise choices I give you, the easier it will be for you to exercise and develop a positive, regular exercise schedule. I have designed two workouts for the plan. These are the two segments that make up your Rx Daily Activity Menu.

1. Denise's Daily Dose
2. The Daily Activity Menu:
   a. aerobic
   b. toning
   c. flexibility

Denise's Daily Dose—Your Minimum Daily Requirement Workout

This five-minute routine is to be done every day. The exercises were designed to provide everyone, no matter what age or physical condition, with the opportunity to achieve and maintain a fit body. It is a series of exercises to improve your flexibility, range of motion, overall strength, and muscle tone. It will mentally trigger you to get your body used to moving, and instill a sense of body awareness. This is one of the greatest benefits of exercise: getting you in touch with your body, becoming aware of what it can do, and its power. This five-minute routine is the minimum you do . . . it's your minimum daily requirement. I do it every day when I wake up. It gets me going. You can do it at night, too. It will help you relax accumulated muscular stress, a great way to wind down and end your day. Regardless of when you do it, the point is that there are no ifs or buts about it. Every day. You can do it. Make my Daily Dose a five-minute daily habit.

Daily Activity Menu—Aerobic Fitness, Muscle Toning and Flexibility

There's no better motivation for maintaining a regular exercise schedule than results. Believe me, the moment you see that waist getting smaller, those thighs getting tighter, those arms firming up, and your old clothes fitting more loosely you will feel so good you won't want to stop. You will be hooked.

The quickest and most effective way to get results is by doing aerobic and toning exercises on alternate days. You need a little of both: aerobics three days a week (minimum) for twenty to thirty minutes; toning/ strength training two days a week for ten to twenty minutes. Recent research has also proven that regular exercise done at a moderate pace is the most beneficial for weight loss, health, and overall conditioning. But consistency is the key.

The JumpStart exercise plan will take no more than 30 minutes of your valuable time Monday through Friday. And for those of you already worried you won't be able to find one half-hour per day, I have the solution to that! Chapter 10 illustrates In-a-Hurry exercises you can build into your regular, daily routine. Here is how your exercise schedule works:

1. Aerobic: Monday, Wednesday, Friday
2. Toning: Tuesday, Thursday

Aerobic Activity

Aerobic exercise improves the cardiovascular system—the heart, blood vessels, and lungs. It uses fat as its main source of energy so it's the best way to burn fat. Today, walking is the most popular form of aerobic exercise, but there are numerous other ways: running, cycling, swimming, cross-country skiing, aerobic dance (low impact and/or step), in-line skating, jumping rope, and so on. Remember to select your aerobic activity by its convenience. If it's convenient, you will stick with it longer. That's why I'm all for home exercise equipment like a treadmill, aerobic rider, or stationary bicycle. It's in the privacy of your own home. You don't have to drive there or find a babysitter. It's always open, and the weather always permits.

Start gradually. Even die-hard aerobic exercisers who have not exercised for a while, for illness or other reasons, don't pick up where they left off. They start gradually. They condition their hearts and lungs over a short period of time until they feel they are ready to reinstate their previous pace and intensity level. That's why I recommend that your aerobic prescription start at just 20 minutes, three times a week (the minimum recommended time for people who have not exercised regularly), and build up to 30 minutes by the third week. Choose an aerobic activity you know you can stick to. If going outdoors is not always possible, go to your local video store. Among my twenty videos there are quite a few aerobic workouts that can be done by people of all ages and fitness levels.

What I like to do is vary my aerobic workouts throughout the week. Two of the days (weather permitting) I go for a 30-minute brisk walk with my girlfriends. It's a perfect way to spend time with my friends and burn fat! The other aerobic activity day I do low-impact aerobics or step aerobics. And on Saturdays, I stay active by playing tennis with my husband, going on a bike ride with my children, or just pushing them in a stroller to get a good aerobic walk out of it. So actually, I make Saturdays an added aerobic activity day because in a perfect world four days a week is best. As you can see, I like to vary my workouts. I cross-train (a variety of different activities) for two basic reasons: to stay motivated and to work all the major muscle groups.

This is your aerobic workout schedule for the next three weeks:

Week 1—Monday, Wednesday, and Friday: Aerobic—20 Minutes
Week 2—Monday, Wednesday, and Friday: Aerobic—25 Minutes
Week 3—Monday, Wednesday, and Friday: Aerobic—30 Minutes

Muscle Toning . . .
Get Flab-Free!

You can go from fat to firm at any age!
—Denise Austin

The other exercise component essential for complete fitness is strengthening. Developing good muscle tone is one of the true secrets to losing weight and keeping it off, because the more active muscle tissue you have the more your metabolism speeds up and increases. Years ago it was believed that only men needed to do strength exercises, which they did mostly in the form of weight lifting. Some women today still fear that lifting weights is going to give them big bulky muscles. This is simply not so because we do not have the level of the male hormone testosterone, which creates big bulky muscles. Your goal is to use light weights (dumbbells) and do several repetitions. Believe me, for those soft spots below the arms and for firming up the chest and shoulders, working with light weights is terrific. And as you build up your muscular strength, you will see inches coming off rapidly. You'll also see defined lines and sexy contours that you didn't know you had.

Of course, there are many ways to develop stronger muscles that do not require weights or machines and that use your own body weight—squats, lunges, and push-ups, for example—to develop stronger muscles. Today, The American College of Sports Medicine recommends a minimum of two toning/strength sessions a week to develop and maintain strong muscles. Research has also proven that a stronger and leaner muscle requires more calories to function. Muscle mass speeds up your metabolism. It is vital to increase your muscle mass as you get older because your metabolism slows down. Firm, toned muscles help slow down the aging process, giving us the chance to have the fountain of youth.

This is your toning workout schedule for the next three weeks:

Week 1—Tuesday, Thursday: Toning—10 Minutes
Week 2—Tuesday, Thursday: Toning—15 Minutes
Week 3—Tuesday, Thursday: Toning—20 Minutes

Flexibility

Stretching is important, and flexibility exercises will be part of every exercise routine. After your aerobic activity and after your toning, I have designed a series of Super Stretches, shown on pages 188–93 that you can choose from to do as a cool-down. Your goal is to do at least 3 minutes worth of stretching after your workout. I believe in stretching at the end of a workout because your body temperature is elevated and your muscles are warm. Don't ever stretch a cold muscle, because you run the risk of tearing muscle fibers. Super Stretches will help reduce muscle soreness, limber your joints, improve range of motion, release tension, and reduce muscular stress.

Warming Up

Before doing any type of activity, even if it's just a round of golf, you must warm up your muscles. A warm-up is a light activity to get the blood flowing, such as walking/marching in place for 2 to 3 minutes. You want your muscles to slowly adapt before more vigorous activity. My warm-up routine is just a slower paced version of whatever my aerobic activity is for the day (I start at 50 percent effort and gradually increase within 5 minutes to 100 percent effort). It's also important to warm up before toning (calisthenics) because you'll be taxing the muscle groups.

Note: Stretching and warming up are two entirely separate processes.

Cool-Down

A cool-down is very much like the warm-up but it comes at the end of your activity. You gradually slow down your pace from the vigorous activity for 3 to 5 minutes.

On the next page is a schedule of your daily fitness for the next three weeks. *Get ready . . . get going . . . you can do it!*

And there you have it. Exercise *is* the answer—the solution. I want

AT-A-GLANCE FITNESS SCHEDULE

	MONDAY	TUESDAY	WEDNESDAY	THURSDAY	FRIDAY	SATURDAY	SUNDAY
Week 1	DDD Aerobics 20 min.	DDD Toning 10 min.	DDD Aerobics 20 min.	DDD Toning 10 min.	DDD Aerobics 20 min.	DDD Free Day	REST
Week 2	DDD Aerobics 25 min.	DDD Toning 15 min.	DDD Aerobics 25 min.	DDD Toning 15 min.	DDD Aerobics 25 min.	DDD Free Day	REST
Week 3	DDD Aerobics 30 min.	DDD Toning 20 min.	DDD Aerobics 30 min.	DDD Toning 20 min.	DDD Aerobics 30 min.	DDD Free Day	REST

Note: DDD means Denise's Daily Dose, which is a 5- minute exercise routine designed to energize you for the day and is your minimum daily requirement.

A little muscle looks marvelous, and works miracles for your metabolism.

you to exercise regularly. It is important to me. Your weight loss is important to me because of the advantages to overall physical and mental health it provides you. Fitness is how we feel when we get up in the morning; how tired or energetic we are after a day's work. *You* will know how great you feel and *everyone* will see how great you look. When you have a healthy body, one that is capable of moving well and feeling good, as well as burning calories and fat efficiently, then you start feeling better about yourself! And when you feel good about yourself, your outlook on the world changes! A positive attitude and an optimistic outlook can awaken you to a wide variety of new possibilities and opportunities that self-doubt and negativity completely miss. There is no better way to reach your goals than through exercise.

Let's Target Those Trouble Zones

If you have specific problem areas (and we all do) that you want to zero in on (like your tummy or thighs) see Chapter 12 for Hit-the-Spot advice on each body part.

In a Hurry

So you say you have no time to exercise? Check out Chapter 13 for In-a-Hurry exercises.

There's a lot you can do to keep your muscles toned and tight that does not require a mate, a quiet room, or a gym. You can exercise at the checkout counter, you can exercise while sitting at your desk, you can exercise while waiting in traffic. Fact is, you can exercise almost anywhere. My In-a-Hurry exercises feature a series of exercises for just about every part of the body to keep it toned. It is so easy to tighten up your tummy while sitting in traffic. Sorry, there are no more excuses! You can do it!

CHAPTER 4

LOOK BEFORE YOU LEAP: SOME THINGS TO KNOW BEFORE YOU GET STARTED!

Dear Denise,

I just want to say thank you for helping me get back on track with my body. I haven't reached my goal yet. I need to lose 33 pounds and I need to lose 32⅜ inches off my body. I've already lost 8 pounds and 8⅜ inches. I'm very proud of myself. Without you, Denise, I would have never gotten motivated. I took Polaroid pictures of myself so I could see the difference, and I can already see changes in my hips and stomach. I'm hoping that by this summer I can wear a two-piece bathing suit and not feel embarrassed. God bless you and your family. Thank you for all your help!

—Rosie, Toppenish, Washington

Measuring Your Success

In this program you will not determine your success by the scale. As a matter of fact, if you can bear to do it, get rid of it! Hide it, give it to a friend, or throw it away! At the very least, promise that you will not weigh yourself until the 21 days are over. We will talk more about this later, but muscle weighs more than fat. Often, the scale provides an inaccurate reading of the changes occurring in your body. Bear in mind that those fat days that we all experience are not figments of your imagination! The female body can fluctuate up and down by four or more pounds over the course of three weeks due to fluid retention and point in the menstrual cycle.

Another reason to get rid of the scale is the negative impact it can have on your mental well-being and self-esteem. One of the reasons that I say this is because of a story one of my girlfriends shared with me about her "dysfunctional" relationship with the scale. Jenny was constantly struggling to lose weight. Diet programs, medically supervised fasting . . . she tried it all. When she put her mind to it, she was often successful at trimming the pounds. Unfortunately, the minute she completed the program, her weight would begin to rise. None of the plans was realistic enough for life-long maintenance.

One of her many diet plans recommended she weigh herself every day. Of all the principles she was taught, this was one that Jenny took to heart. Every morning she jumped on the scale. By Jenny's own admission, she lived and died by that daily reading. If it was down, even a half pound, she felt terrific, confident, and more energetic. She would smile readily, feel good in her clothes, and readily accept social invitations. If it was up, she immediately felt fat, sloppy, and unattractive. On those days she felt and looked depressed and unhappy. She would convince herself that no one could possibly want to be seen with someone like her. When the scale was up, an invitation to a party or night out with the girls was an emotional nightmare. I am talking about heartfelt tears and feelings of utter despair and rejection.

Jenny's emotional response to reading the scale would only sound unbelievable to anyone who had never felt the desolation of excess fat making you feel unwanted and unlovable. I know that there are many of you who ride this emotional roller coaster every day. But now, like Jenny, I want you to get off. After much convincing, Jenny finally gave up her scale. It was not easy on her. She admitted that her deepest fear was that if she did not monitor her weight daily it would spiral upward and forever bury her in obesity. I convinced her to use her clothing, her measuring tape, or have her body fat percentage checked in order to maintain her figure.

You see, the scale fluctuates much more readily than your measurements. Your menstrual cycle, a little extra salt, or how you position yourself on the scale can dramatically affect how much you weigh at a given time. If you are feeling fat on a particular day, your measuring tape will confirm that your dimensions have not changed (or have maybe even gotten smaller), while the scale might read five pounds heavier!

A more accurate means of monitoring your success is with the measuring tape. Before you begin, measure yourself:

1. Around the arm (upper arm)
2. Chest (right across the bust line)
3. Waist
4. Hips (around the fullest point)
5. Thighs (about ¾ of the way to the hip socket)

Record your results on the chart on the next page. Then put these figures away. On Day 21, remeasure the same areas of your body. The results should surprise you! You will find, if you have been faithful, that your body

TAPE MEASUREMENTS			
	DAY 1	DAY 21	INCHES LOST
		2/1	12#
			7/23
Upper Arm:			
Right	11½ in	11 in	___ in
Left	11½ in	11 in	___ in
Chest	38 in	37 in	___ in
Waist	32 in	30 in	___ in
Hips	39 in	39 in	___ in
Thighs:			
Right	21 in	21 in	___ in
Left	21 in	21 in	___ in

Handwritten notes: 37, 30, 38, 21, 21 (in Inches Lost column area); totals below columns: 131   128

is shrinking. In fact, the average woman loses 8 inches from all areas of the body.

As you burn fat and build muscle, your body will actually decrease in size and change shape (Chapter 11 explains more). The neatest thing is that you will feel it happening. The first week of the program you will put on an outfit and it may feel a little snug. Near the end of the second week you will notice that same outfit is much more comfortable. By week three, I'll bet there are places in that clothing that seem baggy! What a terrific achievement!

When I was about eight months pregnant with Katie, I found a great southwestern wrap skirt (in my prepregnancy size 6) on sale. Not being one to pass up a great bargain, I bought it to wear after the baby was born. About two weeks after she was, Jeff and I were invited to a casual get-together at the home of some friends. I was excited by the prospect of wearing my new skirt. It would be perfect! Well, at least it would have been perfect if I could have gotten it around my swollen belly and hips.

I could not imagine why I had trouble . . . I had gained only 35 pounds and increased my waistline from 24 to 44 inches!! I must have been in some kind of denial thinking I could wear a size 6. There was at least an 8-inch gap between button and buttonhole. Well! Let me tell you from that moment on I was focused on getting into that skirt! It became my scale, in a way.

It took over four-and-a-half months of following the dietary and exercise guidelines (I promise I did exactly 30 minutes of exercise per day) I am about to share with you in the 21 Day JumpStart Plan to do it, but it finally happened. After weeks and weeks of watching that gap inch closer and closer, I was finally able to pop that button in the buttonhole. Let me tell you, was I thrilled!! And I am proud to say that it has been a year since the first time I was able to really wear my southwestern skirt, and it continues to fit me perfectly.

Preparation Helps It Happen . . . the Food

Before we get any further, I want you to relax about the meals and menus of the 21 Day JumpStart Plan. I guarantee you these recipes are easy! Quick and easy were important prerequisites, because if it isn't easy, I won't do it. Believe me, I am not a culinary genius. I only learned to heat things up so that Jeff and I would not starve.

My advice for you is to relieve your anxiety right now by taking a few minutes to look at the menus and the recipes. I think you will be quite pleased. Colleen Pierre, a registered dietician and spokesperson for The American Dietetic Association, is nationally respected for her skill in creating nutritionally balanced meals for the everyday cook. When I contacted her and explained my program, Colleen generously agreed to assist me in transforming some of my all-time favorite high-fat meals into low-fat taste sensations! My menu plans and preparation techniques have debunked the myth that eating healthily means boring and tasteless food.

I am confident that there is nothing about these recipes that will make you scrunch up your nose and say diet food. As a matter of fact, these menus are so similar to their fat-filled originals that you should feel free to make them for your entire family (I'll wager that they will not even notice that the entrees are good for them!). Each of the daily menus contained in the JumpStart Plan has 100 percent of your RDA (Recommended Dietary Allowance), a total fat content of approximately 20 percent and a calorie count between 1350 and 1500. At these levels your body can maximize its ability to burn stored fat, particularly during the first three weeks. The menus provide adequate fuel for increased energy and essential nutrients for good health.

I'll mention here that each of the recipes in the 21 Day Plan makes one serving. If you are serving two, double the ingredients in the recipe. In addition, if you are feeding your whole family on these recipes you may want to increase the fat content in your children's portions by adding butter to vegetables and serving whole milk. I know that we all want to pass on healthy eating habits to our children, and that a very logical way to teach them to like low-fat cuisine is to avoid introducing them to such things as buttered vegetables. But the truth is that children need more fat. Fats and oils are actually critical to the adequate development of their brain tissue. If your husband finds himself still hungry after a meal, start doubling his portions. He will have more than enough to eat and still keep his overall diet at 20 percent fat. In addition, my 21 Day Eating Plan is not designed or recommended for pregnant women, since you will have an opportunity to lose weight after your baby is born. If you're a nursing mom, add 500 more calories per day. My doctor recommends adding these calories from dairy products since the breast-feeding mother should have five dairy servings per day (women who are lactose intolerant should use a lactase enzyme product to meet their needs).

Weight loss is a simple matter of calories in and calories burned. If you consume more calories than you burn, your body will store the excess as fat and you will gain weight. If you burn more calories than you consume, your body will be forced to utilize your fat stores and you will lose weight. The more active you are, the more energy your body must supply. A calorie is simply a measure of energy. The amount of calories you require in an average day is determined by how active you are. That is just another of the many reasons that increasing your activity level through regular exercise is so important.

Get Ready to Shape Up

Even if you have never exercised before, you too can follow the workout program in the JumpStart Plan. Just start slowly and listen to your body. If you feel real discomfort—slow down! Before you start thinking up every excuse you can muster to tell me why you can't do aerobics, let me quickly assure you that aerobic activity can be as simple as a 20-minute walk around the block. If you are beginning this program after years of a very sedentary life, a daily 20-minute walk, at a moderate pace, will do wonders for your overall fitness level. Keep up the good work! And use my plan to keep you on track and motivated.

Approach the toning portion of your workout the same way. At first, do all the exercises without weights. And if you can do only one, two, or five repetitions of an exercise, that's okay, just do the best you can. If you can do two full sets (twenty-four repetitions) comfortably, you're ready to add light weights (begin with 1-pound weights in each hand and, as you progress, go to 3- to 5-pound weights). I promise your level of strength and endurance will increase over time. You will also notice that the exercises get progressively more advanced over the three-week period. If Week 2's exercises seem too difficult, simply repeat Week 1. Stay with Week 1's toning routine until you can master two full sets of twelve repetitions of each exercise. Then move to Week 2's routine. Remember, this is *your* program. Adapt it to suit your fitness level. This is not a competition. The only loser is your body fat!

1. Invest in good cookware. Use heavy pans with resilient, nonstick surfaces. A short burst of cooking spray will be enough to keep even the most stubborn food from sticking.

2. Fat carries the flavor in food, so cut back, but don't eliminate, all fat. Use small amounts, just a teaspoon or two, of strongly flavored fats like sesame oil, olive oil, or even butter when flavor really counts.

3. To replace the missing flavor of fat, season foods with just a teaspoon or two of acidic liquids like a dash of white wine, a squeeze of fresh lemon, lime, or orange juice, or a splash of balsamic vinegar.

4. Season foods with fresh or dried herbs instead of big dollops of fat. Basil, dill, cilantro, oregano, tarragon, thyme, freshly ground pepper, and chopped garlic bring out all the best in food . . . and they're fat and calorie free!

5. Trim all the fat from meat before cooking. Chicken can be cooked with the skin on so it stays moist and juicy, but throw the skin away before you sit down to eat.

6. When baking brownies, cakes, or muffins, try substituting pureed fruit for the fat. Use pureed prunes in brownies. Try mashed banana or applesauce in cakes and muffins. Use the same amount of fruit as that of fat called for in the recipe.

7. If a recipe calls for several eggs, eliminate one or two of the yolks, and substitute extra whites.

8. Instead of sautéeing onions and other vegetables in oil, sweat them. Start with a hot pan and a burst of cooking spray. Add vegetables and a small amount of broth, wine, or water. Cover tightly, reduce heat to low and cook gently until vegetables are soft. Watch carefully so they don't burn.

9. Reduce the fat in ground meat. Thoroughly brown meat, drain in a colander, then rinse under hot, running water.

10. Substitute turkey breast or lean ham for fatty luncheon meats like bologna and salami. Use lean Canadian bacon to replace high-fat bacon and provide smoky flavor.

11. Use skim or 1 percent milk or whole, evaporated skim milk in place of cream or half and half, and nonfat yogurt in place of sour cream. Cheese, cottage cheese, ricotta, and sour cream all now come in low-fat and fat-free versions.

Skim the Fat from Your Cooking

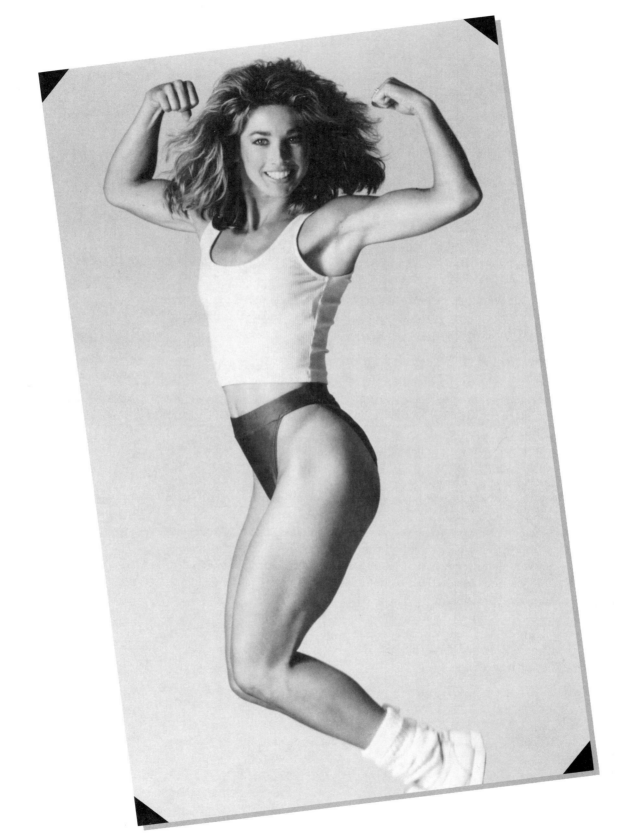

THE 21 DAY JUMPSTART PLAN

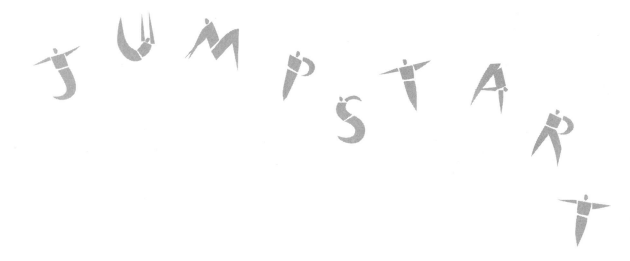

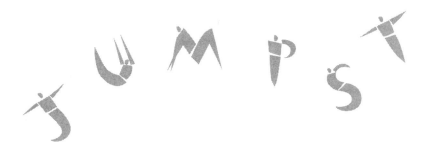

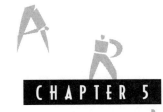
YOUR BLUEPRINT TO A NEW WAY OF LIFE

Dear Denise,

I'm thirty-seven years old, a mother of three, and work full-time as a registered nurse. I got involved with you and your program four months ago, and I feel like a new person! I was always so busy taking care of everyone else that I never had time for myself. I was depressed, always exhausted, and flabby. Because I work during the day, I can't watch Getting Fit *in the morning, so I tape it everyday and exercise with you at night. I have so much more energy, and I feel better about myself. I've actually gained a few pounds but I've lost inches. I look forward to that 30 minutes to myself each day. When I begin to feel nervous or stressed out, I simply do a few stretches and cleansing breaths, or if I'm home, I'll stick one of your tapes in. Sometimes just your positive attitude helps. Thanks for all you've done for me!*

—Cindy, Carlisle, Kentucky

My goal in creating this program was to make the adjustment process as easy as possible in the beginning. I created the Jump-Start Plan to be the blueprint of your new lifestyle. A blueprint provides all the detailed information builders require before they begin construction. It literally eliminates all guesswork. That way the contractor can focus on overseeing the workers, and handling day-to-day problems. A contractor would not even consider hiring workers and beginning construction without a blueprint. He would never achieve the objectives and the project would fail.

How can you be expected to accomplish personal renewal, balanced nutrition and regular exercise without a plan? You can't be. That is the best part about the 21 Day JumpStart Plan! I have done *all the homework for you.*

It is easy to follow and balances the needs of your body and your mind. Now you will be free these first few weeks to concentrate on other daily issues like finding extra time for yourself each day so you can exercise, learning to purchase and prepare healthier, lower-fat foods, and revitalizing your flagging state of mind.

There are three basic components to each day of the JumpStart Plan. Just as a blueprint breaks down a building section by section, part by part, I have designed a daily program that emphasizes the three primary components of good health: the mind (Deniseology), the body (complete menus), and the heart (exercise).

The following 10 tips will help you successfully get through the next 21 days. They are questions that you might ask yourself, so I want to address them before you get started.

1. **Can I make substitutes in my dinner? Be flexible.** The Jump-Start Plan is a blueprint of sorts. Do not hesitate to look in the appendix for great food substitutions and healthy recipes. I don't expect that everyone will prefer the same foods. It does not take a rocket scientist to realize that if you don't like it you won't do it. Now, if you do plan to substitute a meal, make sure you stay in the range of the same calorie and fat allotment. Flexibility and adaptability are a part of the learning process. I also realize there are going to be days when you can't possibly make your own food or stick by my plan. On the days you have to hit the fast-food joints or go to a dinner party or business lunch, look in Chapter 8, "Eating Out," for my smart choices. Take the program and make it your own, one that you can live with each and every day until it becomes a habit for life.

2. **What if I can't do some form of aerobics on Wednesday? Do it on another day.** I want you to do some form of aerobic activity at least three days a week. It's best to do aerobic exercise every other day. Everyone's schedules are different. If it's easier for you to fit it in on Saturday or Sunday, it's okay, just do it then. The same applies for the toning exercises. For instance, one week it might fit your schedule to do it on Tuesday and Sunday. Whatever's better for you. Just remember that you should do the muscle toning twice a week with at least one day of rest in between.

3. **Can I have a drink? Moderation.** While you are trying to lose weight, I recommend avoiding alcohol. Like many of you, I appreciate a glass of fine wine, or an ice-cold beer on occasion. But studies have proven that as little as 4 ounces of wine can slow your body's ability to metabolize your food and burn fat. Alcohol also tends to enhance your appetite while relaxing your resolve, which makes it much more likely

that you will nibble or snack unwisely. In addition, we cannot forget that alcohol is a depressant. We are striving for a *positive attitude.* Consumption of a depressant could constitute an unnecessary obstacle to your long-term goals. Plus, when you think about it, that alcoholic drink is just empty calories.

4. **How can I see results quicker? Be patient.** If for some reason your results seem disappointing, *do not despair!* The program will work! Perhaps you have had some trouble adjusting to the program. That is okay, just stick with it. It will get easier every day. You might also try taking a hard look at your exercise program—were you exercising aerobically or anaerobically? (See Chapter 11 to learn how this difference could negatively affect your results.) Also, were you eating the proper serving sizes of the meals you have prepared? Low-fat foods are not a license to eat unlimited quantities. You may have inadvertently slowed your progress by eating too much. You should eat until you are comfortable, not stuffed. But under no circumstances should you go hungry, that's why I have given you healthy choices for snacks listed in the appendix. Also, I don't want you to think you're going to lose weight more quickly by skipping a meal: That only slows down your metabolism!

5. **Can I have seconds? Keep your portions in proportion.** Even though these meals are low in fat and calories, you still must keep your portions in proportion. It can really throw things if you make a recipe for four—and finish it off at one meal. Read your recipe carefully. Verify how many it serves and eat only one portion! If no one else is eating, save the rest for the next day or freeze it for a day when you have no time to cook. Yes, reducing your fat intake is critical to losing weight, but calories still count! And we need to spread those calories out so that we get the maximum nutrition and energy from every item we eat.

6. **What should I drink? Drink 64 ounces of water per day.** I could not talk about good health and nutrition without addressing the importance of drinking water. It is by far the most perfect, and unequivocally the most important, liquid you can put into your body. While I am sure it has been pounded into you by your mother, your doctor, and now me, you should consume a minimum of eight 8-ounce glasses of water a day! Needless to say, most people do not. An 8-ounce glass is the equivalent of two small juice glasses. (You know, those tiny glasses in your cabinet that you never use because they are way too small.) An iced tea glass, which is the average glass size we usually grab, holds 12 to 16 ounces. Try to drink four of those a day filled with water and you have it made!

I use little tricks to work the appropriate levels of water into my day. Believe me, winging it does not work! I tried that for years. Planning ahead really seems to help. For instance, I always drink one big 16-ounce glassful every morning (even before coffee!). I have water bottles everywhere on my desk while I'm working, in the car for when I drive. And as a rule, I try to drink a glass of water *before* lunch and dinner, as well as throughout the meal. After all, there are plenty of flavors to concentrate on while I am eating. Especially in restaurants—I drive the waiters nuts running back and forth trying to keep my glass full. (My friends tease me and say "Just leave the whole pitcher!") Not only does this practice ensure that I get the water I need, it also takes the edge off my hunger so I don't snack while preparing the meal. I also try to drink only water with my meals.

I try to fit at least one other glass in somewhere throughout the day, usually when I exercise. Of course, sometimes I do not manage to get the minimum 64 ounces, although usually I drink more. But at least by scheduling glasses of water in around my meals and exercise, I am sure that I drink an adequate amount of water every day.

7. **How can I get my kitchen ready? Prepare your kitchen in advance.** Personally, I find a key stress reliever is knowing I have everything I need available. There is nothing more frustrating than rushing home, beginning to prepare dinner, and realizing that you don't have a key ingredient! Talk about transforming what should be a homey experience into a hectic nightmare. That is why I have not only included a shopping list of everything you will need to prepare each week's menus, but an inventory of the necessary kitchen utensils as well. You will probably have many of them if you are already in the habit of cooking meals. If not, most grocery stores carry these basic items. If you are a beginner, acquire the utensils slowly to avoid a big expense. Review the menus for each week to find out what is needed, then determine what items you have and what you need most. Improvising where possible is fine. If you need, speak with a friend whom you consider to be a good cook. I am sure he or she can help you!

8. **What about the groceries and the shopping list? Plan ahead.** The shopping lists have been included at the beginning of every week during the plan for your convenience. Consider them guidelines when you navigate your way through the grocery store. You may not want to buy absolutely everything I have suggested. Once again, I recommend that you familiarize yourself with the menus for the week before you shop. You will need to decide upon the quantities necessary to satisfy the number of people you normally feed. In addition, there may be some meals or ingredients that you do not like or

perhaps cannot eat. It is perfectly all right to modify a recipe slightly or substitute one meal for another. Just remember to adjust your grocery list accordingly.

9. **Do I have to exercise? Yes, keep moving.** The benefits of staying active are endless! Of course, I believe in 20 to 30 minutes of continuous aerobic activity three times a week and resistance training two times per week—but just moving around in general will keep your body burning fat and calories at a higher rate than if you are sedentary all day long. For instance, do you have a friend who seems to eat large quantities of food and never gains an ounce? Well, there could be many reasons for that, but one explanation could be that she just never stops moving! Observe her, if you get the chance. Is she constantly jumping in and out of her chair? Does she tell stories and talk with large motions and expressions? Even when sitting and working or reading does she seem to keep some part of her body moving, like a foot or leg? Well, this type of person is burning as many calories as someone who jogs 3 miles a day. All activity demands energy, which means the body must provide that energy through fat and calories. So keep moving all day long! Take the long way, use the stairs, swing your arms when you walk. Make your body a fat-burning machine.

10. **What about late-night eating? Eat your last meal at least three hours before retiring.** Sleep provides a time of rest for the entire body. When we lay down and recede into truly deep and restful sleep, all of our body processes and functions slow as well. The entire focus of our system changes. The body focuses on functions and organs that it pays less attention to while we are active. It is when we are sleeping that our body can wholeheartedly fight colds and infections, and repair the various microscopic rips, tears, and pulls in our muscles.

The early stages of digestion are a daytime process. This is obvious, because what is digestion but your body breaking food down into energy and nutrients? When do we need energy? During the day when we are active. When we eat just prior to sleeping, the body is not functioning at the proper speed to handle the food efficiently. Also, there are no immediate demands for energy so the body seeks to store this excess into its reserve pile—better known as *fat*.

Clearly, there will be times when you will be starving and need to eat at 9 or 10 P.M. Do so! The night will not be too restful if you are kept awake by a growling stomach. But on those occasions try to eat smart. That is not the time to indulge in a steak dinner or spaghetti. Have a cup of yogurt and fruit, a salad, soup, or steamed veggies. Keep late night meals light.

Don't Procrastinate Another Day!

How often have you said, "I'll do it tomorrow"? How many "next weeks" are in your past? How long have you been making these kind of excuses to avoid doing something?

If you wait until you are in the mood, you'll be waiting forever. Do you really think that you'll ever *really* be in the mood to clean the oven or balance your checkbook? Never. You're never going to feel like it.

All successful people know that the key to getting anything done is to *take action!* Once you get started at something, it will often inspire you to even more action.

The hardest part of any project is getting started and taking those first few steps. It seems that the more you think about it, the more anxiety you have. The more anxiety you have, the more self-doubt you create. Then it is all over. Once you start doubting yourself, chances are you won't take any action.

What's the Key? Don't Think

Thinking alone will never accomplish anything. You can think about getting in better shape, but only thinking about it won't get you there. If you think about it, you can come up with several reasons to start exercising. Be careful, though! If you think too long, too hard, and really use your imagination, you can come up with even more reasons *not* to get in shape.

What's the Key? Don't Think About It! Just Go Do It!

It would be nice if we could all just think our way thin, but we cannot. The only way to get in shape is by getting up, getting your feet on solid ground, and taking action. Thinking + thinking = nothing. Thinking + action = results.

Here Are Some Easy Ways to Break That Nasty Procrastination Habit:

- Pick something easy to get started on. A series of small successes will help you gain the momentum necessary to finish your goal.
- Give yourself a pat on the back for these small successes. Feel good about whatever you accomplish, whether it's running for 30 minutes or walking around the block.
- Remember that you don't have to do something perfectly the first time. Just do the best you can, and if it's not perfect, go back and fix it later.

- Put your goals in writing. This tells your mind that you're committed to make something happen, and will help you take your goals seriously.
- Don't forget that nothing will ever get accomplished without action!

Go clean out your kitchens! No excuses! I don't want to hear, "Oh, that's for my kids" or "My husband likes to eat that." You know as well as I do that if any of those foods are even in the vicinity . . . you'll eat them! How do I know? Because I do it too! The easiest thing to do is not have them around. If your husband complains about not having butter or sour cream on his potato—*too bad!* When your kids whine about having a Twinkie—Tough luck. You'll be doing yourself and your family a world of good by not making those foods an option. Don't leave a half gallon of ice cream in the freezer. If you do, it will call your name all day long!

Fill the Pantry with Healthy Ingredients

I must warn you that a shopping list for Week 1 is quite extensive. It would probably be wise to check your cupboards before setting off to the store to ensure that you don't already have some items on hand. Also, there will be many products purchased during Week 1 that will last throughout the 21 Day Plan. Many of the meals require the same basic fresh ingredients. In fact, you will notice that ground turkey, chicken, fish, and pasta become pantry and refrigerator staples. You may also want to clean out any items that no longer fit your style of eating, like candies, snack foods, real sour cream, mayonnaise, and cheese. Why keep temptation in front of you? It will also create room for your healthy purchases.

KITCHEN ITEMS YOU WILL NEED:

Blender
Can opener
Colander
Cutting board
Hot-air popcorn popper
   (optional)
Food processor (optional)
Wooden spoons
Vegetable peeler

Measuring cups
Measuring spoons
Electric mixer
Mixing bowls
Pastry brush
Rubber spatula
Slotted spoons
Food scale (optional)

Nonstick pots and pans
   (Teflon, for example)
Cookie sheets
Grater
Ladle
Plastic storage containers
Microwave-safe plates
Pot holders

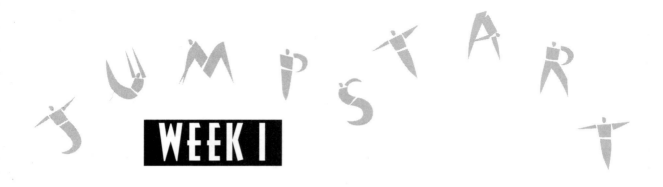

WEEK 1

JUMPSTART WEEK 1 AT A GLANCE							
WEEK 1	MONDAY DAY 1	TUESDAY DAY 2	WEDNESDAY DAY 3	THURSDAY DAY 4	FRIDAY DAY 5	SATURDAY DAY 6	SUNDAY DAY 7
Deniseology	Getting Started	Taking Action	Overcoming Obstacles	Comfort Zones	Confidence Counts	Visualization	Reward Yourself
Fitness	Aerobics	Toning	Aerobics	Toning	Aerobics	Free Day	Rest
Dinner	Pasta	Fish	Beef	Chicken	Pizza	Chicken	Turkey

WEEK 1 SHOPPING LIST

Note: How much you need of the fresh produce and meats will be determined by how many people you are feeding. That's why it is important to look at all of the recipes before you go shopping. Also, look in your kitchen cabinets and refrigerator to make sure which of these foods, spices, and so on you already have.

FRUITS
Cantaloupe
Honeydew melon
Apples
Kiwi fruit
Grapes
Red raspberries
Grapefruit
Pineapple
Lemons
Strawberries

Bananas
Plums
Oranges
Mango
Mandarin oranges (1 can; juice packed)
Peaches (1 can; juice packed)
Raisins
Assorted fruits (for snacks)

VEGETABLES
Bean sprouts
Carrots
Cauliflower
Celery
Cucumbers
Cabbage
Chinese cabbage
Onions
Zucchini
Broccoli

Potatoes
Sweet potatoes
Green pepper
Green onions
Romaine lettuce
Red leaf lettuce
Sweet red peppers
Tomatoes
Chopped garlic in jar
1 16-ounce can tomatoes
  (stewed and sliced)
1 bag frozen fiesta-style
  vegetables
Frozen Italian vegetables
Frozen carrots
Frozen onions
Assorted vegetables

MEATS
Chicken breasts
Ground turkey breast
Beef round steak
Canadian bacon
Turkey ham
Turkey pastrami

FISH
Salmon (3-ounce can)
Orange roughy (or any white
  fish)
Tuna, packed in water

DAIRY
Skim milk
Eggs
Low-fat ricotta cheese
Low-fat or fat-free cottage
  cheese
Nonfat yogurt: vanilla, plain,
  and fruit flavors

Nonfat or low-fat cheddar
  cheese
Nonfat or low-fat Swiss cheese
Nonfat or low-fat sour cream
Butter, margarine, or diet
  spread*

BREADS
Sesame-seed bagels*
Rye bread
Pumpernickel dinner rolls
Whole-wheat or oatmeal bread
Whole-wheat pita pockets
7-grain or Italian bread
Sourdough English muffins
Assorted cereals*
Oatmeal*
Walnuts
Brown rice* (quick cooking)
Tiny pasta shells
Vermicelli (thin spaghetti)
Quinoa
Fat free or low-fat granola bars
Fat free or low-fat cookies
Fat free or low-fat crackers
AK Mak 100% stone ground
  whole wheat crackers
No-oil tortilla chips
Frozen waffles (low-fat)

CONDIMENTS
Light mayonnaise
Canola oil or olive oil*
Cooking-oil spray or olive-oil
  spray
Kraft fat-free ranch dressing
Maple syrup*
Garlic cloves*
Worcestershire sauce*
Garlic powder*

Onion powder*
Ground ginger*
Dried oregano*
Chives*
Curry powder*
Dried parsley*
Spicy brown mustard*
Salsa
Salt and pepper
White pepper*
Dried thyme*
Cinnamon*
Sugar*
Brown sugar*
Chinese five-spice powder*
Cornstarch*

OTHER
Assorted beverages*
Orange juice
1 can garbanzo beans
Guiltless Gourmet Spicy Black
  Bean Dip
1 jar Healthy Choice
  Traditional Spaghetti Sauce*
Boboli Pizza Shell
1 can Progresso Black Bean
  Soup
1 Fantastic Foods "Leaping
  Lentils Over Couscous" or
  Lentil Soup
1 can defatted chicken broth
1 can defatted beef broth

*Could last for entire program, depending on how many people you have to feed.

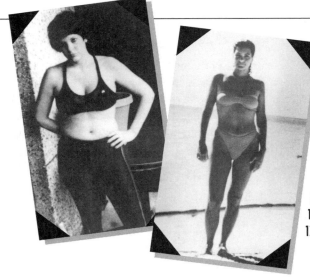

"I felt ugly and had no self-confidence until I did JumpStart. Now I look and feel great. It was worth it. I'm thrilled."
21 day weight loss: 10 pounds and 12 inches

DAY 1: GETTING STARTED

Dear Denise,

I'm 21 years old. As a college student I was constantly enjoying the two most fattening things ever: pizza and beer. The last thing that I found time for was exercise. Your "JumpStart" Plan has helped me to lose 9 pounds and 6 inches in 21 days and it changed my entire lifestyle. I've cut out the beer, started making your fabulous low-fat pizza, and made time to exercise. My boyfriend no longer tells me that I'm "soft"; now he tells me that I'm "fit." Thanks for helping me to get back on track, Denise!

——Mollie, Richmond, Virginia

Deniseology

Congratulations! This is the beginning of a healthier and happier you! You are taking the first step toward discovering all of the wonderful possibilities inside you—just like Mollie. This is not the first day of a diet. It is the first day of a total life change. A revamping of your attitude, your perception of yourself, and your life. This is a time of learning to love what you have while you go after what you want. It is about enjoying life and having fun because you are open to the opportunities it offers. Take an ordinary life and turn it into an extraordinary adventure!

My plan utilizes proper eating habits and regular exercise as tools to improve your confidence, self-image, and energy level. The improvements to your body are important, but not everything. As you journey with me through the 21 Day Plan, consider the concept of total fitness we discussed in Chapters 1 and 2. Think about what you would like to get out of life. Is there anything that you have always wished you could try? Is there a dream you never dared to attempt to realize? What in life brings you, or would bring you, true joy?

The answers to these questions can run the gamut. You may be dreaming of a new career, home, or relationship. If being thinner will bring you joy, then you are on your way. But the point I want to make is this. Use this 21 day period to make an internal declaration to reach your highest goals. Commit to making your deepest, most private wishes come true. Explore your heart, explore your mind. Take the time to *choose your future!* After all, this is not a dress rehearsal, it's the real thing.

As exciting as this prospect may be, it can sometimes be scary and disconcerting as well. Don't worry! We will work through all of those feelings together. Everyone who ever accomplished anything experienced some fear and frustration along the way. The difference is that they never let those feelings become self-defeating. And neither will you because this is a brand-new day. *You can do it!*

Remember these important concepts as we journey these three weeks together:

1. Take each day one small step at a time. Small steps may feel as though you are going nowhere, but, believe me, they will add up over time.
2. Take it easy on yourself if you feel overwhelmed or anxious. It is normal to feel that way in times of change. Talk to a friend, pray, see a professional counselor—do whatever it takes to work through and release your doubts, fears, or anxieties.
3. Each day, take the time to focus on altering the way you *think!* Make a positive attitude and total fitness your ultimate goal.
4. Think of your new food choices as an opportunity to care for your body. Don't be afraid to substitute a menu you prefer for one you don't. All of the recipes are healthy, low in fat and high in fiber.
5. Plan your exercise time on your calendar. That way you are sure to have time. You are worth 30 minutes a day! Often the morning is the easiest—but do what fits your lifestyle.

POSITIVE THOUGHT:

Decide now how you want the rest of your life to turn out. . . . I believe you can have more than you've got and be more than you are. You can do it. I know we are all so absorbed in earning a living that we forget that we can *design* our own life.

EATING TIPS OF THE DAY:

1. The brain requires twenty minutes to register that the body is nutritionally satisfied; therefore, eat slowly. Enjoy your food!

2. Most Americans eat only one-third of the fiber needed in a day. To increase fiber in your diet, cook with brown rice instead of white rice, choose cereals with at least 5 grams of fiber per serving, eat whole fruits and vegetables rather than their juices, and toss kidney beans and garbanzos into your salads.

MENU PLAN DAY 1: MONDAY

Total calories: 1387
Less than 20 percent fat

BREAKFAST
(260 calories)

1 cup cereal (from list)
Small banana
8 ounces skim milk

SNACK
(60 calories)

1 fruit choice (p. 174)

LUNCH
(419 calories)

Salmon pita (p. 156)
Fresh orange

AFTERNOON SNACK OR EVENING DESSERT
(100-150 calories)

Snack List (p. 178) or Dessert List (pp. 179–80)

DINNER
(498 calories)

Garbanzo Pasta (p. 156) with
Italian vegetables
Small slice Italian bread with
1 teaspoon butter or margarine
2 small plums

RX: ACTIVITY PLAN—DAY 1: MONDAY

MINIMUM DAILY REQUIREMENT—5 MINUTES

Start your day off right with "Denise's Daily Dose." It takes only 5 minutes and it's perfect to do in the morning. It will energize you for the day. You can do this separately or before or after your aerobic activity.

See pp. 183-87 for the complete routine.

AEROBIC FITNESS—20 MINUTES

It's an aerobic day. Today you do 20 minutes of an aerobic activity.

Choose from the list on p. 181 for your aerobic options.

For those just starting out, walking is the best form of aerobic fitness. Take a couple of minutes after your aerobics to cool down.

Try at least two of the stretches on p. 188 from my Super Stretches.

When to exercise: The best time that fits your day today.
Time: 20 minutes.
How: Look at your aerobic options on p. 181.
Suggestion: *Walk, walk, walk*—If it's raining, put on your favorite music and march in place, dance, or climb the stairs!

FITNESS TIPS OF THE DAY:

1. Make your workouts fun by listening to upbeat songs. Music keeps you going longer and encourages the mind to wander.

2. Walking energizes, metabolizes, and restores self-esteem. Scientists have found that walking alleviates stress by changing the brain's chemistry.

DAY 2: TAKING ACTION

Dear Denise,

It's about time I wrote you. After being a fat, lonely, and miserable child, I finally decided to do something about it two years ago. I began watching your show and was drawn to your high spirits. Your energy inspired me to take action. So far, I've safely and successfully lost 71 pounds, with approximately 50 more to go. I know I can do it, because as you said, "I'm worth it!" Thank you for making something so difficult so much fun. You are truly my gift from God.

—Brenda, Marcus, Iowa

Deniseology

I know that few things are simply placed in our laps. Everything I have accomplished has been because I had a dream and *I took action*! Those two words are what propelled my career from the early days when I had to rent racquetball courts to teach aerobics classes to the first airing of *Getting Fit* on ESPN.

The road to realizing a national television program was not a series of one success after another either. There were a lot of setbacks along the way. But every time I faced an obstacle I simply looked for another way to take action and make things happen. I cannot even begin to count the number of calls I have placed, letters I have sent, and ideas I have pitched. In the early days of aerobics and fitness, many people thought all that bouncing around was silly and that I was too young to know about business. There must be thousands of people who have hung up on me and refused to talk to me over the years! Often, I would get up at dawn in order to catch a busy executive as he crossed the parking lot to his office building so I could personally give him my promo tapes. Yes, I would get nervous, and, yes, I am sure that many of them thought I was crazy! But the bottom line is that one of them thought I had chutzpah, watched my tape, and gave me the break I had been dreaming of!

What is your dream? Is it a better self-image and weight loss like Brenda? Is it more than that? Do you dream of having your own company? Getting to the top of your division at work? Driving a sports car? Or maybe affording a nice vacation? Whatever it is, *take action*! Start a savings account with your loose change. Start to jot down ideas about the type of business you would like to own. Would it be home-based or need a basic business loan for capital investment? Begin today! Sure, saving loose change sounds like it takes forever, but think of all the change that has passed through your hands over the years. It all adds up. Just like healthy eating, regular exercise, and a positive attitude add up to a more energetic and happier you! You have to take the first step to get to the second. So *take action today*!

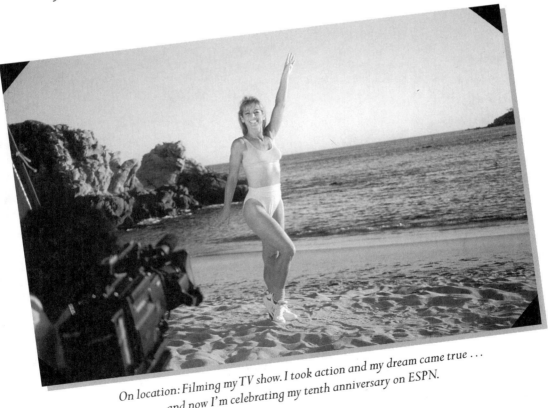

On location: Filming my TV show. I took action and my dream came true . . . and now I'm celebrating my tenth anniversary on ESPN.

Total Calories: 1439
Less than 20 percent fat

BREAKFAST
(255 calories)

Sourdough English muffin
2 slices low-fat cheese (Place cheese slices on muffin halves.
Warm in toaster oven until cheese melts.)
6 ounces orange juice

SNACK
(60 calories)

1 fruit choice (p. 174)

LUNCH
(410 calories)

2 ounces turkey ham with sweet red pepper rings
and romaine lettuce with 1 tablespoon reduced-fat mayonnaise
on 2 slices rye bread
8 ounces skim milk
Small banana

AFTERNOON SNACK OR EVENING DESSERT
(100-150 calories)

Snack List (p. 178) or Dessert List (pp. 179–80)

DINNER
(564 calories)

Poached Orange Roughy (p. 157) with
Ginger Glazed Carrots (p. 157)
Medium baked potato with
1 tablespoon low-fat sour cream and chives
1 cup mixed melon chunks

EATING TIPS OF THE DAY:

1. For a delicious sweet snack try freezing grapes or banana slices. These two frozen fruits will satisfy your sweet tooth and are low in fat and calories.

2. After a meal, stay active. . . . Nothing strenuous, just a light walk or household chores. This will aid in the digestive process and burn those calories.

RX: ACTIVITY PLAN—DAY 2: TUESDAY

MINIMUM DAILY REQUIREMENT—5 MINUTES

Start your day off right with Denise's Daily Dose. It takes only 5 minutes and it will boost your vitality. You can do this separately, or before or after your toning exercises.

See pp. 183-87 for the complete routine.

MUSCLE TONING—10 MINUTES

It's a toning day. Firming your muscles is one of the best ways to reshape your whole body. Your ultimate goal is to do two sets of eight to twelve repetitions of each exercise.

See pp. 195-203 for complete instructions with pictures.

Do the best you can. If you're just starting out, try at least one set slowly (eight to twelve reps) of each exercise. If you do not have light weights (dumbbells), try to hold a can of soup in each hand or use filled water bottles.

Finish up with a few of my "Super Stretches" on p. 188.

TONING—10 MINUTES

Warm-up: 1–2 minutes of marching in place
Back Roll-up (p. 195)
1. **Basic Plies (p. 196)**
2. **Outer-Thigh Press (p. 196)**
3. **Inner-Thigh Press (p. 197)**
4. **Standing Leg Lift to Back (p. 197)**
5. **Basic Stomach Crunch (p. 198)**
6. **Reverse Crunch (p. 199)**
7. **Pec Press (with weights) (p. 200)**
8. **Chest Flys (with weights) (p. 201)**
9. **French Curls (with weights) (p. 202)**
10. **Biceps Curl (with weights) (p. 203)**

FITNESS TIP OF THE DAY:

Muscle toning is important—especially in the tummy region. Your ab muscles are like a girdle—they'll help keep your stomach in. Flatten it and it will keep your internal organs in place. No sagging forward! If you rest, you'll rust. "Use it or lose it."

DAY 3: OVERCOMING OBSTACLES

Dear Denise,

Believe it or not, when I first started working out with you in the mornings, I did it with a cigarette in my mouth! I know—it's gross now to me, too. That was three years, 39 pounds, and 18½ inches ago. I never thought I would stick to a program. Neither did my ex-husband. He left me almost four years ago because he said I made him sick. But after a few weeks of exercise I started to feel so good that I threw the cigs away and never picked up another one! Looking back, I was pretty awful. Now that I have so much energy, I clean the house better, garden, and have even learned how to cook! It's about time, I'm fifty years old! Thank you for your inspiration. My life is the kind of life I dreamed about but never thought could be mine! I guess you can teach an old dog new tricks.

—Sunnie, Charleston, West Virginia

Deniseology

Obstacles can be obstructions to our goals or they can be challenges which force us to expand and grow. I prefer to think of them as challenges, although in the past I have sometimes seen them as obstructions. There have been times when certain situations seemed too large to handle, and my goals got clouded.

Shortly after we were married, my husband Jeff accepted a super position in Washington, D.C., with a sports management firm. It was a great opportunity for him, so I encouraged the move, even though it would mean that I would have to give up everything I had worked for in my own career. I had broken into the television market with my own early-morning exercise show in Los Angeles called *Daybreak L.A.*, and had also started a business in which I (and 25 other instructors that I had trained) would set up fitness programs for corporations. I had worked very hard to create these opportunities, and I loved doing them both.

Taking the job in D.C. meant relocating from our home and families in southern California to D.C., where we knew no one. My family is extremely close. In California, I must have seen one of my three sisters, my mother, or my brother every day. As a matter of fact, even today we burn the phone lines on an almost daily basis. In addition, I was 26 and leaving friendships that I had had for over 20 years! It certainly was hard to leave Los Angeles, where everything seemed to be falling into place for me. But I loved Jeff too much not to support such an important opportunity for him. I have never regretted that decision. Jeff has returned the favor many times in recent years and supported my career by assuming a great deal of responsibility for the children when I have to travel.

However, a new home in a new city was certainly an obstacle. At first I busied myself with unpacking and decorating.. I would call California frequently to try and make Washington seem closer to my family. But as time passed, I became sadder and more depressed about all I had left behind. I wallowed in self-pity by sinking into the couch and watching television. Television had the only familiar faces I knew in this strange city. You know the lineup: *I Love Lucy, Leave It to Beaver,* and *The Andy Griffith Show,* not to mention *Wheel of Fortune* and *Jeopardy!* One day I decided what I really needed to do was get up and do something to make myself feel better. So I did. I made myself some chocolate-chip cookies. They were really good, so I made some more a couple of days later. Pretty soon I was hardly baking the cookies at all because I was eating the dough while watching the tube! I was literally spending my days in a sugar stupor. And believe me, that only made me feel worse.

I knew I had to get a grip on my unhappiness or it would soon become a dark spot in the best part of my life, my marriage. I had made every opportunity I had had in Los Angeles. There was no reason I could not do it again! So that very day I got out the phone book and began to plot my strategy. The moment I *took action* by reaching for that phone book, my *obstacle* became a *challenge!* In retrospect, it was in the process of overcoming the obstacle of moving to D.C. that I was able to focus on my real goal of a national TV show. Had I stayed in Los Angeles, I might have become too complacent with my success in local television, or spent too much time on my corporate business.

What obstacles are you facing? How can those seeming obstructions become challenges and perhaps then open a whole new opportunity? What small steps can you take today to change your circumstances? Remember what we talked about yesterday: *Take action* and make something happen! *Accept life's challenges* as new opportunities! *I know you can do it!* After all, you have already picked up this book and have begun to exercise, eat healthier, and, I'll bet, feel better, too. There ain't no stopping you now!

POSITIVE THOUGHT:

Never underestimate your power to change and improve yourself. You are a good person, with wonderful qualities, and you have the ability to reach your goals.

1. Drink lots of water (at least eight glasses a day!). Cells will not metabolize excess fat without water.

2. Beware of mineral waters! While some can be good sources of calcium, others may be high in sodium.

MENU PLAN DAY 3: WEDNESDAY

Total Calories: 1500
Less than 20percent fat

BREAKFAST
(390 calories)

Small sesame-seed bagel
2 teaspoons jelly
8 ounces nonfat yogurt (plain or Nutrasweetened)
1 cup fresh strawberries

SNACK
(60 calories)

1 fruit choice (p. 174)

LUNCH
(381 calories)

Carrot-Tuna Salad (p. 158) with green pepper rings on
2 slices oatmeal bread
8 ounces skim milk
Fresh pear

AFTERNOON SNACK OR EVENING DESSERT
(100-150 calories)

Snack List (p. 178) or Dessert List (pp. 179–80)

DINNER
(519 calories)

Beef Stir Fry on Brown Rice with Mandarin Oranges (p. 158)

RX: ACTIVITY PLAN—DAY 3: WEDNESDAY

MINIMUM DAILY REQUIREMENT—5 MINUTES

Start your morning off right with Denise's Daily Dose. It takes only 5 minutes and it will energize you for the day. You can do this separately or before or after your aerobic activity.

See pp. 183-87 for the complete routine.

AEROBIC FITNESS—20 MINUTES

It's an aerobic day. Today you will do 20 minutes of an aerobic activity.

Choose from the list on p. 181 for your aerobic options.

Don't forget to do at least 3 "Super Stretches" on p. 188.

When to Exercise: The best time that it fits your day today.
Time: 20 minutes.
How: **Look at your aerobic options on p. 181**
Suggestion: Ask a friend to join you for a walk or hike—how about in a local park or just through your neighborhood?

FITNESS TIPS OF THE DAY:

1. To maximize fat burning, exercise the body before you feed it. For instance, within 1 hour after getting up, go for a walk or do some form of aerobic exercise before having a bowl of cereal or a piece of toast. By doing this you will attack the fat first.

2. To alleviate calf-muscle cramps, stretch the calves by flexing the foot (toes toward the knee). Try not to point your toes.

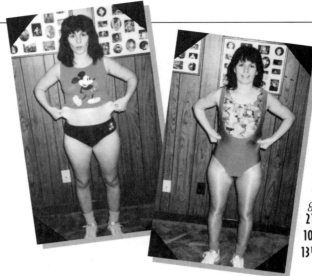

THURSDAY:

DAY 4: COMFORT ZONES

Vicki— Cincinnati, Ohio:
"I've eaten more than I normally do. And look at me: 10 pounds and 13 inches off. I feel great. I'm psyched."
21 day weight loss: 10 pounds and 13¹/₂ inches

Dear Denise,

I am forty years old, a wife and a mother. After 10 years of back pain from a herniated lumbar disc, I finally had surgery. It has been three years since my surgery, but I haven't found an exercise program that doesn't put me off. I forced myself to try keeping up with your low-impact aerobics workout, and I have kept up! I am just starting, but I feel better every time I complete the aerobics; then I take a 30-minute brisk walk, after a short rest. I am grateful for your daily program!

—Diane, Olympia, Washington

Dear Denise,

I first saw your show on ESPN right after my baby was born two years ago. Because of a complication, I could not exert myself at all during my pregnancy and went from 125 pounds to 195 pounds! After only four months of working out with you, four times a week, I had lost half of that. I am now back to my normal weight and like to think that I'm in better shape now than I was before my pregnancy.

—Mary, Mesa, Arizona

Deniseology

Progress always involves a risk; you can't steal second base and keep your foot on first.

Yesterday we talked about obstacles. Today I want to talk about one of the biggest you'll face. No, it is not deciding whether or not to eat cake, or what time to exercise. One of the most difficult obstacles to conquer is that *you are too comfortable!* That couch is great! It's soft and cozy. Your house is familiar and safe. Doing what you have always done, eating what you have always eaten is easy. Why do something hard like learning to cook in a new way? Why venture outside into the *elements* to *walk?*

The only way to take action to get beyond your obstacles is to get *uncomfortable!* Sorry, but it's true. Comfortable means doing nothing. Uncomfortable means breaking away to accept the challenges in your life and doing something. You have probably noticed some achiness in your muscles as you have introduced exercise into your daily routine over the last couple of days. I am sure that it is making your movements *uncomfortable* (but only for a little while). Feel that stiffness! Savor that slightly sore muscle! Congratulate yourself, because you are doing something. You have taken action. You have moved beyond the couch. You have taken control of an obstacle and moved forward toward the opportunity to improve your health, energy, and mental attitude. To be willing to risk a change you must trust yourself. Take all your positives with you as you attempt to change. There's already that comfort zone that you can trust in your new setting.

I don't know about you, but I consider pregnancy one of the most uncomfortable experiences I have ever had! With both daughters I was nauseous, exhausted, and huge. During the early months I lived in the bathroom. Later, the 35 extra pounds I gained and the pressure of the baby on my lower body made it difficult to move around, sit, stand, and sleep but I did work out through both pregnancies. I even filmed a pregnancy workout video during my eighth month. And don't even get me started on labor and delivery. I don't remember one comfortable minute!

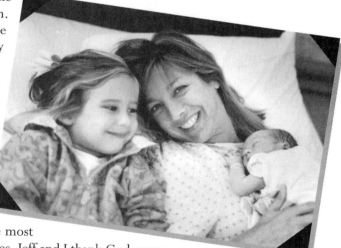

But what a miraculous experience! I can say with all honesty that Jeff and I look back on the birth of Kelly, and, three years later, Katie, as the most wonderful and joyous moments of our lives. Jeff and I thank God every day for our two girls. I would gladly double all of the discomfort I felt for the truly special gifts of our two daughters.

Where else in your life are you allowing your desire to be comfortable outweigh your desire to live a full and vibrant life? Are you avoiding searching for a better job because the current one isn't perfect but at least you are *comfortable* there? Are you dreading attending a social event or joining a club because you would have to meet and talk to people you don't know and that would not be comfortable? Start today to view a little discomfort with pride. Some discomfort can mean you are rising to meet life's challenges. You are not afraid to live life fully and venture beyond your usual parameters. *Take the chance. . . .* The rewards are well worth it!

POSITIVE THOUGHT

Improve your performance by improving your attitude.

MENU PLAN DAY 4: THURSDAY

Total Calories: 1435
Less than 20 percent fat

EATING TIP OF THE DAY:

After finishing dinner,
brush your teeth
so you feel completely
finished and will not
nibble later.

BREAKFAST
(290 calories)

2 slices 7-grain bread
2 slices low-fat cheese
Tangerine

SNACK
(60 calories)

1 fruit choice (p. 174)

LUNCH
(457 calories)

Fantastic Foods' Leaping Lentils Over Couscous
reconstituted with boiling water)
(if not available—lentil soup)
½ cup fresh red pepper strips
8 ounces nonfat yogurt
1 cup fresh grapes

AFTERNOON SNACK OR EVENING DESSERT
(100-150 calories)

Snack List (p. 178) or Dessert List (pp. 179–80)

DINNER
(478 calories)

Curried Chicken Waldorf (p. 159)
Pumpernickel dinner roll
1 teaspoon butter or margarine

RX: ACTIVITY PLAN—DAY 4: THURSDAY

MINIMUM DAILY REQUIREMENT—5 MINUTES

Start your day off right with Denise's Daily Dose. It takes only 5 minutes and it will add a little zest to your day. You can do this separately, or before or after your aerobic activity.

See pp. 183-87 for the complete routine.

MUSCLE TONING—10 MINUTES

It's a toning day. It's time to firm and tone your 640 muscles from head to toe. These trimming and toning exercises can be done anytime during your day. All they take is 10 minutes. Remember the amount of weight is far less important than using proper form.

Turn to pp. 204-11 for complete instructions with pictures.

Try to do two sets of eight to twelve reps of each exercise. For beginners use 1-pound weights and gradually build up to 3–5 pounds in each hand. . . . After all these years, I still only use 5-pound weights. Remember, we're toning, not body-building.

Finish your toning exercises with three Super Stretches on p. 188.

TONING—10 MINUTES

Warm-up: 1–2 minutes of marching in place.
Back Roll-up (p. 204)
1. Basic Squats (p. 205)
2. Pelvic Super Squeeze (standing) (p. 206)
3. Reverse Lunge (p. 206)
4. Basic Outer-Thigh Leg Lift (floor) (p. 207)
5. Basic Inner-Thigh Lift (floor) (p. 207)
6. Beginner Bicycles (p. 208)
7. Crossover Crunches (p. 208)
8. Lateral Side Raises (with weights) (p. 209)
9. Triceps Toner (with weights) (p. 210)
10. Upright Rows (with weights) (p. 211)

FITNESS TIP OF THE DAY:

A hard aerobic workout close to bedtime can lead to a restless night. Instead, exercise earlier in the day and try stretching and toning while listening to soft music at night.

DAY 5: CONFIDENCE COUNTS

Dear Denise,

I am a senior citizen and I just love your JumpStart Plan. I've been getting a lot of attention since I started this program. I have more pep now and I'm having a ball.

—Betty, Orlando, Florida

Dear Denise,

I have a twenty-month-old girl and a five-month-old boy. Needless to say, my body thinks it will always be in the pregnancy stage. I've been exercising with you for five weeks and I've already seen changes. But to me the most important part is inward—I feel better and have more patience with my babies. After having a baby, as you know, your hormones are a roller coaster and I truly believe exercise has helped me. Thanks!

—Julena, Somerset, Kentucky

Deniseology

Do you have a backbone or a wishbone? No, I am not trying to be funny. They are two very different things, and are very important to how well you will succeed in your commitment to change your lifestyle. People I know with a lot of backbone are confident and determined. They believe in themselves and their ability to accomplish things. Those I know with a wishbone are dreamers. You know the type, people always waiting for their ship to come in. They have many grand ideas, but that is what they stay—ideas. They do not believe in themselves enough to take a risk and make something happen.

Wishbones prefer to stay within their *comfort zones.* They spend their time watching others live healthy, full lives while they sit on their couches and moan! They *want* to take action and overcome obstacles, and even have tried, but somehow they end up back on the couch a week or two later. The problem is that *wishbones* do not really believe they can accomplish their goals, whatever they are. Weight loss, a new job, a new car—the obstacles seem too large, the tasks too overwhelming. *Wishbones* lack *confidence!* They are literally paralyzed by a *fear of failure.*

I believe the weight loss industry has contributed to the wishbone fear of failure and lack of confidence. Diet after diet has been marketed as the answer to every weight problem. The Grapefruit Diet, the Popcorn Diet, and, for heaven's sake, the Chocolate Diet! Some diets literally starved people, and others said "Eat whatever you want and still lose weight!" Give me a break! These diets don't work, they never did, and they never will. Innocent people tried one after another, only to succeed in convincing themselves that *they* were the ones who were failing. *They* thought they were the ones who lacked the willpower and self-control. Such experiences are emotionally painful and shatter confidence. Well, I'm here to tell you *it is not your fault! You did not fail!* These diets did not work for anyone. They are unsound and unfair. Stop thinking like a *wishbone!* We are starting fresh!

I know I'm beginning to sound like a broken record, but the only difference between a wishbone and a backbone is a state of mind. *Confidence* is believing in yourself. You can *choose* here and now to believe. Everyone has times when they do not succeed at something, diets or otherwise. But those with backbone keep believing in themselves in spite of those experiences. Just the simple fact that you have picked up this book convinces me that you have a great backbone—it has just been out of action.

Make today (and every day) a brand-new start. Erase all the memories of unsuccessful diets or any other negative experiences. Each time you choose to exercise, eat fruit instead of a high-fat snack, or take action to accomplish a goal, give yourself a pat on the back. Feel that backbone getting stronger and stronger as your confidence and belief in yourself grows. Keep telling yourself how special you are. Remember, *confidence counts!*

POSITIVE THOUGHT:

Work hard to create a good self-image in your children. It's the most important thing you can do to ensure their happiness and success.

EATING TIPS OF THE DAY:

1. To avoid late-night eating, make the kitchen out of bounds. Put a curfew on yourself—you can't go in the kitchen after 8 P.M. Don't even think of going to the refrigerator!

2. To add flavor to food without adding fat, replace margarine with seasonings such as tarragon, thyme, or mustard.

MENU PLAN DAY 5: FRIDAY

Total Calories: 1490
Less than 20 percent fat

BREAKFAST
(290 calories)

One packet instant oatmeal
8 ounces skim milk
2 tablespoons raisins

SNACK
(60 calories)

1 fruit choice (p. 174)

LUNCH
(445 calories)

2 ounces turkey pastrami and 2 slices reduced-fat cheese on
2 slices rye bread with spicy brown mustard
1 cup raw cauliflower with
2 tablespoons fat-free Ranch dressing for dipping
¾ cup fresh pineapple chunks

AFTERNOON SNACK OR EVENING DESSERT
(100-150 calories)

Snack List (p. 178) or Dessert List (pp. 179–80)

DINNER
(545 calories)

Cheese and Bacon Pizza (p. 159)
Temple orange

RX: ACTIVITY PLAN—DAY 5: FRIDAY

MINIMUM DAILY REQUIREMENT—5 MINUTES

Start your day off right with Denise's Daily Dose. It takes only 5 minutes and it will help sculpt and tone your whole body. You can do this by itself, or before or after your aerobic exercise.

See pp. 183-87 for the complete routine.

AEROBIC FITNESS—20 MINUTES

It's an aerobics day. Today you will do 20 minutes of an aerobic activity.

Choose from the list on p. 181 for your aerobic options.

For those just starting out, walking is the best form of aerobic fitness. Just try walking 20 minutes and you will have gone about a mile.

Please finish with three of my Super Stretches on p. 188.

When to Exercise: The best time that fits your day today.
Time: 20 minutes.
How: Look at your aerobic options on p. 181
Suggestion: Here's a chance to alternate your activity—how about going on a bike ride? Tandem is fun, too!

FITNESS TIP OF THE DAY:

For every mile you walk you will burn approximately 100 calories, so get moving!

You're doing great . . . I'm so proud of you . . . keep it up!

DAY 6:
VISUALIZATION

Dear Denise,

When you suggested that I go into the bathroom and look at myself naked from head to toe, front and back, I did it. It almost killed me, but I did it. This was the first time I faced reality about my weight and what I'd let happen to my body. You gave me a reason to keep up the exercise and I did. Six months later and 30 pounds less, I'm no longer ashamed to look at my body. I could never have made the change without knowing what it was that needed changing! Thanks, friend, a dose of reality never hurts (at least not for long).

—Amy, North Bend, Indiana

Deniseology

Visualization is the art of seeing possibilities. If I cannot imagine myself accomplishing a goal, how could I possibly achieve it? Visualize yourself trim and on the beach, or on a European vacation, or exceeding sales quotas. This is part of the process of making things happen in life. There are no limitations to the things you can dream of.

About twelve years or so ago, a girlfriend and I were driving through Los Angeles. I cannot remember where we were going, but it was the first time I had ventured into one of the exclusive neighborhoods of Beverly Hills. I will never forget my astonishment as I gazed at one incredibly huge and beautiful house after another. After passing a particularly amazing home I announced, "Someday, I'm going to have a house just like that!" My girlfriend laughed, responding, "Denise, snap out of it. You are just an aerobics instructor. You will never be able to afford a house like that!" However, from that moment on I saw myself living in a marvelous house with a breathtaking view.

Last year, Jeff and I moved into our dream home on the water. It is by no means a mansion, and is probably one-eighth the size of the house we passed that sunny afternoon, but it is everything I have ever wanted. I have thought back to that day many times throughout my career, and I never lost faith it would happen someday.

Let's test your ability to visualize!
1. Take a moment to picture your childhood home.
2. What color is your kitchen? (If you are in the kitchen, envision another room.)
3. What shape is a banana?

I'll bet all those images came to you very easily! Now let's think of things you want to have in your future. What is your heart's desire? To earn more money, to have more time at home with your children, to run a marathon, or maybe to buy a dress two sizes smaller? Whatever your dream, dream it big and dream it often. *Visualize it, then make it real!*

POSITIVE THOUGHT

Challenge your pessimistic thoughts by visualizing yourself accomplishing your goals, whether it be losing 10 pounds or making a winning presentation to a new client.

EATING TIPS OF THE DAY:

1. You can't eat what you don't have, so avoid buying high-fat foods. . . . Shop smart! Also, never shop when you're hungry.

2. Beware of salt content when shopping because many times salt is increased in low-fat foods to make up for a lack of flavor.

3. To get more vitamin C in your diet, add a little fresh parsley to your rice and vegetables. It's a healthy way to get vitamin C and more great taste!

MENU PLAN DAY 6: SATURDAY

Total Calories: 1478
Less than 20 percent fat

BREAKFAST
(320 calories)

2 Aunt Jemima Low-Fat Frozen Waffles
topped with ½ cup low-fat cottage cheese and
1 cup fresh raspberries.

SNACK
(60 calories)

1 fruit choice (p. 174)

LUNCH
(440 calories)

1 cup Progresso Black Bean Soup
1 sheet (4) Ak-Mak 100% Stone Ground Whole-Wheat Crackers
¼ cup raw sweet potato slices
8 ounces skim milk
Grapefruit half

AFTERNOON SNACK OR EVENING DESSERT
(100-150 calories)

Snack List (p. 178) or Dessert List (pp. 179–80)

DINNER
(508 calories)

Basil Chicken and Zucchini over Quinoa (or brown rice) (p. 160)
½ Mango or
½ cup canned juice-pack peaches

RX: ACTIVITY PLAN—DAY 6: SATURDAY

MINIMUM DAILY REQUIREMENT—5 MINUTES

Start your day off right with Denise's Daily Dose. I know it's the weekend but get your metabolism revved up. You can do this any time today. I like to do it as a morning routine, just like brushing my teeth.

See pp. 183-87 for the complete routine.

FREE DAY!

Saturday is a great opportunity to make up for that aerobics or toning day you might have missed. Also, it's a great add-on day for more physical activity. Make being active fun! The week is so structured and routine that I like to play with my family and friends on the weekends. We enjoy going for longer walks, playing tennis, and, depending on the season, ice-skating or swimming.

FITNESS TIP OF THE DAY

Exercise with friends! Instead of having a cocktail party and dinner, plan a tennis mixer and picnic with your eight closest friends.

SUNDAY:

DAY 7: REWARD YOURSELF

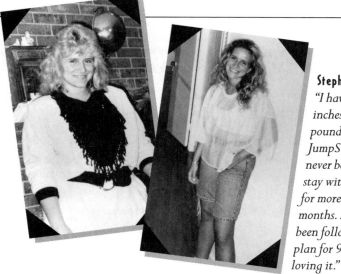

Stephanie—
"I have lost 17 inches and 85 pounds. Prior to JumpStart, I had never been able to stay with a program for more than two months. . . . I have now been following your plan for 9 months and loving it."

Deniseology

Dear Denise,

I am a twenty-five-year-old mother of two preschool-aged children. I have faithfully worked out with you for four months now and have lost 8 pounds and 6½ inches. You and a second honeymoon to Hawaii (without the kids!) were my motivation. Thanks to you, I'm much more toned for my trip! This honeymoon could be as much fun as the first!

—Lynne, Davisburg, Michigan

Whew!! What an eventful week! Give yourself a big pat on the back. You have just completed the six most difficult days of your new life. By far the most arduous aspect of integrating new behaviors into your life is becoming aware of and changing the old ones. Why? Because it really is easy to allow ourselves to do the same old thing day after day. Doing the same things without giving them a second thought allows us to be very lazy! We don't have to think or make decisions, because the status quo seems safe and comfortable. Pretty soon we have developed a rut, with walls so high that even the idea of altering our routine is inconceivable. And often we are so ensconced in our own little world that it becomes impossible to see the possibility of change. Change takes thought, awareness, determination, and evaluation, all of which require us to be mentally and sometimes physically active. And that, as you have discovered this week, is work! As my old friend George Allen, a former coach of the Washington Redskins used to say, "A workout is 75 percent determination and 25 percent perspiration."

That is why you should always take time out to reward your efforts. Treat yourself to something you really enjoy—a little bit of luxury that reminds you of the fact that you are special. You deserve the best things in life, even if you can only afford such an item or activity once in awhile. Make an appointment to get a totally new haircut. Or, if you have been contemplating changing the color of your hair or covering some gray—go for it! How about a manicure, pedicure, full body massage, or facial? If these items are too pricey for your tight budget, create a spa day in your home. Send the children off with your husband or over to a friend's house with strict instructions not to come back for at least one hour! Apply a face mask, fill the tub with a wonderful bubble bath, light a candle for atmosphere and soak! Or invite a friend over and take turns manicuring and pedicuring each other's hands and feet! Bring the spa home.

My favorite indulgence is a full-body massage! I love to have all of the tension released from every muscle by a capable professional. But sometimes the best massages are delivered in my home by my husband and vice versa. I mean, how much more relaxing can it get than being at home with the person you love the most! This could be a great opportunity for you to spend some quality time with your husband. Goodness knows that children really inhibit the ability to focus 100 percent on your spouse!

Whatever you decide to do, the point is to enjoy it. The rewards you reap today will only increase the positive outlook with which you will face tomorrow. Feel as if this is a day of renewal.

As you begin to prepare for next week, the new menus you will sample, the new exercises you will try, and the new challenges you will conquer, remain assured in the success you have already experienced. You deserve to feel healthy, confident, and energetic. *Reward yourself.* You are on your way!

POSITIVE THOUGHT

Overall fitness is a very special key to beauty and a healthy body brings out fresh appeal in everyone. Give yourself a pat on the back!

EATING TIPS OF THE DAY:

1. Remember, you are not on a diet. You are simply eating healthily, which will make you feel great and lose weight.

2. Water is the most valuable nutrient in the body. You know you're getting enough when your urine is clear (if your urine is yellow, you could be dehydrated).

MENU PLAN DAY 7: SUNDAY

Total Calories: 1415
Less than 20 percent fat

BREAKFAST
(380 calories)

2 slices French Toast (p. 161)
2 teaspoons syrup
6 ounces fresh orange juice

SNACK
(60 calories)

1 fruit choice (p. 174)

LUNCH
(475 calories)

1½ ounces no-oil-added tortilla chips (about 33 chips)
½ cup Guiltless Gourmet Spicy Black Bean Dip
1 cup mixed raw vegetables
8 ounces fat-free vanilla yogurt over sliced fresh kiwi fruit

AFTERNOON SNACK OR EVENING DESSERT
(100-150 calories)

Snack List (p. 178) or Dessert List (pp. 179–80)

DINNER
(350 calories)

Turkey Vegetable Soup (p. 162)
Pumpernickel roll with 1 teaspoon butter or margarine
Baked apple

RX: ACTIVITY PLAN—DAY 7: SUNDAY

MINIMUM DAILY REQUIREMENT—5 MINUTES

It's Sunday, a total rest day, it's your day off. But stay active.

Rest! Soak in a hot tub of your favorite bubble bath if your muscles feel achy from the new activity. If you're really sore, the answer is stretching, stretching, and more stretching.

See "Super Stretches" on p. 188.

See "Super Stretches" on p. 188.

FITNESS TIP OF THE DAY

Stretches are most effective when held 15-20 seconds. Never force a stretch and never bounce! Also, make sure you do slow, smooth, and even breathing while stretching.

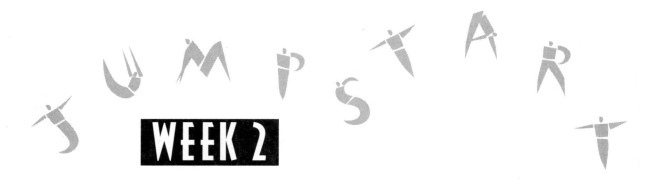

WEEK 2

WEEK 2	MONDAY DAY 8	TUESDAY DAY 9	WEDNESDAY DAY 10	THURSDAY DAY 11	FRIDAY DAY 12	SATURDAY DAY 13	SUNDAY DAY 14
Deniseology	Food A Friend	Enthusiasm	Accentuate Positive	Positive Self-Image	Risk and Achieve	Happiness	Present Yourself
Fitness	Aerobics	Toning	Aerobics	Toning	Aerobics	Free Day	Rest
Dinner	Ham	Pasta	Chicken	Tacos	Turkey Burger	Shrimp	Pork

WEEK 2 SHOPPING LIST

Note: How much you need of the fresh produce and meats will be determined by how many people you are feeding. That's why it is important to look at all of the recipes before you go shopping. Also, look in your kitchen cabinets and refrigerator to make sure which of these foods, spices, and so on you already have.

FRUITS
Lemon
Grapefruit juice
Granny Smith apples
Golden Delicious apples
Golden raisins
Bananas
Navel oranges
Fresh cherries
Cantaloupe
Honeydew melon

Orange Juice
Apricots
Blueberries
Oranges
Kiwi
Apple juice
Tangerine
Nectarine
Dried apricot halves
Dates
Fresh berries

Pears
Pineapple
Assorted fruits (for snacks)

VEGETABLES
Romaine lettuce
Fresh spinach
Sweet potato
Tomatoes
Alfalfa sprouts
Broccoli

Onions
Snow peas and carrots
Red potatoes
Red pepper
Green pepper
Red onions
Zucchini
Yellow squash
Asparagus
Assorted vegetables

MEATS

Sliced chicken breast
Lean, low-salt ham
Steak
Sliced turkey breast
Lean roast beef
Chicken breast with skin
Ground turkey breast
Shrimp
Pork tenderloins

BREADS/GRAINS

Cinnamon raisin bagel
Whole-wheat bread
Dinner rolls
Muesli
Pumpernickel bread
Linguine
Oat-bran English muffin
Sandwich rolls
Cream of Wheat
Multigrain roll
Assorted cereals
Assorted nonfat or low-fat
    crackers, cookies and
    desserts
Corn tortillas
Cinnamon bread
Hearty grains bread

Oatmeal
Rye bread
White rice

DAIRY

Skim milk
Assorted nonfat yogurts
Swiss cheese (low-fat)
Low-fat or nonfat cottage
    cheese
Vanilla nonfat yogurt
Reduced-fat American cheese
Low-fat or nonfat sour cream
Ricotta cheese (low-fat)

CONDIMENTS

Jelly
Chutney
Nutmeg*
Cinnamon
Butter or margarine
Dijon mustard*
Fresh lemon
Pickles
3-inch rosemary branch
Salt and pepper
Black olives
Five-pepper blend
Salsa
Smoky barbecue sauce
Worcestershire sauce
Allspice*
Catalina Fat-free Dressing
Sesame Oil*
Ginger
Bay leaves*
Garlic cloves
Cumin*
Coriander*
Cayenne Pepper

Fresh Lemon Juice
Fat-free Italian dressing

OTHER

Assorted beverages
Progresso White Clam Sauce
Chicken bouillon
Turkey vegetable soup
Vegetarian or fat-free refried
    beans
Peanut butter or reduced-fat
    peanut butter
Campbell's Home Cookin'
    Fiesta Soup
Progresso Split Pea Soup
Chow mein noodles
Aunt Jemima Frozen Waffles
    (Low-fat)
Red lentils
4 cans chicken broth
    (defatted—look for low
    sodium and no MSG)
Whole-wheat mini pitas
Allspice*
"Simply Potatoes" Mashed
    Potatoes or instant potatoes
    (Refrigerated)

*Could last for entire program, depending on how many people you have to feed.

MONDAY:

DAY 8: YOU CAN MAKE FOOD YOUR FRIEND!

Deniseology

Dear Denise,
 Thank you. You got me to stop dieting. I can eat this way forever. I'm a new person, thanks to you.
        —Paula, Denver, Colorado

Dear Denise,
 In four months I lost 25 pounds and untold inches by incorporating your exercise program and videos into my life, along with lowering my fat intake and just being more active. In exercising daily, whether it's a tape or just out riding bikes with my kids, I've understood what doctors, fitness experts, books, and magazines have been trying to tell me for years: If I exercise, I can eat normally! With that knowledge I can give myself permission not to exercise if I'm very tired and eat pizza or cheesecake occasionally. I'm balanced now, and my life is so much fun.
      —Candace, Mission Viejo, California

I want you to take a minute right now to think about your relationship with food. That's right, your relationship with food. How do you *feel* about it? Do you not like food because it makes you nervous, self-conscious, guilty, or miserable? Is food an enemy? Do you feel that certain foods control you? If so, these feelings pose an obstacle to reviving your battered self-esteem. Unlike the alcoholic who can choose to completely eliminate alcohol from his or her life, you must have food for the rest of your life.

 Consider the following about the way you eat. Try to be very honest with yourself. Which, if any, of the following six situations applies to you?

1. Does the thought of sitting down to a meal make you happy? nervous? angry? depressed?
2. Do you eat meals at all? Or do you prefer to nibble without much thought?
3. Do you look at what others are eating and evaluate it? Do you feel others are observing you? Do family and friends ever criticize your food choices or the quantities you eat?
4. When you're feeling bored, sad, lonely, frightened, worried, or anxious, do you find comfort in eating? How about when you are happy or feel like celebrating?
5. Do you calculate every calorie and fat gram?
6. Have you ever turned down a social or business invitation because you know you will not have complete control over what you eat?

If any of these thoughts or feelings are familiar to you, then perhaps it would be a good idea to evaluate your relationship with food. Is it positive or negative? If more than one of these situations apply to you, chances are food has become something you fight.

As I mentioned in the earlier sections of this book, food is our life's sustenance. It is meant to nourish us by allowing our bodies to generate essential fuel.

Meals are also about sharing. Think about it. All of our holidays revolve around festive, succulent feasts. When a hostess plans a party she dedicates most of her time to deciding upon a menu to serve her guests. And of course, there are the countless times we call to friends, "Let's get together for lunch," "dinner," "breakfast," or "coffee." When I am visiting home, my mother uses food to tell me how excited she is to see me! I feel the pressure to eat one rich meal after another of my childhood favorites in order not to hurt her feelings. But truly, I do love it. . . . And I do eat it, just in smaller portions. Then I go for a quick 10-minute walk or I add 10 minutes to my walk.

Once, to help a friend who was struggling to lose weight, some of my girlfriends and I decided that we would get together in situations that did not involve food. It was really hard! We went for a walk to the park by the river and the smell of grilling burgers and hot dogs almost overwhelmed us.

Food is everywhere! By learning as much as you can, by planning ahead, by not being afraid of food, you can make food your friend. Over the 21 Day Plan you're learning to make food a healthy and positive part of you life. After all, food is fabulous and having a good relationship with it will make you healthy and happy.

POSITIVE THOUGHT:

Be realistic when setting goals and develop a specific plan of attack. Drastic lifestyle changes are simply not maintained.

EATING TIPS OF THE DAY:

1. Eat a variety of foods to ensure that you are getting all essential nutrients.

2. Do not feel guilty if you've eaten something that is extremely high in fat or calories—you should enjoy everything you eat. Just make sure you get back on track with your next meal.

MENU PLAN DAY 8: MONDAY

Total calories: 1499
Less than 20 percent fat

BREAKFAST
(332 calories)

Small cinnamon-raisin bagel
2 teaspoons jelly
8 ounces skim milk
6 ounces grapefruit juice

SNACK
(60 calories)

1 fruit choice (p. 174)

LUNCH
(485 calories)

Cold sliced chicken breast with 1 tablespoon chutney on
2 slices whole-wheat bread with romaine lettuce
Granny Smith apple
8 ounces nonfat yogurt

AFTERNOON SNACK OR EVENING DESSERT
(100-150 calories)

Snack List (p. 178) or Dessert List (pp. 179–80)

DINNER
(472 calories)

3 ounces lean, low-salt ham steak
Fresh Spinach with Golden Raisins (p. 162)
Small microwaved sweet potato with
cinnamon and 2 teaspoons butter or margarine
Small dinner roll

RX: ACTIVITY PLAN—DAY 8: MONDAY

MINIMUM DAILY REQUIREMENT—5 MINUTES

Start your week off right with Denise's Daily Dose. It's Monday, but these exercises will get you back on schedule. You can do this separately or before or after your aerobic exercise.

See pp. 183-87 for the complete routine.

AEROBIC FITNESS—25 MINUTES

It's an aerobics day. Today you will do 25 minutes of an aerobic activity.

Choose from the list on p. 181 for your aerobic options.

Finish with three of your favorite Super Stretches on p. 188.

When to Exercise: The best time that fits your day today.
Time: 25 minutes.
How: **Look at your aerobic options on p. 181.**
Suggestion: Exercise along with one of my videos or *Getting Fit* on ESPN.

FITNESS TIPS OF THE DAY:

1. **Food isn't the enemy. Sitting still is.**

2. **Avoid becoming bored with your fitness regime by varying your activity. Different activities will also ensure that all muscles are used.**

DAY 9: MAINTAIN ENTHUSIASM

Deniseology

Dear Denise,

I am sixty-five years old. I eat healthily and walk every day; however, my body still needed toning up. I discovered your program and have stayed with you through thick and thin for the last six weeks. I've not only enjoyed it but have noticed how my body has toned up; plus, your routines are getting easier for me. Thank you so much for your sunny disposition, encouragement, and excellent programs.

—Jeanette, Beach Haven, New Jersey

People have always said to me, "Denise, I wish I could bottle your positive energy!" "Denise, you are always in a great mood! How do you stay so up all of the time?" or, my favorite, "Denise, don't you ever get depressed?" Well, the honest answer is I am up most all of the time because I *choose* to be! Sure, I have things in my life that have made me unhappy (remember the move to D.C.?), but I try to be enthusiastic about everything that happens in my life. I like to think of enthusiasm as the momentum I build when things are going great—so that when I hit a bump in the road I can fly right past it without feeling low.

When I was a little girl, I was involved in all sorts of activities. I wasn't always the fastest, the most talented, or the best athlete, but I always had the most enthusiasm. My shelves were packed with trophies, but not many were for "Most Valuable Player." They were almost all "Most Spirited" and "Best Sportsmanship." (I have always been a bit of a cheerleader.) My mother used to joke that she could never tell if my team had won or lost by the way I would bound into the house full of stories. I just loved the whole experience of being on a team, and it showed!

One of my favorite ways to stay enthusiastic is to think of every day as a new and exciting adventure! Katie and Kelly have made that even easier, since there is nothing more exciting than watching your children develop and grow. I am constantly amazed by how quickly they learn new things, not to mention how thrilled they are when they manage to do something new, even the simplest of everyday tasks, like vacuuming. Katie's face just filled with glee when she learned how to push the button on our Dust Buster and it sucked up her Cheerios! Just watching her made me get excited and jump up and down, too.

Enthusiasm is contagious! I always prefer to be around other enthusiastic people. It makes every experience much more fun. Think of all the friends and coworkers you know. Are there one or two individuals who particularly stick out in your mind? I'll bet that they are people you like to have near you. Try to make today an extra-enthusiastic day. From your first cup of coffee to the end of the day, relish each experience with the freshness and energy of a child. See if those around you don't start responding with a little more enthusiasm too. I promise you, you'll see that it works! Enthusiasm breeds enthusiasm.

POSITIVE THOUGHT:

Become the most positive and enthusiastic person you know. Learn to show enthusiasm and cheerfulness even when you don't feel like it.

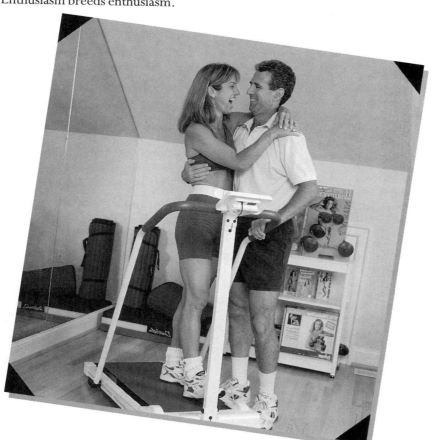

"One of the first things that struck me about Denise when I met her was that whatever we did it was always the greatest. She had enthusiasm for everything. Everything was wonderful, everything was the best she'd ever seen. She had a real joy for life with whatever it was we did. It was obvious, it set her apart from just about everyone I had ever met. Her enthusiasm was really the most striking thing about her."

—*Jeff Austin, Denise's husband*

Total calories: 1421
Less than 20 percent fat

BREAKFAST
(300 calories)

⅔ cup Muesli
8 ounces skim milk
Small banana

SNACK
(60 calories)

1 fruit choice (p. 174)

LUNCH
(411 calories)

2 ounces sliced turkey breast with 1 ounce low-fat Swiss cheese
and romaine lettuce, tomato, sprouts, and Dijon mustard on
2 slices pumpernickel bread
Fresh navel orange

AFTERNOON SNACK OR EVENING DESSERT
(100-150 calories)

Snack List (p. 178) or Dessert List (pp. 179–80)

DINNER
(500 calories)

½ cup Progresso White Clam Sauce over
3 ounces fresh linguine (¼ package)
Large broccoli spear, steamed, with squeeze of fresh lemon
12 fresh cherries

EATING TIPS OF THE DAY:

1. To avoid heavy snacking while preparing meals, keep cut-up raw vegetables in the refrigerator.

2. Pasta is a great source of complex carbohydrates, which results in lower fat intake, fewer calories, and more fiber. Avoid the creamy sauces!

RX: ACTIVITY PLAN—DAY 9: TUESDAY

MINIMUM DAILY REQUIREMENT—5 MINUTES

Start your day off right with Denise's Daily Dose. These extra 5 minutes every day are designed to invigorate you. You can do this separately or before or after your toning exercises.

See pp. 183-87 for the complete routine.

MUSCLE TONING—15 MINUTES

It's a toning day. It's time to strengthen your arms, your abs, your thighs, and buttocks. Remember, the more toned muscles you have, the more calories you burn, even while you sleep. Muscles work miracles on your metabolism.

For complete instructions and pictures turn to pp. 212-20.

You will notice these exercises are progressively more difficult than Week 1 but they continue to target all the major body parts.

After toning those muscles don't forget to do three Super Stretches of your choice on p. 188.

TONING—15 MINUTES

Warm-up: 1—2 minutes of marching in place
Back Roll-up (p. 212)
1. Butt Taps (p. 213)
2. Bent Knee Butt Lift (p. 214)
3. Front Leg Lift (p. 214)
4. Standing Calf Raises (p. 215)
5. Super Sit-up (with chair) (p. 215)
6. Double Crunch (p. 216)
7. Oblique Crunch (p. 217)
8. Overhead Presses (with weights) (p. 218)
9. Upper-Back Firmer (with weights) (p. 219)
10. Underarm Firmer (with weights) (p. 220)

FITNESS TIP OF THE DAY:

When doing buttocks exercises, imagine you're squeezing the last drop of water from a wet sponge.

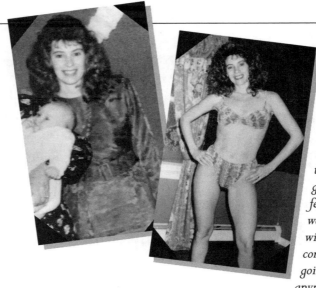

WEDNESDAY:

DAY 10: ACCENTUATE THE POSITIVE

**Kelly—
Scotch Plains,
New Jersey:**
"The excess pounds started to drop and my body started to tone. It was the greatest feeling.... I feel great and I can wear anything I want without feeling self-conscious. I don't dread going to the beach anymore either."

Dear Denise,

My main goal is to trim down my tummy and waistline. I know I will eventually reach my goal since you give me so much confidence to continue working out with you. I have surprised myself by exercising at least four days a week. Your program has variety and, most important, is a whole lot of fun!"

—Debra, Houston, Texas

Deniseology

We hear a lot of talk these days about attitude. "She has a great attitude!" "I wonder how she keeps this job with that attitude!" A popular phrase recently has been "Do it with attitude!" Even I opened this book by telling you it was one of the single most important changes we would be working on together. Why? Because your attitude illustrates how you feel about yourself, how you perceive things, and your response to the circumstances you face. Your life, your job, your body image, and your success—all relate directly to attitude.

Let's face it, bad things do happen to good people! From cars breaking down and pressure on the job to financial worries and serious family or personal crises, there will always be something in life to worry about. We all go through tough and trying times. However, it is up to you to decide how such circumstances will affect you. There is a positive and a negative side to every situation. Only you can decide which you would rather dwell on. You can choose to complain about the rain, or be thankful for the green grass, shady trees, and fresh flowers it waters. Your attitude about your situation, your day, and your life is a choice! Think about it! If you are convinced that you live life under a black cloud, then you probably do!

For instance, two years ago I lost a sponsor for my television show right before taping for the next season was to begin. Without this particular company's support I could not afford to begin production. So here I was about to lose my television show. However, instead of crying over the company's withdrawal or canceling of all our plans, I decided that this was a perfect opportunity to meet new people and find new and different organizations to help me. I spent weeks poring through magazines. Every time I came across an ad or article that I thought might be fitness-related I called the company (sometimes even the president!) and asked them to sponsor *Getting Fit*. Many times I would have to call again and again to talk to a decision maker. I was turned down repeatedly. Finally, after two and a half months, I found a company that was interested, and before I knew it there were two—and they both wanted to help keep my show on the air! I was thrilled, and I was proud of myself for keeping a positive attitude!

Make adjusting your attitude the focus of today. Try to see the positive or humorous side of everything that happens. Ask yourself how you can benefit or learn from a situation. It's all in how you look at it! It's your choice! You can control your actions and your attitudes. Isn't that great? With all the things in life we can't control, here's something you can: your attitude—make it positive!

POSITIVE THOUGHT:

Your mind can only hold one thought at a time. Make it a positive and constructive one. When you arrive somewhere—at your job, at someone's house— let the first thing you say brighten everyone's day.

EATING TIPS OF THE DAY:

1. Trim all visible fat from steaks, chicken, and roasts before cooking.

2. Your fat intake should never exceed 30 percent of your daily calories. A good way to ensure that you're staying within this limit is to consume no more than three grams of fat per 100 calories.

MENU PLAN DAY 10: WEDNESDAY

Total calories: 1446
Less than 20 percent fat

BREAKFAST
(392 calories)

Oat-bran English muffin with 2 teaspoons jelly
½ cup low-fat cottage cheese mixed with
1 cup cantaloupe cubes and 1 teaspoon cinnamon

SNACK
(60 calories)

1 fruit choice (p. 174)

LUNCH
(401 calories)

2 ounces lean roast beef on sandwich roll with
lettuce, tomato, pickle, onions, and mustard
8 ounces orange juice

AFTERNOON SNACK OR EVENING DESSERT
(100-150 calories)

Snack List (p. 178) or Dessert List (pp. 179–80)

DINNER
(443 calories)

Rosemary Chicken (p. 162)
Elegant Peas and Carrots (p. 163)
Microwaved red bliss potato with 2 teaspoons butter or margarine
2 fresh apricots

RX: ACTIVITY PLAN—DAY 10: WEDNESDAY

MINIMUM DAILY REQUIREMENT—5 MINUTES

Start your day off right with Denise's Daily Dose. Get over the hump with this quick routine. You can do this separately or before or after your aerobic exercise.

See pp. 183-87 for the complete routine.

AEROBIC FITNESS—25 MINUTES

It's an aerobics day. Today you will do 25 minutes of an aerobic activity.

Choose from the list on p. 181 for your aerobic options.

It's important to cool down after your aerobic activity with at least three "Super Stretches" on p. 188.

When to Exercise: The best time that fits your day today.
Time: 25 minutes.
How: Look at your aerobic options on p. 181.
Suggestion: Go to a gym and try something for the first time, like a stair-climbing machine, a stationary bike, a treadmill, or a rowing machine. Usually clubs allow one free visit.

FITNESS TIPS OF THE DAY:

1. One of the quickest ways to boost your metabolism and consequently to lose fat and weight is to exercise twice a day. For instance, do calisthenics—Denise's Daily Dose—in the morning and then in the late afternoon or evening, walk, swim, or bike.

2. Exercise for your mental well-being. I like to call it my "mental filter" since exercise filters out excess stress and helps give me a tranquil feeling.

DAY 11: BUILDING A POSITIVE SELF-IMAGE

Deniseology

Dear Denise,

With your help and a healthy diet, I've lost a grand total of 82 pounds! There are lots of tapes and exercise programs out there. Too many, if you ask me. But yours are more fun than any of them. You laughed and giggled me from a size 18 to a size 6! I hope you know I'm not laughing now when I say thank you from the bottom of my heart.

—Joyce, Fort Worth, Texas

Few women have escaped the experience of trying on half a dozen outfits before a special date or activity, only to be confronted with a bulging tummy or some other undesirable body part that defies all effort to camouflage it. From rear ends that seem to spread unendingly to thighs that are the opposite of svelte, most women at some time or another regard their mirror image as the enemy. We stare and we scrutinize with a critical glare as intense as a laser gun, as we will our perceived imperfections to vaporize!

Believe it or not, the mirror is not the most accurate reflection of your true appearance, and that is why we use measurements as part of the 21 Day Plan. Not only can your reflection vary from one mirror to another (ever heard of fat mirrors and thin mirrors?), but the mind is also not a very objective observer. The fact is, the longer we stare into that mirror the more distorted our image becomes. The more we focus attention on our thighs, tummy, or buttocks, the more exaggerated that feature appears.

When I was much younger and far more critical of my appearance, I learned a little trick. Try it and see if it works for you. Take a break from the mirror for a while. Later, close your eyes and step in front of the mirror. Now open them, very quickly assess the body image reflected there and immediately step away. The thought behind this exercise is that the most accurate perception we get from the mirror is in the first 20 to 30 seconds. After that, our mind begins to "edit" the picture by focusing on and magnifying those areas we dislike. The mirror, in essence, becomes a mind game.

Let me tell you a story to illustrate how obvious our flaws are to us, and how unaware of them most other people are. When Jeff and I were ready to have our first child, we knew that scheduling would be very important to accommodate my professional commitments. Luckily, Kelly cooperated, and was conceived almost immediately, allowing me plenty of time to finish my spring schedule, take off the summer (she was due at the end of August), and be ready for filming *Getting Fit* by October.

The only thing that was a concern was that the ESPN bigwigs meet every spring to discuss what the new fall lineup will be. It is the annual meeting where television shows get picked up, moved to more or less favorable time slots, or canceled completely. I was invited, as I am every year, to pitch my ideas for the next year's run and convince them that *Getting Fit* should stay on the air. Normally, this meeting is quite routine for me. After all, I have been with ESPN for many years. But this particular April, I was five months pregnant and my stomach was definitely protruding. No one at ESPN was aware of my pregnancy.

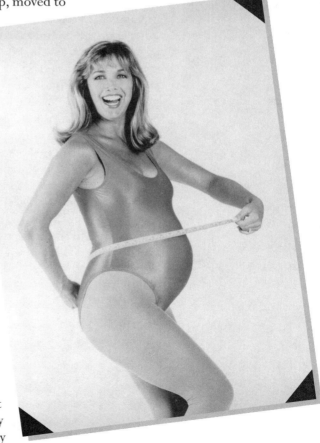

The closer the date for the meeting came, the more petrified I became that if they found out I were pregnant, they would assume I could not fulfill my commitments and would cancel my show! Night after night I tossed and turned, sure my career was over. Before I knew it, I had convinced myself that the only way I would keep my TV show was to camouflage my tummy and keep my pregnancy a secret. I shopped and I shopped for the perfect outfit. Finally, I came across a double-breasted suit with a short skirt that I bought in a very baggy size. I knew that the skirt would emphasize my legs, but to be on the safe side I also got a pair of dynamite earrings to keep all attention away from my midsection!

The day of the meeting I dressed nervously. When the time of my appointment arrived, I marched in and presented my spiel as if nothing was the matter. There was not a hitch and they promptly told me I had been renewed for another year. I was jubilant! But then I felt I must come clean. I told them about my pregnancy (sure that they had all noticed that I had gained a bit of weight). They were completely clueless. The ESPN executives were amazed and delighted at my good news! When I revealed my fears prior to the meeting they were surprised and assured me that it would not have occurred to them that I would not make good on my professional commitments. (And yes, by the way, all my shows were perfectly on schedule.) Here I had spent months worrying about this meeting, and they were positively ecstatic about my new baby!

Sometimes we create our own stress through the games our minds allow us to play. In this case, I had clearly allowed the doubt and negativity gremlins to overtake my common sense. I had allowed my imagination to exaggerate the circumstances way beyond their normal proportions, as we do with our mirror images. Certainly I was much more conscious of my changing body and the executives were too preoccupied with their own stresses and details to worry about mine.

It just goes to show that you will always be much more aware of your figure flaws (or anything else about you, for that matter) than anyone else around you. For the most part, human beings are so absorbed with family, work, finances, and who knows what else, that they hardly have time to concentrate on what you look like. Release yourself from the power you are giving your mirror and those around you. Take control of who you are and what features others will remember about you. They will only remember your "negative" ones if you draw their attention to them. So think positively, speak positively, and believe positively about yourself, and so will everyone around you!

POSITIVE THOUGHT:

Have good posture. Enter a room with purpose and confidence. You are a unique person; no one in this world is exactly like you. Isn't that great? You are special in your own way.

MENU PLAN DAY 11: THURSDAY

Total calories: 1410
Less than 20 percent fat

BREAKFAST
(260 calories)

1 cup cooked Cream of Wheat
¾ cup fresh blueberries
1 cup nonfat vanilla yogurt

SNACK
(60 calories)

1 fruit choice (p. 174)

LUNCH
(390 calories)

1½ cups Homemade Turkey Vegetable Soup (p. 164)
Multi-grain roll
8 ounces skim milk
Fresh temple orange

AFTERNOON SNACK OR EVENING DESSERT
(100-150 calories)

Snack List (p. 178) or Dessert List (pp. 179–80)

DINNER
(550 calories)

2 Soft Bean Tacos (p. 163)
Kiwi fruit

EATING TIPS OF THE DAY:

1. Some toppings and sauces add ridiculous amounts of calories to otherwise low-calorie healthy foods (such as sour cream on baked potatoes, bacon bits in salads, butter-lemon sauce on fish). Use lemon, vinegar, mustard, and herbs to replace butter and sauces.

2. It takes two to three weeks to reset your eating habits . . . so don't give up, your appetite will adjust.

RX: ACTIVITY PLAN—DAY 11: THURSDAY

FITNESS TIP OF THE DAY:

When exercising make sure the workout room is well-ventilated. Also, exercise in a room that is between 65-75 degrees; fresh air is much better than air conditioning.

MINIMUM DAILY REQUIREMENT—5 MINUTES

Start your day off right with Denise's Daily Dose. It takes only 5 minutes and will keep you motivated. You can do this routine by itself or as a warm-up before or after your toning exercises.

See pp. 183-87 for the complete routine.

MUSCLE TONING—15 MINUTES

It's a toning day. It's time to firm those thighs, tighten your tummy, and achieve sexy-looking arms. The main reason we get fatter as we get older is we lose our muscle tissue. The only way to fight it is to build more muscle . . . so get pumped up!

Finish the muscle toning routine with 3 Super Stretches of your choice on p. 188.

TONING—15 MINUTES

Warm-up: 1—2 minutes of marching in place
Back Roll-up (p. 221)
1. Walking Lunges (weights optional) (p. 222)
2. Plies with Heel Raises (weights optional) (p. 223)
3. Biceps Curl (with weights) (p. 223)
4. Front Lateral Raises (with weights) (p. 224)
5. Overhead Presses (with weights) (p. 224)
6. One-Arm Row (with weights) (p. 225)
7. Pelvic-Tilt Stomach Crunch (p. 226)
8. Lower-Tummy Tightener (p. 226)
9. Rear-View Shaper (p. 227)
10. Back Extension (p. 228)

DAY 12: RISK A LITTLE, ACHIEVE A LOT!

Dear Denise,

Four years ago I quit smoking and gained 40 pounds. Two years later, at the age of forty, I gave birth to twin girls and put on an additional 20 pounds! Finally, I got thoroughly disgusted and decided to do something about it. After reading up on nutrition at the library, I started eating 1,300 healthy calories a day. I also tuned in to your show and found it so much fun, I invested in your workout tapes as well. Now, ten months later, I've lost 45 lbs! Thank you, thank you, for inspiring me, keeping me motivated, and being my personal trainer! I'm healthy, I'm fit, but best of all, I can keep up with my two little girls!

—Vickie, Hemet, California

Deniseology

Some of the greatest rewards in life include some measure of risk. Falling in love and getting married is a great joy, but we risk a lot emotionally within such an intimate relationship. Taking a new job or promotion means that we might make some mistakes, but the financial rewards and personal fulfillment can make the cost of a couple of errors worth it. Leaving a secure career to start your own business is certainly a risk, but there is no greater feeling than becoming your own boss!

I decided to launch my own business creating fitness programs for the corporate environment. As I look back, it is amazing that I managed to get that business off the ground. After all, I had no business experience. All I had was the conviction that exercise really was good for everyone, and the tenacity to keep calling people until they said *yes!*

I started by meeting with the human resource directors of many of the numerous large companies based in Los Angeles. At appointment after appointment, I pitched them on the benefits of improving the health of all employees through exercise. My goal was to convince them that I could design an exercise program and teach the classes within the building. The classes would be offered as an employee benefit. My first client was Kaiser Permanente. Their program was a hit. Everyone was amazed that exercising in the cafeteria after hours was so much fun! And, as I had promised, productivity and morale increased and tension levels decreased.

From there my business grew. More and more companies wanted my program. I was forced to recruit and teach my friends how to instruct classes in order to keep pace with the demand. Pretty soon, I was paying 25 young women to travel around Los Angeles conducting corporate aerobic classes. Life was good, but I was already looking for ways to expand.

One day in 1990, I read in the newspaper about a dinner being held for the President's Council on Physical Fitness in Washington, D.C. Anyone who was anyone in the fledgling field of fitness would be there. I called immediately to see if I could be included among the attendees.

Eventually I was referred to Dr. Richard Keelor, who happened to be from the UCLA-Long Beach area, which is where I had earned my teaching credentials. I explained my business to him and my background in gymnastics (I had attended college on a full scholarship in gymnastics and had ultimately ranked tenth in the NCAA) and fitness. He reassured me that I was welcome as long as I was willing to pay for a ticket, my expenses for overnight, and travel from California. Needless to say, the arrangements were completed in a heartbeat.

Then I began to get nervous. Here I was, twenty-three years old, attending a big, formal event in Washington D.C. Would I be dressed appropriately? Would anyone talk to me? And, for that matter, what do they talk about at a formal business dinner? I had never been to one before. Was I nuts? I was putting myself out there. . . .

About thirty minutes after arriving for the President's Council dinner, I spotted the famous Jack LaLanne across the room. I gathered all of my courage, put a big smile on my face, and walked straight up to him. Within minutes I was telling him all about myself, how my mother watched his show, and explaining my business back home. I even made him feel my rock-hard tummy (if you can believe it)! Then I blurted out, "Will you have me as a guest on your show?" He was so kind! He just laughed and said "Sure!" and told me whom to call. I was euphoric! I could hardly wait for Monday.

It did not take long to get an appearance date. I was so excited! On the appointed day, I arrived at the studio bright and early. Talk about fate. It turned out that Jack's second regular partner on the show besides his wife, Elaine, was stricken by morning sickness and would be unable to go on that day. My heart almost skipped a beat when they asked if I would mind doing the whole show! Mind? It was my dream! From that day on I was a regular on *The Jack LaLanne Show.* And from that experience I was able to launch my own local fitness show, *Daybreak L.A.*

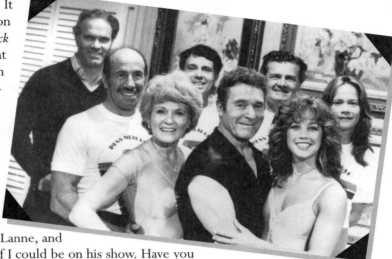

Certainly, luck and timing were important to everything falling into place as it did. But before any of it had a chance of happening I had to risk creating a business, risk going to a dinner in a far-off city, risk walking up to Jack LaLanne, and risk asking him right up front if I could be on his show. Have you missed any opportunities in life because you were afraid to take a risk? Are you considering making a change in your life, but avoiding a final decision because you are afraid to leave your *comfort zone?* Don't forget, as we discussed before, dreams are just wishes unless you apply a little backbone. Take a chance. Take a risk. Take the initiative. Make your wishes a reality. Make your dreams come true.

EATING TIPS OF THE DAY:

1. When you're going to a party that starts at 8 P.M. or later, eat dinner beforehand so you won't be tempted to overindulge in fattening foods.

2. Eating one serving of something will not make you fat. If you must eat something you crave, try to eat three bites of it only, then throw the rest away.

MENU PLAN DAY 12: FRIDAY

Total calories: 1474
Less than 20 percent fat

BREAKFAST
(370 calories)

2 slices cinnamon toast topped with
½ cup low-fat ricotta cheese
4 ounces apple juice

SNACK
(60 calories)

1 fruit choice (p. 174)

LUNCH
(454 calories)

Peanut butter and jelly sandwich
8 ounces skim milk
Tangerine

AFTERNOON SNACK OR EVENING DESSERT
(100-150 calories)

Snack List (p. 178) or Dessert List (pp. 179–80)

DINNER
(440 calories)

Turkey Burger on Sandwich Roll (p. 165)
with lettuce, tomato, pickle, onion and Dijon mustard
1 cup Campbell's Home Cookin' Fiesta Soup
Medium nectarine

RX: ACTIVITY PLAN—DAY 12: FRIDAY

MINIMUM DAILY REQUIREMENT—5 MINUTES

Start your day off right with Denise's Daily Dose. Thank God it's Friday! Give yourself these 5 minutes so you will be energized for the weekend. You can do this by itself or before or after your aerobic exercise.

See pp. 183-87 for the complete routine.

AEROBIC FITNESS—25 MINUTES

It's an aerobics day. Today you will do 25 minutes of an aerobic activity.

Choose from the list on p. 181 for your aerobic options.

An aerobic workout is the best way to burn fat, so burn that butter!

After your activity, pick three Super Stretches from p.188 to cool you down.

When to Exercise: The best time that fits your day today.
Time: 25 minutes.
How: Look at your aerobic options on p. 181.
Suggestion: Try step aerobics. If you don't have a step bench, just use the bottom step of your staircase. Try a step class at a local club or try one of my step workout videos.

FITNESS TIPS OF THE DAY:

1. Don't forget to cool down for at least three minutes after exercising, then stretch.

2. Decide to get up 30 minutes earlier each day for a year; and you'll add a little over a week to your waking world.

Give yourself a pat on the back. . . . You're doing great!

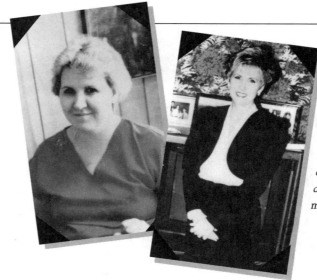

DAY 13: HAPPINESS IS NOT A DRESS SIZE

Joyce— Watauga, Texas: "Thanks to you I went from 214 pounds and a size 24 to 145 pounds and a size 10. You're a great inspiration to me."

Dear Denise,

Before I started exercising with you, I had lost my self-esteem. What happened was that I woke up one day and realized I had gotten fat! I thought I was so ugly that I didn't even bother putting on make-up or fixing my hair. One day I saw my husband looking at another woman and that was all I needed to begin to change. I wanted to be that girl! I cut out nearly all of the junk I'd been eating and turned on Denise Austin. You and I have been working out five days a week for several months and what a difference it has made! I've got so much energy now I enjoy doing everything—and the best is—I'm doing everything with my husband!! Thank you for giving me my life back."

—April, San Diego, California

Deniseology

How many times have you caught yourself thinking, "When I get down to a size____, then I will really feel great. I am sure I'll be truly happy and attractive then. I can see it now! The promotions, the friends, the romances . . . " and on and on and on. Don't feel bad, because every woman in America has probably subscribed to that point of view at some point or another. Even me!

Immediately following my delivery of Kelly, after they propped me up so I could hold her, I looked down at my tummy in utter shock! I stared at the doctor in bewilderment and asked "Are you sure that there isn't another one in there?" (I know all mothers know exactly what I mean— and for those of you who aren't, get prepared!) My stomach was still huge! I didn't expect to walk out of the hospital with my prepregnancy rock-hard tummy, but I at least thought it would be a little smaller than at nine months! Even worse, at least it was firm when Kelly was in there. Now it was just a mass of bloated mushy stuff!

Jeff and my mother tried to be encouraging, but all I could think was "I want to be a size six! I'll never fit into my clothes again! And I'll look ridiculous in leotards." I was so depressed! I just knew I would never be happy again and that my career was ruined. And to add to my misery, I had a filming deadline, leotards and all (without tights, mind you) in six weeks!!

Needless to say, my worries were unfounded. Another baby later and I am still going strong professionally. However, the point of this story is that size is relative and often temporary. First of all, size in the world of fashion is not uniform. Every manufacturer varies slightly on how it interprets and cuts a size. Some cut full (allow more fabric) and some cut narrow. When I was young, skin-tight jeans were the rage and Jordache jeans were the brand to have. Well, Jordache was also cut so slender and narrow that you had to have hips and thighs that were shaped like a young boy's, that is, with no shape. If you were built with any type of curve, as I was, you could forget even squeezing your big toe into those stupid jeans. To have worn Jordache I would have had to buy at least a size twelve, if not fourteen. Forget that! Thank heaven Calvin Klein came out with jeans for the female figure soon after.

Even more than that is how you feel. What you wear or the size of it is not a reflection of your goodness or worthiness. Size is only a tool of measurement, not an evaluation of your value as a person. Rather than buying into the Madison Avenue version of beauty, cultivate your own good-sense standards!

Today's focus is to take time to embrace the qualities that make you special, unique, and remarkable as an individual. In a word, we call it self-esteem. The word *esteem* means favorable opinion, regard or respect. Respect is not offered to people who simply look good—admiration, perhaps, but not respect. We earn respect by the manner in which we live up to our values and remain true to our beliefs. Self-respect is your personal evaluation of how you feel about yourself and all that you have chosen to define as important. Your sense of self communicates to the world how you feel about who you are; inside and out.

Here are some ideas for you to think about as you contemplate your sense of self.

1. Take advantage of life now! Be aware of the dangers of postponing opportunities because you think things will be better tomorrow. Let me tell you a secret . . . tomorrow never comes. Tomorrow is always tomorrow, never today. For instance, I have a friend who wanted a

POSITIVE THOUGHT:

You are your own worst critic. How should you deal with the inner voice contributing negative thoughts? Be kind to yourself and do something positive for yourself.

mother and daughter portrait taken, since her resemblance to her daughter was positively striking. But she felt the picture would be better if she just waited a little longer and she was just a few pounds thinner. Well, before she knew it her toddler was a young lady preparing to graduate from high school! She forfeited something very valuable that she will never get back. Make sure you don't miss out on any of your personal adventure in this world!

2. Refocus your concentration on how your body feels versus how it looks. Do you have more energy? Can you walk up a flight of steps without huffing and puffing? Are you calmer and less stressed? Have you been more positive at work and with friends? Do you eat good food with the sense that you are nurturing and protecting a healthy body? When you feel good, you look better too. It is much easier to smile when we feel good. Our steps have more bounce when we feel good. And it is definitely easier to love ourselves wholly and completely when we feel good!

3. Don't waste time and energy fixating on the small stuff. Keep your energy for accomplishing your dreams! One of my girlfriends evaluates the success of an event, her day, and practically her life by whether or not she feels she was dressed appropriately. Now, I will admit there is value to good hygiene, and certain times when common sense and decorum should rule as far as clothing goes, but she takes it way too far. She is literally wasting her life. First of all, she shops constantly—when she is not shopping, she is returning. And when she is not en route to the mall or home, she is dressing! It takes her two hours to dress to go out! Amazing! I cannot even imagine how she could draw the process out so. Even if I had the luxury of all that time, I could never be so preoccupied by my appearance. (And I know that those of you with small children and babies will agree—we just hope our clothes are clean and that nothing gets spilled or wiped on us in an obvious spot!) She obviously has weak self-esteem. I keep telling her that if she would spend even a fraction of the time she uses to shop and dress to exercise, she would feel so much better about herself. She would also rely less on the perfect clothing to prove her worth to the world.

Remember, you are valuable for reasons that go far beyond the superficiality of appearance. Know it and believe it because it is true!

MENU PLAN DAY 13: SATURDAY

Total calories: 1476
Less than 20 percent fat

BREAKFAST
(310 calories)

1 cup cooked oatmeal with 7 dried apricot halves (chopped), 8 ounces skim milk, and pinch of Allspice

SNACK
(60 calories)

1 fruit choice (p. 174)

LUNCH
(445 calories)

*1 cup Progresso Split Green Pea Soup
1 slice rye bread with
1 slice melted low-fat American cheese
2 cups tossed green salad with
½ chopped Golden Delicious apple,
2 chopped dates, and
2 tablespoons Catalina Fat-Free Dressing*

AFTERNOON SNACK OR EVENING DESSERT
(100-150 calories)

Snack List (p. 178) or Dessert List (pp. 179–80)

DINNER
(511 calories)

*Shrimp Stir Fry (p. 165)
1 cup mixed cantaloupe and honeydew melon*

EATING TIPS OF THE DAY:

1. Our bodies need lots of calcium (RDA, 800 mg). A great source is dark green leafy vegetables which have few calories and no fat—but watch the dressings.

2. Never skip breakfast! Juice, skim milk, and hot or cold cereals with fruit provide about one third of your RDA of vitamins and minerals.

RX: ACTIVITY PLAN—DAY 13: SATURDAY

MINIMUM DAILY REQUIREMENT—5 MINUTES

Start your day off right with Denise's Daily Dose. Whew, it's finally Saturday, but don't just sit there! Get going with this 5-minute routine. You can do this any time of the day. This is the only must for the day

See pp. 183-87 for the complete routine.

FREE DAY

It's the weekend. This is your day to improve at a sport you love, or try a new activity. Once again, if you missed a day of exercise during the week, take advantage of Saturday to make up for it. Saturdays are also great if you're a mom, because you can ask your husband to watch the children while you exercise.

FITNESS TIP OF THE DAY:

Exercise is a great way to combat low self-esteem. It's hard to feel bad about yourself when you're doing an activity that is good for you.

DAY 14: PRESENT YOURSELF

Dear Denise,

I am thirty-seven years old and have been through dieting, workouts, and so on, and nothing has made me as happy as the results I get from you. I went from a size 13 down to a size 5. I now wear shorts and crop tops— for the first time in my life I actually bought two form-fitting A-line dresses. I received tons of compliments on how great I looked in my dresses. Thank you for touching my life and bringing me happiness.

—Elaine, Arlington Heights, Illinois

Deniseology

I know we discussed the concept that "you are your own architect" in the introduction to the 21 Day Plan. Let's revisit that idea, since it is an important point about your body and how it responds to your design choices. I am not talking about physical design—I realize that if we really had input into the physical design of our own bodies we would probably exchange a few things. I know that I, and every one of my friends, have a couple of body parts we would be delighted to trade in for new models. However, since that is impossible, it is our responsibility to make the very best of the body we have been given. I am referring to the design qualities of the outward persona we select to represent who we are to the world.

The principle underlying the concept of thinking of yourself as the architect of your body is the fact that you determine how you present your physical self to the world. How you stand, sit, walk, move, gesture, speak, touch, and use facial expressions is completely under your control. Your skeleton supplies the frame and your muscles the tools; your mind constitutes the driving force behind the person others see. The manner in which you incorporate the features of your body communicates a message to those around you. It is called *body language*.

Body language is probably the only system of communication that is universally understood throughout the world. I have traveled a lot, and even in countries where I had no understanding of the language, I was able to understand a great deal through body language.

Here's a story about what happened to me in Russia in 1985. Twenty women in professional fields were chosen to represent the United States in a delegation to the Soviet Union. I was honored to have been chosen in the field of fitness. While there I did a live broadcast for the *Today Show* on the state of Russian fitness. I was the first woman at NBC to do a live broadcast from the Soviet Union. As I was about to go on live, three Russian soldiers entered and stood rigidly with arms folded directly behind the camera. Their body language clearly communicated to me that I had better watch what I said about Russia. Just as I was able to understand the Russian soldiers, I was able to communicate to the local people through body language as well. As I traveled to other countries of the Soviet Union, through gesture and expression the local people could generally tell if I was distressed, excited, impressed, or frustrated. They would usually respond accordingly, whether it was to try and help me find my way, or simply rejoice along with my euphoria in experiencing their country and its history. It really is quite amazing to share an experience with another human being, and yet not understand a single spoken word.

The body is also an effective communicator among people who speak the same language. For instance, you can tell almost immediately upon entering a room how the individuals within it feel about where they are. Are their expressions and bodies relaxed or uptight? Are people mingling close together or are they isolated? One quick glance can usually provide enough information for you to decide if the people are happy, angry, frightened, or sad. This intuitive response affects how you behave upon joining the group.

The same principles apply in my work. People respond to me because I am happy, energetic, optimistic, and upbeat. I communicate those qualities in the way I speak, my posture as I move, sit, and stand, and the way I look at people. Imagine that you came to see me during a live appearance and I looked melancholy and rarely smiled. Say that on top of that, my shoulders were slumped, my hips jutted out to one side, my hands and arms were crisscrossed over my midsection, my head drooped forward, and you could not understand a word I said because I was speaking into my chest. Well, I can assure you that you would not be impressed! First, you would wonder what in the world was wrong with me. Then, you would begin to doubt anything that I said was true because, heck, believing in fitness sure didn't seem to be doing me any good! You would leave that event depressed! Why? Because the messages my body language sent were those of an unhappy, unsure woman.

You can affect your own audience the very same way! Maybe you do not go on stage for your living, but you do present yourself to people in a similar way every minute of every day. Think about some people you know who are quite popular and enjoyable to be around. Watch them. How do they move, speak, hold their bodies? How do they make you and others feel? Take what you see and apply it to your own body language. It is very important to be yourself in this process; you do not want to act in a way that is unnatural to you. But do try to modify your body language to communicate positive messages to others that say you believe in yourself and your own unique abilities. Even if you are very shy, quiet, or reserved, you can still illustrate, simply by standing straight, proud and tall, that you are happy with the person you are.

Remember the smile experiment we tried in the first chapter? People find it very hard to resist someone who approaches them with a big smile and a friendly face. Besides, it is easier to smile than frown— a frown uses forty-three muscles and a smile only thirteen. So go ahead! *Present yourself!* Put that best face forward, and I bet you will see immediate change in the way others respond to you. *You are the architect!* Construct a body that communicates how wonderful you are!!

POSITIVE THOUGHT:

Overall fitness is a very special key to beauty. . . . and a healthy body brings out fresh appeal in everyone.

EATING TIP OF THE DAY:

Keep a basket filled with
sugar-free candy and gum
in the kitchen. When
you're craving something
sweet, reach into the
basket instead of the
refrigerator or pantry.

MENU PLAN DAY 14: SUNDAY

Total calories: 1416
Less than 20 percent fat

BREAKFAST
(250 calories)

Waffle Danish (p. 166)

SNACK
(60 calories)

1 fruit choice (p. 174)

LUNCH
(470 calories)

Homemade Lentil Soup (p. 166)
2 toasted whole-wheat mini-pitas
Tossed green leaf lettuce, zucchini, and yellow squash with
2 tablespoons fat-free Italian dressing, and
1 ounce low-fat Swiss cheese chunks
Bosc pear

AFTERNOON SNACK OR EVENING DESSERT
(100-150 calories)

Snack List (p. 178) or Dessert List (pp. 179–80)

DINNER
(486 calories)

3 ounces BBQ Pork Tenderloin (p. 167)
⅔ cup Simply Potatoes (found in refrigerated section)
1 cup steamed fresh asparagus
2 teaspoons butter or margarine
¾ cup fresh pineapple

RX: ACTIVITY PLAN—DAY 14: SUNDAY

It's Sunday, it's a total rest day, it's your day off. But stay active.

Rest! Reward yourself! You have made it through two weeks of living healthily. You're getting closer to a new way of life.

Option: Remember, you can use your rest day on another particularly busy day during the week. Just don't forget to complete the routine on Sunday!

FITNESS TIPS OF THE DAY:

1. Take some time to plan your workouts and menus for the next week. Thinking ahead is your best defense against a busy schedule!

2. Laughter is the best medicine. It can get your blood circulating and produce the same body chemicals that a runner experiences during a runner's high.

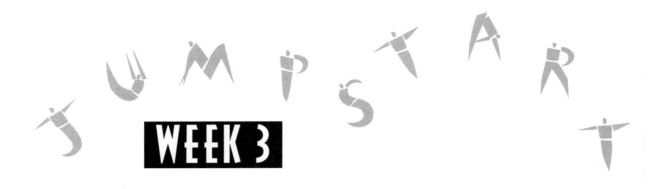

WEEK 3

WEEK 3	MONDAY DAY 15	TUESDAY DAY 16	WEDNESDAY DAY 17	THURSDAY DAY 18	FRIDAY DAY 19	SATURDAY DAY 20	SUNDAY DAY 21
Deniseology	Sharing	Positive Relations	Positive Self-Talk	Thanks for Blessings	Optimism	On Target	Goals for Success
Fitness	Aerobics	Toning	Aerobics	Toning	Aerobics	Free Day	Rest
Dinner	Chicken	Beef Salad	Turkey	Chicken	Tuna Salad	Egg-Baked Potato	Beef

Table title: JUMPSTART WEEK 3 AT A GLANCE

WEEK 3 SHOPPING LIST

Note: How much you need of the fresh produce and meats will be determined by how many people you are feeding. That's why it is important to look at all of the recipes before you go shopping. Also, look in your kitchen cabinets and refrigerator to make sure which of these foods, spices, and so on you already have.

FRUITS

Assorted fruits
Orange juice
Cranberry sauce
Winesap apples
Watermelon
Fresh raspberries

Seedless grapes
Mango
Canned juice-pack peaches
Tangerines
D'Anjou pears
Dried figs
Bananas

Canned juice-pack pineapple
Grapefruit juice
Honeydew melon
Oranges
Apples

VEGETABLES

Assorted vegetables
Carrots
Green peppers
Romaine lettuce
Fresh-cut green beans
Mushrooms
Mixed greens
Broccoli
Snow peas
Water chestnuts
Brussels sprouts
Onions (regular and red)
Corn on the cob
Cucumber
Celery
Alfalfa sprouts
Fresh asparagus
Potatoes
Avocado
Fresh spinach

MEATS

Sliced turkey breast
Boneless chicken breast
Lean beef
Tuna (water-packed)
Turkey Breast cutlets
Tuna steak
Smoked chicken
Lean beef cubes

BREADS/GRAINS

Low-fat granola bars
7-grain bread
Orzo (rice-shaped pasta)
Assorted cereals
Whole-wheat pretzels
Bugs Bunny Graham Snacks
Vermicelli
Corn tortillas
"Simply Potatoes" Mashed
    Potatoes (refrigerated
    section)
Oatmeal
Ak-Mak Whole-Wheat Muffins
Rye bagels
Whole wheat pitas
Raisin bran English muffins
Buckwheat pancake mix
Couscous
Fat-free or low-fat assorted
    crackers, cookies, and
    desserts

DAIRY

Nonfat yogurt
Skim milk
Low-fat string cheese
Reduced-fat cheese slices
Nonfat or low-fat sour cream
Muenster cheese
Eggs
Ricotta cheese (part-skim)

CONDIMENTS

Spicy brown mustard
Chicken broth
Olive oil*
Toasted sesame seeds
Soy sauce*
Sugar*
Garlic cloves
Ground ginger*
Red-pepper sauce
Peanut oil
Fresh lime juice
Fresh cilantro
Salsa
Cooking spray*
White wine (or nonalcoholic
    white wine)
Dried tarragon*

*Could last for entire program, depending on how many people you have to feed.

DAY 15:
SHARING

Dear Denise,

Never would I have believed it, had someone said, "Pat, a year from now you'll be 56 pounds less and wearing a size 12 (I was a 20!)." In six months, Denise, working out faithfully with you, and following your eating plan, I lost the 56 pounds, sizes, and inches. Our small-town society made me the talk of the town for a while! I've kept the weight off for six months now and have decided to go for a size 10! My husband gave me your Super Stomachs video for Valentine's Day and I love it. I've had encouragement from all my family and friends which has been a huge help. I just wanted to say thank you. Your workouts are always so personal and the settings are beautiful. No one else rates with me.

—Pat, Athens, Georgia

Deniseology

Have you ever noticed that some of our best memories and our best feelings about ourselves occur when we have shared something with others? Our time, money, insight, knowledge, understanding, or maybe just our ears for listening are all ways in which we can give of ourselves to others. Sometimes the best way we can learn to feel better about ourselves, who we are, and what we have, is by reaching out to those in need: emotionally, physically or financially. For instance, my favorite appearances are those for charitable organizations. I cannot possibly commit to every organization that asks, but over the years I have found a few that I truly believe in. For over seven years I have been an "ambassador" for the March of Dimes. I have also volunteered my time for the Juvenile Diabetes Association (earning $275,000 for them just last year).

Jeff and I also believe, since we have been blessed in so many ways, that it is very important to share all we have. We try to be generous with our time for friends who need us, and we are always willing to help our families in any way possible. As a matter of fact, the moment in which I was most aware that all of my hard work was truly worth it was when Jeff and I surprised my mother with a brand-new Toyota Camry for Christmas a couple of years ago. There is no greater joy than in being able to spoil your mother!

I want my whole family to share in my success. I often invite one of my sisters or my mother to join me when I travel for *Getting Fit* to one of those beautiful resort locations. It allows them to get away from the day-to-day routine of their own lives, and it makes things a lot more fun for me!

This past year I treated "the girls," my mom and my sisters, to a week-long vacation. We traveled from New York City to Martha's Vineyard (and every place in between). Believe me, other than tourist walking, it was not a fit vacation! Our itinerary was literally one meal after another. I am not sure I can recall some of the more historical sites we saw, but if you need some recommendations on restaurants—I know them all! It may not have been low fat, but it certainly was fun. And it made me feel great that I could offer my family such a wonderful vacation.

> **POSITIVE THOUGHT:**
>
> For every person you see today that you deeply care about, I want you to smile and give one compliment to each. It could be your spouse, brother, sister, child, best friend, whomever. If you do, you will feel such joy.

The old adage, "It is better to give than to receive," continues to ring true today. Some of life's greatest rewards come not from what we get but from what we give. Giving of yourself not only makes others feel good, it builds self-worth. Sharing money and material goods enables you to become spiritually richer, while increasing the means of those with less. You are happier with yourself, and those you help are happier because they have received some much-needed attention or relief. It is a win-win situation.

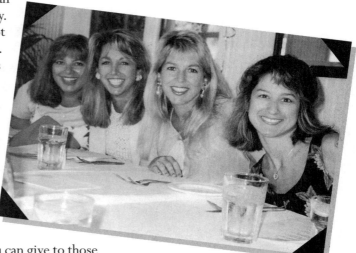

My sisters and I spending time together . . . and, of course, eating!

Today, I would like you to consider at least one small way in which you can give to those around you. Volunteer in your community. Help out in the local schools. Tutor a neighborhood child. Take a prepared meal to a friend who is alone or particularly busy and probably not eating well, and if your friend seems lonely, stay for a while and talk. Offer to take a friend's child for an afternoon, a day, or a weekend if a couple is in need of some time together. Or maybe even agree to baby-sit one evening a week for a single parent who needs a break! The list of possibilities is endless. Be creative! I promise, the greatest rewards will be yours!

MENU PLAN DAY 15: MONDAY

Total calories: 1368
Less than 20 percent fat

EATING TIPS OF THE DAY:

1. Have a midafternoon snack to keep yourself from raiding the refrigerator when you get home from work or school. Great choices are plain popcorn, pretzels, or cut-up vegetables. Watch the portion size.

2. When eating out, try to order foods that are steamed, grilled, roasted, or poached.

BREAKFAST
(310 calories)

6 ounces orange juice
Low-fat granola bar
8 ounces nonfat yogurt

SNACK
(60 calories)

1 fruit choice (p. 174)

LUNCH
(330 calories)

2 ounces sliced turkey with
2 tablespoons cranberry sauce and romaine lettuce
on 2 slices 7-grain bread
Winesap apple

AFTERNOON SNACK OR EVENING DESSERT
(100-150 calories)

Snack List (p. 178) or Dessert List (pp. 179–80)

DINNER
(518 calories)

Chicken Moutarde (p. 167)
with French-cut green beans and mushrooms
over orzo (rice-shaped pasta)
1¼ cup watermelon cubes

RX: ACTIVITY PLAN—DAY 15: MONDAY

MINIMUM DAILY REQUIREMENT—5 MINUTES

Start your week off right with Denise's Daily Dose. You're in the home stretch—you're doing great. You can do this routine by itself or before or after your aerobic exercise.

See pp. 183-87 for the complete routine.

AEROBIC FITNESS—30 MINUTES

It's an aerobics day. Today you will do 30 minutes of an aerobic activity.

Choose from the list on p. 181 for your aerobic options.

Walking is one of the best forms of aerobics, but this week pick up the pace. Walk briskly, pump those arms, and tighten that tummy!

Don't forget, you need to stretch those muscles after exercising so do at least three of my Super Stretches on p. 188.

When to Exercise: The best time that fits your day today.
Time: 30 minutes.
How: Look at your aerobic options on p. 181.
Suggestion: Try interval training. Walk in speed intervals: Walk slowly for 5 minutes, walk quickly for 5 minutes, walk slowly for 2 minutes, walk quickly for 5 minutes, walk slowly for 2 minutes, walk quickly for 5 minutes, and gradually slow down the pace for 6 minutes (until finished). If you would like, I have a TrimWalk audio tape that helps you walk to the beat of the music while guiding you through the intervals.

FITNESS TIPS OF THE DAY:

1. Walking raises the body's metabolism to 5 or more calories per minute (cpm). The average person burns 1 cpm at rest (sleeping.)

2. If you must work long hours and cannot possibly fit in 30 minutes to take a brisk walk or jog, then concentrate on tightening your stomach and buttock muscles while sitting at your desk. Also, always take the stairs.

DAY 16: CHOOSE POSITIVE RELATION- SHIPS

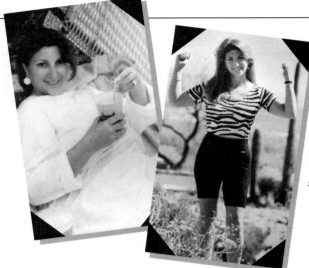

Marilyn— Birmingham, Michigan:
"I did it. I dropped those awful pounds and inches . . . all thanks to you. It feels so good."

Dear Denise,

About four months ago I started working out with you. I have stuck with it because it makes me feel great, not physically as much as mentally. I finally figured it out: Exercising just to look great doesn't work for me. It never did. Since we've been exercising I've got a nice relaxed body, and tons of confidence. Exercise has really adjusted my attitude. I have excelled so much in the past few months. All of my relationships have improved and I'm so much more comfortable with myself. I don't look like a model, but I don't want to. I'm me, and I can only look and be the best me. Thank you!

—*Becky, Benicia, California*

Deniseology

One aspect of life that fascinates me is how people choose with whom they spend their time, and even their lives. I can't tell you how many people I have met who are unhappy due to the way those around them make them feel. What I am referring to is negative relationships. A *negative relationship* is one in which one member of the relationship does the majority, if not all, of the giving, and the other just takes and takes.

Negative relationships can occur when a person is emotionally needy, or perhaps just particularly self-centered (also called *narcissistic*). Sometimes people are overly selfish, depressed, belligerent, or unnecessarily critical of others. Negative relationships can be found anywhere and everywhere. They occur in families, marriages, dating, work, and social relationships. You may think this is an unusual way to view things, but every relationship we engage in is an investment of our valuable time and energy. Perhaps we should evaluate those around us in terms of the returns received from the time invested.

Don't get me wrong; I'm not down on relationships and friendships.

As a matter of fact, just the opposite! I think family and friendships are essential to providing the love and support we need and desire. God did not create human beings to live alone. Instinctively our prehistoric ancestors formed communities and social environments. Humans thrive on interaction and exchange. Other people make things more interesting and certainly much more fun. After all, what is a party other than a group of people gathering to enjoy each other?

Negative relationships adversely affect you because people like this have a parasitic effect. They latch on, often very innocently, to others for strength, support, positive reinforcement, superiority, control . . . the list could go on and on. Such personalities can be very draining physically and emotionally, particularly for someone striving to maintain a positive attitude. The desire to satisfy their personal needs far outweighs any concern they may have for those around them, even if they are completely unaware of it. As a matter of fact, the most extreme form of a negative relationship is termed abusive. Other negative relationships can be just as complex, but a lot more subtle.

Jeff and I have had friends over the years tell us how much they love to spend time with us because we are so positive and upbeat. (Jeff and I truly enjoy each other: Even after twelve years of marriage, each of us finds that our favorite person to spend time with is the other!) Our friends say that the warmth and laughter generated by the two of us make them feel happy, too!

What I can say is this: If you have a positive attitude about yourself, your life, and your relationships, you will be empowered to triumph over the negative people who attempt to influence you. Focus your time and energy on spending time with people you consider to be inspiring and optimistic.

Ever heard the saying "One bad apple spoils the whole bunch"? Well, negative people breed negative energy. Even the most upbeat personalities get dampened by pessimistic, derogatory, or parasitic behavior. Think of it as a contagious disease. Sure, these people need our care and often our help; just remember to protect your own emotional center. If you meet a friend who drains you emotionally one day, make an extra effort to get in contact with a positive, upbeat person very soon.

Take a moment right now to think about the people who surround you at home, work, and socially. Would you categorize them as optimists (those who see the glass as half full) or pessimists (those who see the glass as half empty)? Try to focus on how you feel when you are with these people or after you leave them. Do you feel happy or sad? Better about yourself or worse? Relationships should be a positive and invigorating force in our lives.

POSITIVE THOUGHT:

A person's greatest emotional need is to feel appreciated.

MENU PLAN DAY 16: TUESDAY

Total calories: 1376
Less than 20 percent fat

BREAKFAST
(260 calories)

1 cup cereal (p. 177)
8 ounces skim milk
1 cup fresh raspberries

SNACK
(60 calories)

1 fruit choice (p. 174)

LUNCH
(400 calories)

1 ounce low-fat string cheese
1 ounce whole-wheat pretzels
1 cup seedless grapes
13 Bugs Bunny Graham Snacks

AFTERNOON SNACK OR EVENING DESSERT
(100-150 calories)

Snack List (p. 178) or Dessert List (pp. 179–80)

DINNER
(506 calories)

Thai Beef Salad with Sesame Noodles (p. 168)
Mango half or
2 halves canned juice-pack peaches

EATING TIP OF THE DAY:

Many times people cannot tell if they are hungry, or just stressed or bored. To make sure hunger is what you're satisfying and not stress or boredom, try taking a walk, playing the piano, or calling a friend. After that activity, if you're still hungry, then eat.

RX: ACTIVITY PLAN—DAY 16: TUESDAY

MINIMUM DAILY REQUIREMENT—5 MINUTES

Start your day off right with Denise's Daily Dose. It takes only 5 minutes and it will boost your energy level for the day. You can do this separately or before or after your toning exercises.

See pp. 183-87 for the complete routine.

MUSCLE TONING—20 MINUTES

It's a toning day. It's time to firm those thighs, tighten your tummy, and achieve sexy-looking arms. Today you will use your weights for almost all the exercises. All these exercises require a chair (make sure chair does *not* have rollers). A step or bench would be great! Today you will spend 20 minutes, so I want you to take your time on each exercise—concentrate and focus on proper form.

It's important to finish with at least three of the Super Stretches on p. 188.

You're on your way to a better body!

TONING—20 MINUTES

Warm-up: 1–2 minutes of marching in place
Back Roll-up (p. 229)
1. Thigh and Bun Firmer (p. 230)
2. Lean Legs (with chair) (p. 231)
3. Lower Body Toner (weights optional) (p. 232)
4. Kickbacks (with weights) (p. 233)
5. Shoulder Raises (with weights) (p. 234)
6. Push-ups (p. 235)
7. Thigh and Tush Tightener (p. 235)
8. Bottoms Up (p. 236)
9. Waistline Slimmer (p. 237)
10. Advanced Bicycle (p. 238)

FITNESS TIPS OF THE DAY:

1. You cannot change your bone structure—your skeleton—but you *can* change your fat content and muscle tone.

2. Do you want to know what the true fountain of youth is? Toned muscles! Turn back your time clock with firm muscles. Each muscle is made up of millions of tiny cells; to keep the skin from sagging you must work these cells.

DAY 17: POSITIVE SELF-TALK!

Deniseology

First, let's talk about the opposite of *positive self-talk*. I like to call it *stinky thinking*. Stinky thinking results from giving credence to the negative thoughts and ideas about yourself that sometimes settle in our minds. Like, "I'm not even going to try for the promotion because the boss has never liked me and Sally is much more talkative and popular. I am not going to waste my time. I'm not even sure I have enough experience, maybe I would screw up and get fired—besides, nothing good ever happens to me." Or maybe, "Diet and exercise have never worked for me. I am just meant to be fat." And possibly, "Why should I bother to go to the party? No one ever notices me and I never have anyone to talk to." Pretty soon, stinky thoughts become comments as we start to verbalize them, usually without hearing ourselves. Stinky thinking makes you feel bad about yourself, your job, and your life.

Stinky thinking can be, and often is, debilitating. At the very least it frequently succeeds in making you unhappy. And in its worst form it allows feelings of self-hatred to evolve. I consider it a modern phenomenon that women, in particular, choose to hate themselves. This most commonly takes place in regard to our bodies and how we feel we rate compared to a national standard. (I suppose that would be the one-to-ten scale.) We feel we are judged by the sexiness of our bodies, the stylishness of our clothes, and the structure of our faces.

But just like our discussion earlier regarding self-imposed rules, who the heck created this standard? Who is in charge? Who defined the difference between a one, a five, or a ten? I guess Bo Derek is the most famous ten. However, I would bet any amount that if you talked to her she would share her personal doubts about that rating. I am sure that she, like many other women I know, thinks that her body is flawed and that she is personally lacking in some critical qualities. So even a nationally recognized ten does not think she is a ten.

After all, the definitions of beauty are as fleeting as the seasons. The attractiveness of a beautiful heart, however, has never changed. You are worth loving—no matter what you look like or what you think you look like.

I know for certain that in order to truly believe you deserve to be happy, you must learn to acknowledge your goodness. Personally, I have never met a person who couldn't contribute something valuable to the world. I am convinced that all of your wonderful talents and abilities are just waiting for you to let them shine!

If you are truly in doubt on this point, then try this simple exercise. Choose someone you trust who cares about you, and set up an informal interview. Explain that you are in the process of transforming your life from your head down to your toes. Ask your friend or family member to tell you what it is they like about you, and what qualities particularly stand out that make you special and unique. Your job is to listen. Write their comments down on a small piece of paper or index card. Review it every night before you go to bed or pull it out when stinky thinking attempts to infiltrate your mindset. The only rule, if you will, to this exercise is that this conversation must only focus on your gifts. No criticisms are allowed—no matter how constructive.

I remember a saying that was popular ten or fifteen years ago: "I'm lovable because God don't make junk." It was true then and it is true now. Learning to love yourself starts with you. It starts with reprogramming that little voice way down inside you. I try to program my little voice with positives. And so can you! Do not forget that you are in control here. You can make a *choice*. Tell that little voice to cease and desist with those negative thoughts. Stop all that stinky thinking immediately. Introduce *positive self-talk* into your life today!

Okay, I realize that everyone has days on which they feel less attractive than others—for instance, a bad hair day. But that does not mean you must dwell on that negativity. Maybe you cannot control feeling or thinking a negative thought here and there, but you have 100 percent control regarding the thoughts you choose to save and focus on. From now on, I want you to make a conscious effort to eliminate from your conversation and your mind negative self-talk and stinky thinking, even as a joke. Resist any temptation to put yourself down. When your mind, or your mouth for that matter, says "I'm so fat" or "I'll never make it," replace those words immediately with "I can do it!" "I'm worth it!" "I'm getting healthier and stronger every day!" and "God don't make junk!" Whenever that old familiar stinky thinking rears its ugly head, douse it with a strong dose of positive self-talk.

POSITIVE THOUGHT:

When you feel good about yourself, you're more likely to stick to your healthy ways, so take a minute to sit down and make a list of things you like about yourself. For instance, you have a great smile, you have toned arms, or you're a great friend.

Sometimes the most difficult aspect of this transformation in thinking is becoming aware of how often we allow stinky thinking or negativity to rule our conversation and our thoughts. A good way to increase your consciousness is by incorporating the assistance of some close family members or friends. Ask those close to you to help you be more aware of the negativity that creeps into your daily conversation. In the beginning, you will be surprised how often they interrupt you. Soon though, those negative thoughts will be a thing of the past! When that happens you will know that positive self-talk is firmly entrenched in your life.

MENU PLAN DAY 17: WEDNESDAY

Total calories: 1496
Less than 20 percent fat

BREAKFAST
(370 calories)

Healthy Choice Breakfast Sandwich
(Egg on Muffin)
8 ounces skim milk
Tangerine

SNACK
(60 calories)

1 fruit choice (p. 174)

LUNCH
(410 calories)

2 Tuna-Salsa Tortillas (p. 169)
D'Anjou pear

AFTERNOON SNACK OR EVENING DESSERT
(100–150 calories)

Snack List (p. 178) or Dessert List (pp. 179–80)

DINNER
(506 calories)

3 ounces Turkey Cutlet Tarragon (p. 170) with
¼ cup fat-free brown gravy
⅔ cup Simply Potatoes (in refrigerated section)
1 cup brussels sprouts steamed with onion slices
2 teaspoons butter or margarine
Fresh or juice-packed canned pears (2 halves)

EATING TIPS OF THE DAY:

1. Many times restaurants serve portions that should be for two. As soon as your meal comes, divide it and eat only half. If you can't stand to see it go to waste, ask the waiter for a doggie bag.

2. When buying dairy products, choose the most nutritious but least fattening. Some good choices are skim milk, low-fat buttermilk, nonfat yogurt, low-fat cottage cheese, and ice milk.

RX: ACTIVITY PLAN—DAY 17: WEDNESDAY

FITNESS TIP OF THE DAY:

Swimming can be a great aerobic workout. It involves a large number of the major muscle groups in the body and the threat of injury is minimal, because the buoyancy reduces stress on the bones and joints.

MINIMUM DAILY REQUIREMENT—5 MINUTES

Start your day off right with Denise's Daily Dose. It takes only 5 minutes and it will give you energy for the day. You can do this separately or before or after your aerobic exercise.

See pp. 183-87 for the complete routine.

AEROBIC FITNESS—30 MINUTES

It's an aerobics day. Today you will do 30 minutes of an aerobic activity.

Choose from the list on p. 181 for your aerobic options.

Finish off your activity with at least three of your favorite Super Stretches on p. 188.

Smile, you're burning fat!

When to Exercise: The best time that fits your day today.
Time: 30 minutes.
How: Look at your aerobic options on p. 181.
Suggestion: Try in-line skating (rollerblading)! It's fun and a great aerobic workout. Remember to wear a helmet and all the pads for extra safety.

DAY 18: GIVE THANKS FOR YOUR BLESSINGS EVERY DAY

Dear Denise,

In April of 1990 I had my first child. A day under ten months later I had my second child. Twenty-three months later our third child was born. Things were getting pretty bad with the extra "baby fat" that wasn't coming off, the bad marriage, and depression. But one day I just got up and did it! With a sore body the next day, I did it again. Things started changing. I've lost 10 pounds, changed my diet, fit into a smaller pair of jeans, and got a whole new way of doing things. With the added problems of a divorce and moving out, lots of anger and stress came to me but you helped me learn how to release everything. I have rough days but I take you very seriously as my personal trainer and keep my morning routine. I feel better, my energy is higher, and I get my day going.

—*Tracy, Southside, Alabama*

Deniseology

Have you ever been in a situation that forced you to reevaluate your priorities in life? Such experiences certainly are not much fun, but they truly provide a new, and often much-needed, change in perspective. We all know that life has many ups and downs. There isn't one soul on earth who hasn't, at some point, felt the sting of rejection, pain of a broken heart, frustration of delay, and anger at themselves or an uncontrollable situation. I believe that these incidents and circumstances are supposed to happen to us. I think of them as God's way of opening our eyes to all of the blessings and joys He has bestowed upon us.

I fall into the same traps you do. My life is so busy that it is easy to become preoccupied with things that may or may not be all that important. For instance, when I began to emerge as a television personality, I could easily have been wrapped up in the seductions of fame. In many ways it was very hard to avoid, because suddenly people began treating me differently.

Even though it takes years of hard work, once you become famous (*marketable* is probably the more accurate word) you become a VIP and get treated very nicely. And then you start hobnobbing with all sorts of other famous people (some of whom have forgotten that we all put our pants on one leg at a time!) and you think "maybe I really am one of them."

If you are not careful it is tempting to buy into the press and the hoopla. After all, you are in demand! People want photos and autographs. Your picture appears in magazines and you are offered spots on television. For me it is a constant schedule of zipping back and forth across the country to appear on radio and TV shows, to film *Getting Fit,* and to make guest appearances. There are limos, hotel suites, and fruit baskets . . . and on and on. Suddenly, even without really realizing it, you start to expect such treatment.

Thankfully, my day of reckoning came early in my career. Once, while I was flying to an appearance in New York City, the plane I was on experienced some mechanical difficulties and we were forced to make an emergency landing. All of the passengers were asked to assume the crash position by a flight attendant who worked very hard to remain calm in a cabin full of panic and fear. I will never forget that, even among the noise of those who vented their anxiety vocally and the roar of the engines, it seemed deafeningly silent. Through those long few minutes as the plane touched ground and skidded over the runway to a stop, all I could do was pray that we survived. All of my thoughts focused on my family. I was thinking about Kelly (I didn't have Katie yet), Jeff, my mom, my dad, my sisters, my brother, and my closest friends. I kept trying to remember the last time I had told them all how much I loved them and appreciated all of the special joy they had brought to my life.

When the plane stopped, everyone cheered, and even began cracking jokes as we began to evacuate the fuselage. Once on the ground, I made my way as quickly as I could to a pay phone to call my husband and family. I could barely describe what had happened as I tearfully and joyfully told them how much I loved them. I knew then and there that no career was worth my life. I wanted to live a quality life filled with normal and balanced friendships in an average neighborhood with children. The gilded towers of Los Angeles and Hollywood were not for me! I decided fame was an occupational hazard to be eyed with caution and handled safely.

Surviving that near plane crash enabled me to count my blessings thankfully and reestablish my priorities in short order. Never again will I judge my success by whether or not my products sell or how many magazines contain stories on me. No, my true successes are in my household.

My strong marriage, our happy children, a foundation in faith, and the good health we all enjoy are my greatest blessings. Do I value my professional achievements? Of course! But if I ever had to choose—my family would come first.

What are your blessings? Take a moment today and list them. I'll bet that the things you value most have nothing to do with your job, money, or appearance. In spite of the emphasis society puts on it, money is a commodity, a system of exchange—nothing more. Friendship, love, health, energy, enthusiasm, joy are the things that make life worth living, worth exploring. When you are feeling down, depressed, or pessimistic, whip out your list and give thanks for the blessings you share every day.

POSITIVE THOUGHT:

Don't use time carelessly for it can never be retrieved. Life is precious.

MENU PLAN DAY 18: THURSDAY

Total calories: 1368
Less than 20 percent fat

EATING TIP OF THE DAY:

A salad bar can
be a high-fat and
high-calorie nightmare.
Avoid sauces, bacon bits,
and pre-made salads
containing oil and mayo;
go for the vegetables,
beans, and fruit.

BREAKFAST

(300 calories)

1 cup cooked oatmeal with
2 chopped dried figs
8 ounces skim milk

SNACK

(60 calories)

1 fruit choice (p. 174)

LUNCH

(400 calories)

1 cup Homemade Lentil Soup (p. 166)
2 sheets Ak Mak 100% Stone Ground Whole-Wheat Crackers
8 ounces nonfat yogurt
Small banana

AFTERNOON SNACK OR EVENING DESSERT

(100-150 calories)

Snack List (p. 178) or Dessert List (pp. 179–80)

DINNER

(458 calories)

Chicken Stir Fry with Pineapple (p. 171)

RX: ACTIVITY PLAN—DAY 18: THURSDAY

MINIMUM DAILY REQUIREMENT—5 MINUTES

Start your day off right with Denise's Daily Dose. It takes only 5 minutes and will keep you motivated. You can do this routine by itself or as a warm-up before or after your toning exercises.

See pp. 183-87 for the complete routine.

MUSCLE TONING—20 MINUTES

It's a toning day. It's time to firm those thighs, tighten your tummy, and achieve sexy-looking arms. Today you will use your weights for most of the exercises except for the abdominals. Get pumped up for 20 minutes of reshaping your body!

End the toning routine with at least three Super Stretches of your choice on p. 188.

TONING—20 MINUTES

Warm-up: 1—2 minutes of marching in place
Back Roll-up (p. 239)
1. Power Lunge (weights optional) (p. 240)
2. Bun Firmer (weights optional) (p. 241)
3. Upright Rows (with weights) (p. 242)
4. Bust Builder (with weights) (p. 243)
5. Underarm Tightener (with weights) (p. 244)
6. Triceps Press on Bench/Chair (p. 245)
7. Super Crunches (with chair) (p. 246)
8. One Legged V-sit (p. 247)
9. Ab Presses (p. 247)
10. Back Strengthener (p. 248)

FITNESS TIP OF THE DAY:

Exercise with a buddy. An exercise partner helps keep you focused and motivated. It's also harder to skip workouts. Find a committed partner and I can almost guarantee you success.

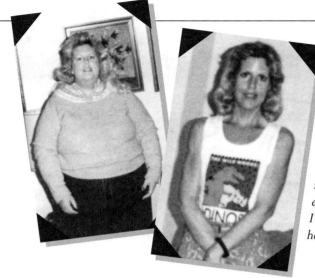

**Lee Ann—
Springfield, Illinois:**
*"Thanks for
JumpStarting me!
Your plan gave me
the confidence I
needed to lose all my
excess weight . . . and
I've kept it off. I'm
hooked."*

DAY 19:
OPTIMISM

. . . Optimism is more than finding the sunny side of any circumstance. It means savoring each moment of life as one would relish the sweetest fruit or the most breathtaking sunset, understanding this moment of bliss might never come again.

Optimism is more than smiling at everyone we meet. It means treasuring others as you would treasure the rarest gem or the finest painting. It means building relationships that prosper and endure.

Optimism is more than a philosophy of life; it is a philosophy of living. It is the acknowledgment a life is only lived when it is lived to its fullest. Optimism is more than just a way of thinking. It is a way of being. . . . It is unimportant whether or not a 'philosophy of optimism' has impacted my life. What is important is whether or not it has impacted the lives of others.

—*Optimist International*

Deniseology

Contrary to what you may believe, I have not been successful at everything I have tried. Nothing I have accomplished was handed to me on a silver platter. What did happen to me, fortunately at a very early age, was that I failed to achieve something I really wanted. (I truly believe that even bad things happen in life for positive reasons!) At the tender age of twelve years old, I experienced a failure that changed me forever. That temporary setback helped me to realize that reaching a goal required hard work, focused energy, and optimism.

One day, as I was heading to swim-team practice at the local YMCA, I cut through the gymnasium. It so happened that their gymnastics team was practicing. I stood there spellbound. They were wonderful! I loved the way their bodies gracefully swung through the air, the strength, poise, and discipline with which they moved, and the assured beat on the mat as they landed. I just knew I was meant to be a part of the team.

Like most young girls, I played gymnastics with my friends in our backyard. We would try all of the moves we saw on TV, you know, cartwheels, backbends, walkovers, and even some flips. I was always considered the best since I was pretty athletic and such moves came easily to me. I quickly mastered one-handed cartwheels, walkovers without hands, and standing up out of a backbend. I could even do the splits!

When I heard that there would be tryouts for the team, I was one of the first to sign up. I wasn't nervous, my backyard gymnastic tricks had been a breeze to learn. Surely the judges would see my ability as well. On the big day I gave it all I had! I flipped, flopped, and rolled with all the energy and enthusiasm I could muster.

But it wasn't enough. My name was not among those who had been selected for the team. I remember running home to bury my head in my pillow and cry my eyes out. I was devastated. How could the judges not have chosen me? For weeks I had dreamed of nothing but gymnastics!

Not being one to be down for too long, my grief soon turned into plans to change the situation. If I wasn't good enough to make it this time, then I would prove to them how good I could be at the next tryout. Since we did not have much extra money, I knew that a private coach was out of the question. If I wanted to learn more about gymnastics, I would have to hang around the team.

I badgered and badgered my mother to drive me to the gym. She finally agreed to drop me off, even though she was worried because she had to work and would not be able to pick me up. In my mind, that was a minor obstacle. I assured her I would get someone to take me home. Which I did, every day.

Day after day, for that entire school year, I showed up at gymnastics practice. They would see me scrutinizing their moves and attempting them on my own. There was so much to each movement! I had never realized the skills involved. Sometimes I would ask a coach to observe my movements and to give me pointers on how to improve. I must admit I was relentless. Soon, I made friends with the coaches and many of the team members. The coaches were so impressed at my commitment and dedication that after a while they let me practice along with everyone else.

The following year when gymnastics tryouts rolled around, I was ready. But this time I was really nervous! When my turn came, I did my best to show the judges all I had learned over the past year.

It was with crossed fingers and a great deal of apprehension that I checked the list of new team members. My name was there. I had made the team! I ran home full of excitement at my accomplishment. My mother had tears in her eyes when I shared my news. Of course, she was happy I had made the team, but she said her tears were from the deep pride she felt in how hard I had worked to make my dream come true. I now know that she was aware of something that I was simply too young to appreciate fully. This experience of dedicating myself to achieving a goal would be an asset for the rest of my life.

And it has. Not making the gymnastics team the first time taught me that it is not the things we don't accomplish in life that matter. Our success in life stems directly from how we choose to learn from all of our experiences, how we focus our energy and drive to move forward by thinking positively. Nothing was ever achieved by giving up or standing still.

Optimism is your ability to reach beyond your disappointments and to visualize alternative possibilities. Optimism allows you to embrace life as an adventure where every challenge represents the future joy of victory. Optimism is the confidence to risk potential failure because the road to triumph is the path of growth and fulfillment. Optimism is believing in yourself because God don't make junk!

As you approach the end of these first 21 days, take a moment to reflect back on your past experiences. What good things have come from situations that brought sadness or disappointment? Have you ever come through a negative experience only to be stronger or better prepared for something that happened later? How can you turn life's lemons into the best lemonade you have ever tasted? Optimistic thinking is the most *positive habit* I know!

POSITIVE THOUGHT:

Judge your success by the degree to which you're enjoying health, peace, and love.

MENU PLAN DAY 19: FRIDAY

Total calories: 1498
Less than 20 percent fat

BREAKFAST
(340 calories)

*Small rye bagel with
2 slices low-fat cheese
6 ounces grapefruit juice*

SNACK
(60 calories)

1 fruit choice (p. 174)

LUNCH
(435 calories)

*Turkey Gyro (p. 171)
1 cup seedless grapes
8 ounces skim milk*

AFTERNOON SNACK OR EVENING DESSERT
(100-150 calories)

Snack List (p. 178) or Dessert List (pp. 179–80)

DINNER
(513 calories)

*Grilled Tuna Salad (p. 172)
2 ears corn on the cob with 2 teaspoons butter or margarine
1 cup honeydew melon*

EATING TIPS OF THE DAY:

1. Make a habit of including one fruit with breakfast and at least one vegetable with both lunch and dinner.

2. One of the best ways to flavor vegetables without fatty sauces is to boil or steam your veggies in defatted chicken broth. I use just one can of broth and a little water for two handfuls of vegetables.

RX: ACTIVITY PLAN—DAY 19: FRIDAY

FITNESS TIP OF THE DAY:

A 20-30 minute
walk three times a week
may be just enough to
save your life. . . . every
step you take protects
your heart! Active women
in their fifties have
the heart and lung
function of sedentary
women in their thirties
and even twenties.

You're almost there . . .
yes . . . you did it. . .

MINIMUM DAILY REQUIREMENT—5 MINUTES

Start your day off right with Denise's Daily Dose. You made it! It's the weekend. Don't stop now—you're shedding those pounds. You can do this 5-minute routine separately or before or after your aerobic exercise.

See pp. 183-87 for the complete routine.

AEROBIC FITNESS—30 MINUTES

It's an aerobics day. Today you will do 30 minutes of an aerobic activity.

Choose from the list on p. 181 for your aerobic options.

Whatever you choose to do, finish the activity with your three favorite Super Stretches on p. 188.

When to Exercise: The best time that fits your day today.
Time: 30 minutes.
How: Look at your aerobic options on p. 181.
Suggestion: If you have children and cannot leave them alone while you exercise, go to a school track and walk around it (four times around most tracks equals a mile) Your children can play in the center of the track or if they're small, push them in a stroller.

- Give it all you've got today.
- It's Friday.
- The weekend is here.
- Burn those calories.
- Lose the fat.

DAY 20: NOW YOU ARE ON TARGET!

Dear Denise,

I thank God for you every day. Before I started working out with your show and videos, I weighed 192 and now I weigh 125! I've gone from a size 16 to a size 5/6. Can you believe it? Your encouragement is what got me fit and healthy. I cut out the picture of you from your Super Stomachs video and put it on my mirror. Every day I said to myself, "That's what you can look like!" Well, I don't look like you, but I look the best I ever have. Thanks, Denise, for everything you've done for me. I feel wonderful!

—Karen, Connelly Springs, North Carolina

Deniseology

Congratulations! Now you are on target! The key to maintaining all of the positive habits you have acquired is to keep living them every day. Staying on track and remaining in control of your decision to eat healthy, exercise regularly, and think positively should now be a habit for life. The whole point of this program was to introduce you to some simple strategies that could be incorporated into any normal person's lifestyle.

If you feel overwhelmed by all the information I shared during the program, then post these basic tips in an obvious place as a simple reminder.

1. Everything in moderation. Should you choose to indulge yourself by eating a rich meal or dessert, skipping exercise one day, or taking time out for a pity party, relax, and enjoy it. I do it, too! Life is full of experiences, moods, and emotions. Feeling, tasting, and resting are also an important part of this overall journey! After all, your new habits are the habits of a lifetime. And a lifetime is a lot longer than an occasional piece of cheesecake! Try to think of my 80 percent–20 percent trick.

Eat well 80 percent of the time and enjoy (I mean *really* enjoy) eating 20 percent of pure indulgences.

2. Try not to eat late at night. Try to allow yourself three hours to metabolize your final meal before bed. If you generally do not go to bed before 11:00 P.M., then dinner by 7:30 or so is best. As always, however, never practice any of these guidelines to extremes. If you get home late one night and are hungry, then eat something! Don't forget what starving does to your metabolism.

3. Drink plenty of water. Water is critical to the body's ability to function and flush itself of toxins. It is an important component to a committed exercise program, not to mention that it is the consummate thirst quencher!

4. Be a smart shopper. Think about shopping the perimeters of the grocery store first (that is where all of the fresh produce, meats, fish, and low-fat dairy can be found). Read all labels before you buy. Remember the quick method of determining the fat content of foods I taught you.

5. Do not be afraid to ask questions when dining out. There is no reason to be embarrassed! Now that you are aware of the hidden sources of fat, take control. Ask if the fish or chicken is grilled in butter. Request all dressings and sauces be served on the side. And order your salads and sandwiches with mustard instead of mayonnaise.

6. Keep moving. We have discussed many creative ways to exercise, from walking with friends to venturing off to roller skate or ice skate as a family outing. Just remember to schedule those activities into your calendar, and to keep the activity going for at least 15 to 20 minutes (longer if you can).

7. Be positive, be proud! Each day you practice your new habits will make you healthier, happier, stronger, and more energetic. Confidence in yourself and your abilities will do more to help you keep that weight off forever than any diet ever could. You are a unique, beautiful, and rare individual—the one and only you!

MENU PLAN DAY 20: SATURDAY

Total calories: 1500
Less than 20 percent fat

BREAKFAST
(322 calories)

Raisin-bran English muffin with 2 teaspoons jelly
8 ounces skim milk
Fresh orange

SNACK
(60 calories)

1 fruit choice (p. 174)

LUNCH
(484 calories)

2 ounces sliced smoked chicken and
1 ounce Muenster cheese, on
2 slices multigrain bread with
1 tablespoon honey mustard, and lettuce
1 cup broccoli florets
Red delicious apple

AFTERNOON SNACK OR EVENING DESSERT
(100-150 calories)

Snack List (p. 178) or Dessert List (pp. 179–80)

DINNER
(484 calories)

Egg-Baked Potato (p. 172)
1 cup cooked frozen asparagus
Fresh pear

EATING TIPS OF THE DAY:

1. To prevent belly bloatedness:
   - don't chew gum
   - eat slowly
   - don't sip from a straw
   - don't drink carbonated beverages

2. When ordering pizza, I order half pizza with cheese for the kids and the other half with just sauce and veggies.

RX: ACTIVITY PLAN—DAY 20: SATURDAY

MINIMUM DAILY REQUIREMENT—5 MINUTES

Start your day off right with Denise's Daily Dose. It takes only 5 minutes and it will energize you for the day. You can do this separately or before or after your stretching exercises.

See pp. 183-87 for the complete routine.

FREE DAY

It's the weekend. Have fun and stay active! You did great, just keep it up! Go ahead. Get up and push yourself. Walk that extra mile, swim another lap, and ski hard down that slope. It takes guts and persistence to keep going!

FITNESS TIPS OF THE DAY:

1. Take a few minutes each day to relax. It's easy and takes barely any time. Close your eyes, take deep breaths, and just let go. These few minutes will give you energy and help to reduce tension/stress.

2. Exercise is the fountain of youth! It lowers your cholesterol and blood pressure, raising your metabolism to prevent weight gain.

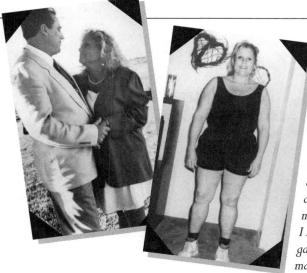

Debbie—
"I love the JumpStart Plan. I got so much confidence I asked my boyfriend to make a commitment after 2½ years of dating and he asked me to marry him! … I lost weight and gained a wonderful man!"

SUNDAY:

DAY 21: MAKE GOALS THAT SET YOU UP FOR SUCCESS

Deniseology

Congratulations! For the past three weeks you have worked very hard to transform your negative habits into new healthy ones. Some of you are feeling a little nervous about the coming weeks as you face the prospect of planning your own menus and exercises. Don't be! Over the past three weeks, I have established small goals for you to focus on every day. Some of them were probably more difficult than others. But all of them were *achievable!* Each day you had the chance to succeed, even if only in a very small way. Each small success contributed to the next small success; each was a separate building block toward your overall goal of positive habits.

Now that you are ready to move beyond the blueprint of the 21 Day Plan, you will have the opportunity to set your own daily, weekly, and monthly goals. So let's take a minute and examine the word *goal*. Personally, I define a goal as a commitment, no matter how private. You make an oath with yourself to accomplish something when you set a goal.

That prospect can be very exciting and also a little scary. Goals are necessary because they keep us motivated and moving forward. Goals also include some measure of risk. Failing to reach your goals too often (such as your past efforts at dieting) can be demoralizing and discouraging. And very soon you want to just quit!

I felt it was very important to discuss this concept because, while we all know that I encourage you to make your dreams a reality by seeing them as a goal to accomplish, some goals are of such major proportions they can take years to reach. And the prospect of ever getting close to them can seem overwhelming and remote. Without some successes along the way to keep us motivated, human beings become bored, distracted, and frustrated by an effort that appears futile.

Here are a few hints for good goal setting:

1. Set a goal. It could be a goal for this year, five years from now, or for life. The object here is to clarify what the goal really is and then to brainstorm all the roads that could take you there. Don't worry about realism here, think and dream.

2. Take time to learn. This is the step most often skipped by people setting a goal. But it only makes sense. How can you expect to succeed at anything unless you have a clear grasp of what it will take to get you there? Ask your friends and colleagues how they would go about accomplishing a similar goal. Call friends who may be professionals in a related field, if necessary, and ask their advice. Will you need additional education? If so, is it something you can do yourself, or will schooling be required? For instance, when I wanted to start my business after college, I asked everyone I knew how they would approach large businesses and how they would market the idea, who to talk to, what type of legal requirements there were, and on and on.

3. Draw up a plan of action. A *plan of action* is the articulation of a particular goal you would like to achieve and a general outline of the path you think will get you there. The best plans of action are those that are written down and posted somewhere where you can see them frequently. At this point, you can still be somewhat general, but try to keep it realistic. Even though you have a job that you just can't stand and you think your boss is a jerk, it might be a little difficult to just go out and find another job. If you set some short-term goals for yourself the task will seem much easier. Today, buy a paper and look through the want ads. Tomorrow, start to put the information together to write a new resume. Next week have your resume typed. In two weeks send it out to all the companies that you want to work for, then the week after, follow up and start to go on some interviews. Before you know it, you'll have a great new job, you'll love getting up in the morning to go to work, and it will all have started with a couple of small goals that turned into small successes!

4. Create realistic benchmarks. It is important, particularly when reaching for large goals, to set up benchmarks. *Benchmarks* are the achievable baby steps, or little successes, that keep you motivated as you march forward toward your secondary goals, and your ultimate goal. The difference is that a benchmark can be accomplished over a relatively short period of time. Say schooling is involved in your goal. The first benchmark could be researching a school that best fulfills your criteria. From timing to location to cost, you need to find the institution that suits your requirements and fits into your budget. The second benchmark might be requesting the application. The third benchmark would be completing the application. See? I think you have the idea.

5. Reward yourself. Every time you accomplish a benchmark, a secondary goal, and, of course, the ultimate goal, take the time to give yourself a reward. It does not have to be much. Maybe a special outing with friends if you have had your nose to the grindstone. Whatever it is, make sure it is something that you enjoy and makes you feel good about all that you are accomplishing!

It is no surprise that I think setting a goal is one of the most critical aspects to achieving all you want to in life. Remember the backbone and the wishbone? The wishbone only dreamed of what could be; the backbone made it happen through concrete steps and commitment.

We would all love it if life delivered everything we wanted like the genie in Aladdin. (Can you tell I'm a mom?) But we also learned from that movie that even having our wishes granted instantly does not solve all of our problems. I believe that every process, every path we forge in life, is a valuable lesson. Our journey on this earth is meant to have peaks and valleys, deserts and streams, rough and easy roads. Each step only prepares us further for the next bend in the road. As difficult as our road may seem, wouldn't life be really boring if everything were easy?

Setting and attaining goals in life is a valuable and wonderful positive habit. You are now well on your way to reaching your goal of a fit, energetic body, healthy eating habits, and a positive attitude. Now try to branch out with the principles behind these habits into other areas of your life. As I said in the very beginning, this is not a dress rehearsal! Dare to dream and dare to make things happen. You are the creator of your own destiny. Set your goals and realize your heart's desire!

POSITIVE THOUGHT:

Focus! Time is our most valuable asset, yet so many of us tend to waste time and kill time. Time is something you can never get back—it's more valuable than money. We need to learn to focus, to concentrate, and to stay directed.

Give yourself a big hand. You did it.

EATING TIPS OF THE DAY:

1. To cut fat and reduce your food bill, replace one quarter to one half of the meat in a casserole or meat sauce with cooked brown rice, couscous, or cooked dried beans.

2. To thicken soups and sauces, use pureed cooked vegetables instead of cream or butter.

MENU PLAN DAY 21: SUNDAY

Total calories: 1499
Less than 20 percent fat

BREAKFAST
(356 calories)

2 3-inch buckwheat pancakes, from mix
$\frac{1}{4}$ cup part-skim ricotta cheese
2 tablespoons apricot jam

SNACK
(60 calories)

1 fruit choice (p. 174)

LUNCH
(418 calories)

2 ounces sliced turkey breast
$\frac{1}{8}$ avocado, thinly sliced
Sliced fresh mushrooms
Sliced red onion
Alfalfa sprouts on
2 slices 7-grain bread
8 ounces skim milk
Fresh navel orange

AFTERNOON SNACK OR EVENING DESSERT
(100-150 calories)

Snack List (p. 178) or Dessert List (pp. 179–80)

DINNER
(515 calories)

Beef Shish-Ka-Bab over Couscous (p. 173)
1 cup mixed fresh fruit

RX: ACTIVITY PLAN—DAY 21: SUNDAY

Yes, you did it. . . . Give yourself a big hand. It's time to buy a new outfit for your new body.

It's Sunday, it's a total rest day, it's your day off. But still stay active and keep moving those 640 muscles. The more you move, the more calories you burn.

Rest!

Option: Remember, you can use your rest day on another particularly busy day during the week. Just don't forget to complete the routine on Sunday!

FITNESS TIPS OF THE DAY:

1. Exercise is worth it, because you are worth it. Exercise is the best energizer in the world.

2. One way to stay motivated to work out: Train like an athlete . . . feel like an athlete in training!

JUMPSTART

THE 21 DAY JUMPSTART PLAN RECIPES

Here are the recipes for the dishes in the 21 Day JumpStart Plan. Remember, you can be creative! Look at pp. 331–87 for more recipes and meal ideas!

Taste is important to me as well as eating healthily; therefore, I have included low-fat mayonnaise, low-fat cheeses, and even a little butter, instead of all nonfat products. However, please feel free to exchange the low-fat with nonfat choices if you prefer less fat in your diet. When opting for nonfat, you will save some fat, but you might sacrifice some taste.

My goal with these recipes is to introduce you to a life of healthy eating. These menus are set for you to follow for 21 days; however, I know that dinner parties and important lunch meetings are a part of life. Try to stick to the set menu as much as possible, but when confronted with these events check my options on pp. 266–71 for healthy alternatives (that is, sandwiches for lunch and the right choices when dining out). Also in the 21 day plan, if you dislike any of the choices or don't feel like eating chicken or fish on a certain day, feel free to replace a meal with one of your favorites, either from the 21 day plan or from my other recipes on pp. 331–77; just try to choose a meal with similar fat and calorie allotments.

SALMON PITA

Menu Plan Day 1

2   ounces canned salmon
1   ounce low-fat cheese, cut in chunks or shredded
1   cup tossed salad
1   tablespoon fat-free Italian dressing
1   large whole-wheat pita pocket

Combine salmon and low-fat cheese with salad. Toss with one tablespoon fat-free salad dressing and stuff into whole-wheat pita pocket.

*You can always substitute tuna or white chicken for salmon.

Makes one serving
Calories: 359
Fat: 8g

GARBANZO PASTA

Menu Plan Day 1

1   ounce dry vermicelli (very thin spaghetti)
1   cup frozen Italian vegetables
½   cup canned garbanzo beans (chick peas)
½   cup Healthy Choice spaghetti sauce
1   tablespoon Parmesan cheese

Cook vermicelli about five minutes, to the *al dente* stage. Add one cup frozen mixed Italian vegetables and one half cup garbanzo beans to the cooking pasta. Cook about two minutes until vegetables are tender but crisp. Drain thoroughly in a colander.

Serve topped with one-half cup Healthy Choice spaghetti sauce and 1 tablespoon grated Parmesan cheese.

Makes one serving
Calories: 339
Fat: 4g

GINGER-GLAZED CARROTS

Menu Plan Day 2

1   *cup frozen carrots*
½   *cup defatted chicken broth*
1   *teaspoon brown sugar*
¼   *teaspoon ground ginger*
     Pinch white pepper
¼   *teaspoon lemon juice*
1   *teaspoon butter or margarine*

Combine defatted chicken broth with brown sugar, ginger, and a pinch of white pepper.

Boil carrots in this liquid uncovered, about 8 minutes, or until carrots are soft and liquid evaporates. Stir in lemon juice and butter or margarine.

Makes one serving
Calories: 103
Fat: 4g

POACHED ORANGE ROUGHY

Menu Plan Day 2

3½   *ounces orange roughy fillet*
½   *cup white wine*
      Ginger-Glazed Carrots (see above)

Bring white wine to a boil in a shallow pan. Reduce to simmer.

Gently add an orange roughy fillet. Simmer gently for about 5 minutes until fish turns white and flakes easily with a fork.

Gently remove fish to dinner plate. Top with carrots.

Makes one serving
Calories: 161
Fat: 5g

CARROT-TUNA SALAD

Menu Plan Day 3

2   ounces water-pack tuna
¼   cup grated carrots
1   tablespoon light mayonnaise

Mix tuna with grated carrots and light mayonnaise.

**Makes one serving
Calories: 131
Fat: 6.5g**

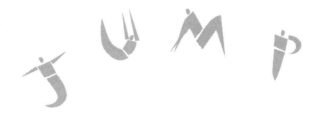

BEEF STIR-FRY ON BROWN RICE WITH MANDARIN ORANGES

Menu Plan Day 3

3½   ounces beef round steak
1   teaspoon sesame oil
2   cups salad vegetables (celery, green onions, bean sprouts, broccoli,
     cauliflower, carrots, Chinese cabbage)
½   cup beef broth or bouillon
1   teaspoon cornstarch
¼   teaspoon Chinese five-spice powder
1   cup quick-cooking brown rice, cooked according to package directions
½   cup juice-pack mandarin oranges

Slice beef round steak into thin slivers. Heat a heavy, nonstick pan over high heat until very hot. Add sesame oil. Coat pan, then quickly sauté beef just until pink. Add salad vegetables.

Reduce heat to low, and stir in beef broth or bouillon mixed with cornstarch. Stir, then simmer gently until vegetables are tender but crisp. Season with Chinese five-spice powder.

Spoon stir-fry over one cup quick-cooking brown rice. Top with mandarin oranges, drained.

**Makes one serving
Calories: 519
Fat: 12g**

CURRIED CHICKEN WALDORF

Menu Plan Day 4

- 1   boneless skinless chicken breast
- 1   red delicious apple, cored and cubed but not skinned
- ¼   cup diced celery
- 1   tablespoon light mayonnaise
- ½   teaspoon curry powder
- 4   walnut halves, coarsely chopped
      Salt and pepper
      Red-leaf lettuce

Broil chicken breast. Allow to cool, then cut into bite-sized chunks. Mix with apple, celery, light mayonnaise, curry powder, walnut halves, and salt and pepper to taste.

Serve on a bed of red-leaf lettuce.

Makes one serving
Calories: 328
Fat: 11g

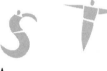

CHEESE-AND-BACON PIZZA

Menu Plan Day 5

- 1   small Boboli pizza shell
- 1   ounce Canadian bacon
- 2   fresh mushrooms, sliced thin
- ¼   teaspoon dried oregano
      Black pepper
- ½   teaspoon garlic powder
- 2   fresh plum tomatoes, sliced thin
- 2   ounces reduced-fat mozzarella cheese

Preheat oven to 450 degrees.

Top pizza shell with Canadian bacon, fresh mushrooms, dried oregano, freshly ground black pepper to taste, and garlic powder. Cover with thin slices from two fresh plum tomatoes, and top with the mozzarella cheese. Place directly on oven rack and bake for 8 to 10 minutes, until cheese melts.

Makes one serving
Calories: 485
Fat: 13g

BASIL CHICKEN AND ZUCCHINI OVER QUINOA

Menu Plan Day 6

Cooking spray
2   *boneless, skinless chicken breasts*
2   *teaspoons olive oil*
1   *medium onion, sliced*
1   *small zucchini, sliced*
1   *clove fresh garlic, chopped*
2   *tablespoons fresh basil leaves, chopped, or 1 teaspoon dried*
1/3 *cup quinoa* or brown rice*
2/3 *cup water*

To prepare chicken: Spray a heavy, nonstick pan with cooking spray. Over high heat, brown chicken breasts. Remove chicken. Reduce heat to medium. Add olive oil. Add onion and zucchini to pan. Add garlic. Add salt and freshly ground pepper to taste, then top with basil. Place chicken breasts on top of vegetables, then cover pan with tight-fitting lid. Reduce heat to simmer and cook until zucchini is translucent, onions begin to brown, and chicken is cooked through, 10 to 15 minutes.

Refrigerate one chicken breast for Monday's lunch.

To prepare quinoa: Rinse quinoa thoroughly in a strainer. Place grain in a small saucepan with water. Bring to a boil, reduce to simmer, cover and cook 10 to15 minutes, until all water is absorbed. Fluff with a fork. Top with chicken breast. Spoon vegetables over all.

*Quinoa (pronounced keen-wa) is a quick-cooking, high protein "whole" grain with a very mild flavor which makes a good base for a spicy dish.

Makes one serving
Calories: 448
Fat: 16g

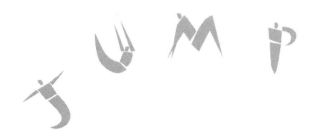

FRENCH TOAST

Menu Plan Day 7

Cooking spray
1   egg
½   cup skim milk
1   teaspoon vanilla
½   teaspoon cinnamon
1   teaspoon sugar
2   slices stale bread

Preheat a nonstick pan sprayed with cooking spray, over medium heat.

In a wide, shallow bowl, beat together with a fork the egg, skim milk, vanilla, cinnamon, and sugar. Soak bread in liquid until all is absorbed. Spray heated pan with cooking spray.

Cook toast, turning once, until both sides are nicely browned and centers are custard-like.

**Makes one serving
Calories: 260
Fat: 6g**

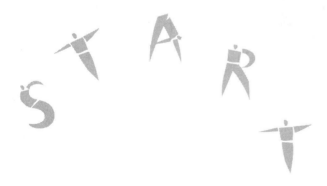

FRESH SPINACH WITH GOLDEN RAISINS

Menu Plan Day 8

> 5 ounces fresh spinach
> 2 tablespoons golden raisins
> Nutmeg
> Salt and pepper

Wash spinach until water is clear of sand. Remove tough stems.

Place spinach, with only the water that clings to the leaves, in heavy saucepan with tight-fitting lid. Add golden raisins. Cover. Bring to a boil. Reduce heat to simmer.

Cook just until spinach is wilted, 5 minutes or less. Drain well. Season with a dash of nutmeg. Add salt and pepper to taste.

Makes one serving
Calories: 102
Fat: 0g

ROSEMARY CHICKEN

Menu Plan Day 10

> 1 medium chicken breast with skin
> 1 3-inch branch rosemary
> Salt
> Five-pepper blend

Place chicken breast, skin side down, in a heavy, nonstick skillet with a tight-fitting lid. Place rosemary on the breast. Cover. Cook on high heat, without turning, until chicken is cooked through (20 to 30 minutes). Remove skin. Season with a pinch of salt and freshly ground five-pepper blend.

Makes one serving
Calories: 142
Fat: 3g

ELEGANT PEAS AND CARROTS

Menu Plan Day 10

¾ cup frozen sugar snap peas
⅔ cup frozen whole baby carrots
½ teaspoon chicken bouillon granules
½ cup water

Combine sugar snap peas and whole baby carrots in a heavy saucepan. Add water and chicken bouillon granules. Cover. Cook just until tender, about 5 minutes.

Makes one serving
Calories: 55
Fat: 0g

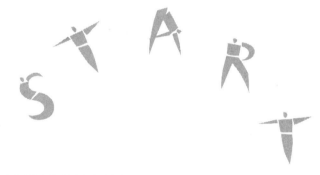

SOFT BEAN TACOS

Menu Plan Day 11

2   small corn tortillas
½ cup fat-free refried beans
2   slices reduced-fat American cheese or 6 tablespoons low-fat shredded cheese
4   tablespoons chopped fresh tomato
    Shredded lettuce
4   tablespoons salsa
2   tablespoons sour cream or light sour cream (optional)

For each taco, place tortilla in a heavy skillet over medium heat. Spread with refried beans. Top with one slice American cheese or shredded cheese. Cover. Heat 1 to 2 minutes, until cheese begins to melt.

Remove to plate. Top with 2 tablespoons each tomato, lettuce, and salsa. Serve with sour cream, if desired. Repeat for second taco.

Makes one serving
Calories: 245
Fat: 8g per taco

TURKEY VEGETABLE SOUP

Menu Plan Day 11

½   pound ground turkey breast
1   cup chopped fresh or frozen onions
¼   cup chopped celery
2   tablespoons chopped garlic (fresh or from a jar)
3   cups water
1   bag frozen Rancho Fiesta Style vegetables
2   tablespoons dried parsley
1   16-ounce can stewed tomatoes
½   cup shredded cabbage
½   teaspoon dried thyme
½   cup tiny pasta shells

Brown turkey in a large, nonstick soup pot over medium-high heat. Add onions, celery, and garlic. Cook and stir until vegetables begin to soften.

Add water, vegetables, parsley, tomatoes with liquid, cabbage, and thyme. Cover. Bring to a boil, then reduce heat. Simmer 20 minutes.

Add pasta shells. Cover and simmer 10 more minutes until shells are cooked but still firm.

Makes six servings
Calories: 165
Fat: 3g

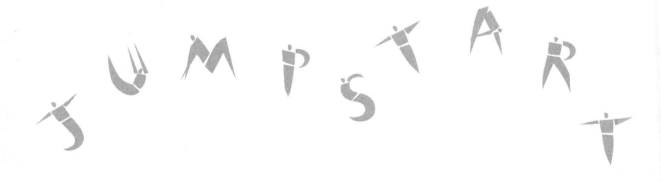

TURKEY BURGER

Menu Plan Day 12

3 ounces ground turkey breast
1 tablespoon smoky barbecue sauce
1 teaspoon Worcestershire sauce

Combine turkey with barbecue sauce and Worcestershire sauce. Form into patty and broil 5 minutes on each side.

Makes one serving
Calories: 190
Fat: 2g

SHRIMP STIR-FRY

Menu Plan Day 13

1 teaspoon sesame oil
3 ounces frozen cooked, peeled deveined shrimp, thawed
½ teaspoon ground ginger
1 cup sweet red pepper strips
1 cup snow peas
½ cup chicken bouillon
1 teaspoon cornstarch
1 cup steamed white rice
¼ cup chow mein noodles

Heat a heavy skillet until very hot. Add sesame oil. Swirl to coat pan. Add shrimp. Stir just until shrimp are warm.

Add sweet red pepper strips, snow peas, and ground ginger. Cook, stirring, until vegetables are tender but crisp.

Stir in chicken bouillon mixed with cornstarch. Stir until thickened.

Serve over steamed white rice. Top with ¼ cup chow mein noodles.

Makes one serving
Calories: 451
Fat: 10g

WAFFLE DANISH

2   *Aunt Jemima Low-fat Frozen Waffles*
½   *cup low-fat ricotta cheese*
1   *cup fresh berries*
    Ground cloves

Toast waffles. Top each with ¼ cup low-fat ricotta, ½ cup berries, and a pinch of ground cloves.

Makes one serving
Calories: 250
Fat: 4g

HOMEMADE LENTIL SOUP

1   *cup dried red lentils*
4   *cups defatted chicken broth*
1   *bay leaf*
2   *garlic cloves, chopped*
1   *teaspoon ground ginger*
1   *medium carrot, grated*
¼   *cup chopped green pepper*
1   *cup chopped red onion*
1   *fresh tomato, chopped, or 1 cup canned*
1   *teaspoon ground cumin*
2   *teaspoons ground coriander*
    Pinch cayenne pepper
1–2   *tablespoons fresh lemon juice*

In a soup pot over medium-high heat, combine lentils with chicken broth. Add bay leaf, garlic, ground ginger, carrot, green pepper, and onion. Bring to a boil. Stir.

Lower heat, cover, and simmer about 15 minutes, or until lentils are tender. Remove bay leaf. Add tomato, cumin, coriander, and cayenne pepper. Cook, stirring, about 2 minutes. Stir in lemon juice.

*Freeze remaining portion for Thursday's lunch (Day 18).

Makes four 1-cup servings*
Calories: 115
Fat: 0g

BBQ PORK TENDERLOIN

Menu Plan Day 14

2   *2-ounce pork tenderloin slices*
2   *tablespoons honey Dijon barbecue sauce*

Brush pork tenderloin with barbecue sauce. Broil 2 to 3 minutes on each side, until just done.

Makes one serving
Calories: 210
Fat: 6g

CHICKEN MOUTARDE

Menu Plan Day 15

1   *boneless skinless chicken breast*
     Spicy brown mustard
½   *cup orzo*
1   *cup chicken broth*
1   *cup frozen French-style green beans with mushrooms*
2   *teaspoons olive oil*
     Five-pepper blend

Preheat broiler.

Brush chicken with mustard and broil three minutes on each side, until done (juices should run clear). Slice across the grain into narrow strips.

Cook orzo in chicken broth according to package directions. Drain.

While orzo is cooking, heat olive oil in sauté pan over medium heat. Add green beans and mushrooms, and cook, stirring occasionally, 5 minutes.

Place beans in center of plate, and season with five-spice blend. Top with chicken, and surround with orzo.

Makes one serving
Calories: 458
Fat: 10g

THAI BEEF SALAD

Menu Plan Day 16

½ ounce vermicelli
1 teaspoon sesame seeds, toasted
2 cups mixed greens
1 cup mixed frozen broccoli, snow peas, and water chestnuts (or use your own fresh veggies, blending ⅓ cup of each)
3 ounces lean beef (tenderloin or sirloin)
2 tablespoons soy sauce
1 tablespoon sugar
2 cloves chopped garlic
½ teaspoon ground ginger
   Dash red-pepper sauce
1 teaspoon peanut oil
   Fresh lime juice
   Fresh cilantro

Cook vermicelli according to package directions. Drain. Rinse with cold water to chill. Toss with sesame seeds. Place in center of plate on mixed greens.

Cook broccoli, snow peas and water chestnuts, until tender but crisp. Rinse to cool. Drain. Place on noodles.

Trim all fat from beef. Slice into thin strips. Combine soy sauce, sugar, garlic, ginger, and red pepper sauce to taste in a small bowl. Toss beef slices in bowl and marinate for 5 minutes.

Heat a heavy, nonstick pan until very hot. Add peanut oil. Saute beef until barely done.

Place beef on top of vegetables. Squeeze fresh lime juice over beef and garnish with cilantro.

Makes one serving
Calories: 446
Fat: 18g

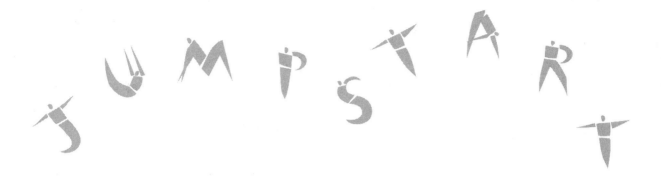

TUNA-SALSA TORTILLA

Menu Plan Day 17

2   ounces water-pack tuna
4   tablespoons salsa, well drained
2   small corn tortillas
2   slices reduced-fat cheese
2   tablespoons light sour cream

Mix tuna with salsa.

For each tortilla, warm one tortilla in a heavy skillet over medium heat. Top with a cheese slice. Allow cheese to melt. Remove to plate.

Top with half the tuna-salsa mixture. Top with 1 tablespoon sour cream. Roll. Repeat for second tortilla.

Makes one serving
Calories: 175 each tortilla
Fat: 3g each tortilla

TURKEY CUTLET TARRAGON

Menu Plan Day 17

1	cup fresh brussels sprouts
½	cup sliced onions
2	fresh turkey breast cutlet*
	Cooking spray
⅔	cup fresh mashed potatoes or Simply Potatoes (in refrigerated section)
½	cup white wine
½	teaspoon dried tarragon
	Fresh pepper
¼	cup fat-free brown gravy

Place brussels sprouts in steamer basket in a heavy pot with tight-fitting lid. Add one cup water to pot. Top sprouts with sliced raw onion rings. Cover and steam until tender, about five minutes.

Place turkey cutlets on cutting board. Pound with a mallet or the edge of a heavy plate until cutlet is thin.

Spray a heavy, nonstick pan with cooking spray and heat until very hot. Brown cutlets one minute on each side. Remove from heat. Place one cutlet on dinner plate next to potatoes and brussels sprouts. To the turkey pan, add white wine, tarragon, and freshly ground pepper. Bring to a boil and add gravy. Stir until hot. Pour over turkey cutlet.

* Save and refrigerate second cutlet for Friday's lunch.

Makes one serving
Calories: 380
Fat: 11g

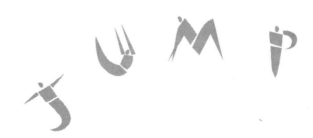

CHICKEN STIR-FRY WITH PINEAPPLE

Menu Plan Day 18

3   *ounce boneless skinless chicken breast*
2   *teaspoons peanut oil*
8   *ounces Hanover Vegetable and Rice Stir Fry with ½ sauce packet or other vegetable-rice stir-fry combination*
⅓   *cup juice-pack pineapple*

Slice chicken breast into strips. In a heavy pan over high heat, heat peanut oil. Brown chicken in oil. Stir in vegetable and rice stir fry and ½ of sauce packet. Cover and cook on medium high heat for 5 to 6 minutes, stirring frequently. Stir in pineapple.

Makes one serving
Calories: 458
Fat: 13g

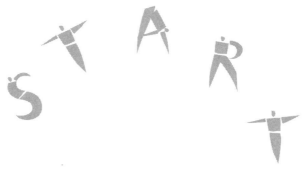

TURKEY GYRO

Menu Plan Day 19

2   *ounces cooked turkey cutlet*
2   *tablespoons sour cream (or light sour cream)*
½   *teaspoon oregano*
½   *cup sliced red onion*
    Romaine lettuce
½   *cup sliced tomato*
1   *large whole-wheat pita pocket*

In a small bowl, combine all ingredients except pita. Halve and open pita pocket, and stuff with turkey mixture.

Makes one serving
Calories: 295
Fat: 7g

GRILLED TUNA SALAD

Menu Plan Day 19

$3\frac{1}{2}$ ounces tuna steak
     Soy sauce
2   cups spinach and lettuce leaves
     Cucumbers, tomatoes, onions, celery, alfalfa sprouts
     Fat-free Italian dressing

Brush tuna steak on both sides with soy sauce. Grill over charcoal or broil in oven, until tuna flakes easily. Cut into strips or crumble on top of salad.

Toss vegetables with salad dressing and top with tuna.

Makes one serving
Calories: 287
Fat: 5g

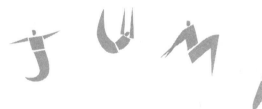

EGG-BAKED POTATO

Menu Plan Day 20

1   medium baking potato
2   eggs
$\frac{1}{4}$ cup skim milk
1   slice reduced-fat American cheese, cut in strips

Bake potato in microwave.

Meanwhile, beat eggs with skim milk. Add cheese. Cook over low heat until cheese is melted and eggs are done to your taste.

Split potato open, serve topped with eggs.

Makes one serving
Calories: 380
Fat: 13g

BEEF SHISH-KA-BAB OVER COUSCOUS

Menu Plan Day 21

3	ounces lean beef cubes
½	cup balsamic vinegar
3	small whole onions
3	cocktail or cherry tomatoes
3	sweet green pepper chunks
2	teaspoons olive oil
½	cup defatted beef broth
¼	cup couscous (Moroccan pasta)

Marinate beef in balsamic vinegar to cover for about 10 minutes. Thread beef chunks on skewers, alternating onions, tomatoes, and pepper chunks. Brush with olive oil. Grill over charcoal or broil in oven until beef is pink and vegetables are tender.

Meanwhile, bring beef broth to boil in a small covered pan. Add couscous, stir, cover and remove from heat. Let stand 5 minutes. Fluff with fork. Place on center of dinner plate. Top with beef and vegetables.

**Makes one serving
Calories: 455
Fat: 17g**

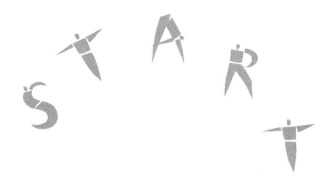

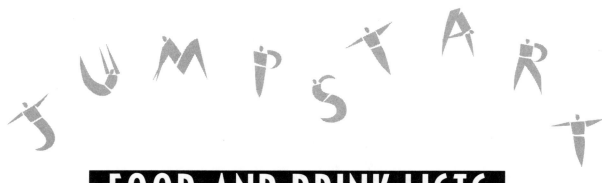

FOOD AND DRINK LISTS

60 CALORIE FRUIT LIST

(You may substitute for any fruit on the menu from this list.)

1 apple
2 apricots
1 small banana
¾ cup berries (boysenberries, blackberries, raspberries, blueberries)
1 cup cantaloupe
12 cherries
1 cup unsweetened cranberries
2 fresh figs
½ grapefruit

½ cup grapefruit juice
15 grapes
⅓ cup grape juice
1 guava
¼ honeydew melon
1 kiwi fruit
¾ cup mandarin oranges
½ mango
1 orange
½ cup orange juice
½ papaya

1 peach
1 pear
½ pineapple
½ cup pineapple juice
2 plums
2 prunes
⅓ cup prune juice
2 tablespoons raisins
1¼ cup strawberries
2 tangerines
1¼ cup watermelon

VEGETABLE LIST

One-half-cup cooked vegetables or one cup raw vegetables from this list can be substituted for any vegetables in the meal plan, for about 25 calories per serving.

Alfalfa sprouts
Artichoke
Asparagus
Bamboo shoots
Wax beans
Green beans
Italian beans
Beets
Bok choy
Broccoli
Brussels sprouts
Cabbage
Carrots
Cauliflower
Celery
Cucumber

Eggplant
Green onion
Collard greens
Mustard greens
Turnip greens
Beet greens
Swiss chard
Jicama
Kale
Kohlrabi
Leeks
Mushrooms
Onions
Snow peas
Sweet green pepper
Sweet red pepper

Sweet yellow pepper
Raddichio
Radishes
Rutabaga
Sauerkraut
Spinach
Yellow squash
Patty pan squash
Tomatoes
Tomato juice
Turnips
Vegetable juice
Water chestnuts
Zucchini

The following leafy greens can be eaten as often as you like.

Endive
Escarole
Iceberg lettuce

Green-leaf lettuce
Red-leaf lettuce
Romaine

Frisée
Spring salad mix

These starchy vegetables can be substituted for one slice of bread, or one-half cup rice or pasta (80 calories per serving).

½ cup corn
6-inch corn on cob
½ cup lima beans
½ cup peas

½ cup mashed plantain
1 small baked potato
½ cup mashed potato

¾ cup acorn or butternut
 squash
⅓ cup sweet potato

VEGGIE TIP:

To retain the nutrients in your vegetables, keep them covered in plastic bags because you can lose vitamins and minerals through exposure to air. For instance, broccoli left uncovered for four days lost 30 percent of its vitamin C, but sealed in plastic lost just 15 percent and retained more beta-carotene.

FREE BEVERAGE LIST

You may have noticed that there are no beverages listed on the menus for my 21 Day JumpStart Plan. I know everyone enjoys drinking something different with their meals. As you are certainly aware by now, I strongly recommend water with every meal, even if you drink something else as well. An eight-ounce glass of water before you begin eating will (among other things) help fill your stomach and make you less likely to overindulge. Here is a list of other liquids you can enjoy as much as you'd like (unless stated), with minimum calories and no fat.

Bottled water

Tap water

Flavored water (sugar-free)

Carbonated water

Decaffeinated coffee

Herbal tea

DRINKS IN MODERATION

Coffee or tea (2 cups a day)

Sugar-free soft drinks (1 a day)

Sugar-free punch (Crystal Light)

Sugar-free Snapple Iced Tea

Iced tea

Watered-down lemonade

Nonfat milk

Sugar-free Tang

Assortment of your favorite juices (½ juice and ½ water; grapefruit and orange juice are best for vitamin C and potassium)

If you would like a glass of wine, you may treat yourself once a week.

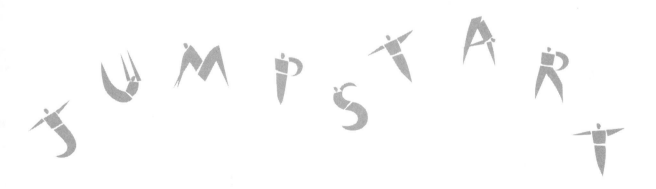

CEREAL LIST

When buying cereals, look for:

- **Whole Grain Cereals.** Make sure some type of grain (wheat bran, wheat, corn, oats, etc.) is the first ingredient listed; these cereals contain more fiber.
- Choose cereals with less than 2 grams of fat per serving.
- Choose cereals with less than 300 milligrams of sodium per serving.
- Choose cereals that are free of the preservatives BHA and BHT.
- Below are just a few examples of my favorite cereals (if you like others, check the labels).

Product	Serving Size (cup)	Fat (g)	Fiber (g)	Calories
Kellogg's All-Bran (with extra Fiber)	½	0	14	100
General Mills Fiber One	½	1	13	60
Kellogg's All Bran	⅓	1	9	71
Kellogg's Bran Flakes	¾	.5	5	93
Post Bran Flakes	⅔	.5	5	90
Kellogg's Fruitful Bran	⅔	0	4	110
Kellogg's Raisin Bran	¾	1	4	120
Kellogg's Nutri-Grain Wheat	⅔	0	3	102
Post Grape Nuts	¼	0	3	110
Kellogg's Corn Flakes	1¼	0	1	100
Kellogg's Product 19	1	0	1	100
Special K	1⅓	0	1	110
Kellogg's Rice Krispies	1	0	0	110
Shredded Wheat	1 biscuit	1	3	90
Corn Chex	½	0	0	110
Healthy Choice	1	0	3	100

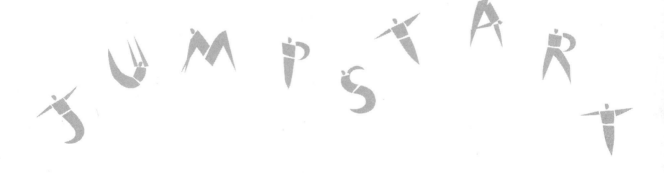

SNACK LIST

If you feel like you can't even stop to peel an orange, "fast" doesn't have to mean fat.
You can grab a piece of fruit, a bagel, a fat-free muffin, or a bag of pretzels.
For traveling—in traffic, road trips, airplane trips—or just going anywhere, reach for a healthy snack.
Here are my favorites:

Chewy dried fruits
Pretzels
Apples
Air-popped popcorn
Raw vegetables

Cereal snack mix (honey nut
Cheerios, shredded wheat
and oat squares or Chex)
(Sometimes I add graham
crackers for flavor and break
them into pieces.)

Here are more of my favorites. If you like others, just check the labels . . . watch the fat content.

Product	Serving Size	Calories	Fat
Fat-free pretzels	20 (small)	100	0 gm
Air-popped popcorn	1 ounce	120	2 gm
No Oil Tortilla Chips	22 chips	110	1.5 gm
Baked Tortilla Chips	13 (big) chips	110	1 gm
Fat Free Potato Chips	1 ounce	100	.5 gm
Crackerjack	1 cup	100	0 gm
Hains:			
Mini Rice Cakes:			
Plain Rice Cakes	7 cakes	60	0 gm
Honey Nut Rice Cakes	7 cakes	60	0 gm
Popcorn Cakes	7 cakes	60	0 gm
Generic Rice Cakes	1 cake	50	0 gm
Health Valley Vegetable Crackers	5 crackers	45	0 gm
Snack Well's:			
Wheat Crackers	5 crackers	60	0 gm
Cheese Crackers	19 crackers	60	1 gm
Cracked Pepper	5 crackers	60	0 gm
Lavosh Crackers, Any Flavor	3 crackers	60	0 gm

DESSERTS

This is a list of my favorites. I'm a big dessert lover but I want zero guilt. These choices are hand picked by me and guaranteed to be great tasting and low in fat and calories.

Product	Serving Size	Calories	Fat
Frozen Yogurt, Ice Cream and Sorbet			
Breyers:			
Fat-Free Frozen Yogurt	½ cup	90	0 gm
Healthy Choice:			
Low-Fat Ice Cream	½ cup	110-120	2 gm
Bananas Foster	½ cup	110	1.5 gm
Häagen-Daz:			
All Fruit Sorbets	½ cup	100	0 gm
Real Fruit:			
Non-fat Chunky Sorbet	½ cup	90-100	0 gm
Breyers:			
Fat Free	½ cup	102	0 gm
Sealtest:			
Fat-Free Chocolate	½ cup	100	0 gm
Lucerne:			
Fat-Free Ice Cream	½ cup	96	0 gm
Nonfat Yogurt	½ cup	92	
Borden:			
Fat-Free Ice Cream	½ cup	90	0 gm
Stonyfield Farm:			
Nonfat Yogurt	½ cup	113	0 gm
Yoplait:			
Fat-Free Yogurt	½ cup	95	0 gm
Light Chocolate Mousse	½ cup	103	1.5 gm
Vanilla	½ cup	103	1.5 gm
Colombo:			
Nonfat Shoppe Style	½ cup	117	0 gm
Lowfat Shoppe Style	½ cup	127	1.5 gm
Mattus'			
Lowfat Ice Cream	½ cup	160	3 gm

Product	Serving Size	Calories	Fat
Frozen Yogurt, Ice Cream and Sorbet			
Häagen-Daz:			
Frozen Yogurt Bars	1	90	0 gm
Creamsicle:			
Frozen Yogurt Bar	1	66	.5 gm
Weight Watchers:			
Orange Vanilla Treat Bars	1	30	.5 gm
Treat Bars	1	100	1 gm
Good Humor:			
Sugar-Free Fudgesicle	1	35	1 gm
Klondike:			
Light Ice Cream Sandwich	1	100	2.5 gm
Cake			
Angel Food Cake	1 sliver	100	0 gm
Cookies			
Snackwells:			
Devils's Food	2	100	0 gm
Mini Chocolate Chip	10	100	3 gm
Cinnamon Grahams	20	110	0 gm
Chocolate Sandwich	2	100	2.5 gm
Creme Sandwich	2	110	2.5 gm
Double Fudge	2	100	0 gm
Entenmann's:			
Chocolate Chip	2	80	0 gm
Oatmeal	2	80	0 gm
Nabisco:			
Fat Free Newtons	2	100	0 gm
Nilla Wafers	4	70	2.5 gm
Ginger Snaps	2	60	1.2 gm
Graham Crackers	4	60	1.5 gm
Frookie:			
Fat-Free Fruitins	2	90	0 gm

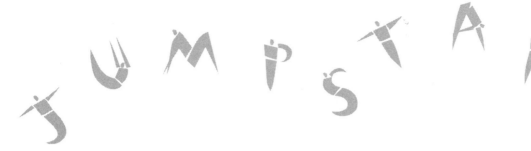

AEROBIC ACTIVITY OPTIONS

Walking

Stair Climbing (on a machine or stairs at home)

Jogging

Running

Hiking

Swimming

Bike riding (Stationary Bike)

Rowing Machine

Step aerobics

Water aerobics

Aerobics (low- or high-impact aerobics)

Aerobic riders

Dancing

Cross-country skiing or cross-country skiing machines

Ice skating

Glide slide (slide board)

Roller skating/Roller Blading/In-line Skating

Jump rope

Rebounding/Mini Trampoline

TIPS FOR SUCCESS

- Work at least 12 minutes; go for 30 minutes.

- Try varying the activities to stay motivated.

- Cross train to work different muscle groups—for instance, I like to do a fast walk on Monday, step aerobics on Wednesday, and my aerobic rider on Friday.

JUMPSTART

DENISE'S DAILY DOSE

Here is Denise's Daily Dose . . . your minimum daily requirement. It only takes 5 minutes, and there are only 10 moves to this quick routine. Ten *very effective* movements that tone all the major muscle groups. Do them in sequence, memorize them, and I promise you they'll become second nature.

DEEP BREATH

1. Take a deep breath.
2. Inhale through the nose as your arms flow out to the sides and up overhead. Exhale out the mouth as your arms slowly come down to your sides.
3. Take 3 deep breaths.

LOWER BACK STRETCH—PELVIC CURL

1. Stand with feet shoulder-width apart, knees slightly bent and hands on thighs for support.
2. Keep back flat and inhale.
3. Exhale as you contract your abdominals, round your back, and curl your pelvis. You should feel a stretch in your lower back.
4. Move slowly, holding each move for at least 2 counts, to make it really count.
5. Repeat. Inhale flat back, exhale, round back 3 times.

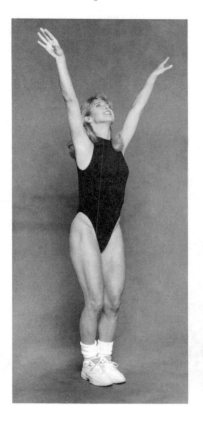

Great to get that oxygen flowing!

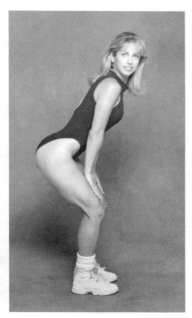 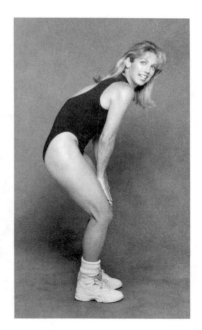

Stretches the muscles of the back and also strengthens the abdominals.

SIMPLE SQUAT AND REACH

1. Stand with your feet slightly wider than your hips. Your back should be straight and your abs tucked in.
2. Begin bending your knees to a partial squat. Try to sit back (hips behind your heels). Simultaneously, let arms flow down close to your body.
3. As you stand up, squeeze the buttocks and reach your arms up overhead (as high as you can), even up on your toes, feeling your entire body reach, stretch, and elongate.
4. Continue squat and reach sequence 10 times. Move slowly, holding each move for 2 counts. Exhale on squat; inhale on reach.

A slimming exercise for your hips, thighs, and buttocks. Look great from behind! The reach is a fantastic full-body stretch that makes you look tall.

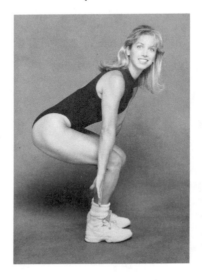

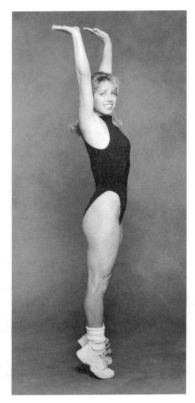

CALF STRETCH

1. Place one foot in front of the other. Bend your front knee and rest your hands on your thigh.
2. Keep your back heel flat on the floor, holding the stretch for 10 to15 seconds.

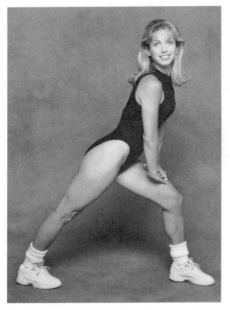

This is a wonderful stretch for the lower legs and to relieve achy leg muscles.

LUNGE

1. From calf stretch position bend and then lower your back knee toward the floor. Hold for a count of 2 (stretching hip flexors), then come back up. Go down and up (bending knees) for 10 dips (keep your front knee aligned with your front ankle).
2. Switch legs and repeat calf stretch, then hold hip flexor stretch, then do 10 up-and-down dips (lunges).

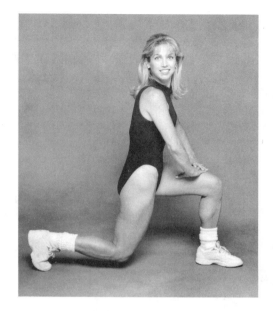

One of the best exercises to reshape your thighs and buttocks.

SIMPLE SIT-UP

1. Lie on your back with your knees bent and your feet on the floor. (If you are a beginner, or have neck problems, use a pillow under your neck and head.)
2. Press your lower back firmly into the floor. There should be no arch in your back at all.
3. Rest your head in your hands but keep your neck and shoulders relaxed.
4. Tighten your abdominals and slowly lift your shoulders up off the floor as you exhale (about 6 inches).
5. Exhale as you lift up. Keep your elbows back and chin up as if you have an apple between your chin and chest.
6. Slowly lower your shoulders back to the floor and repeat. Continue for 10 sit-ups.

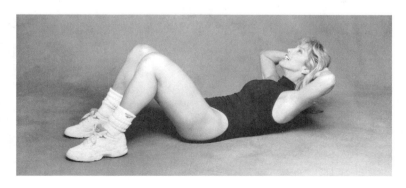

Get that rock-hard tummy you've always wanted.

LOWER TUMMY TIGHTENER

1. Lie on your back on the floor, and place your hands palms down just beneath your buttocks. This allows you to keep your lower back on the floor during the exercise.

2. Bend your knees and elevate your legs (cross your ankles).

3. Using the lower abdominals, lift your hips off the floor just a few inches and then release.

4. Exhale as you lift your bent knees toward your chest. Your knees should stay bent at the same angle throughout the exercise. Continue for 10 lower tummy tighteners. This exercise is a very small movement. Try to control the lift using the abdominals; don't rely on momentum.

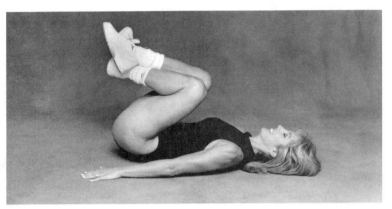

Great to tighten the muscles below the belly button!

PUSH-UP

1. Kneel on the floor, with your hands out in front of you.

2. Keep your back straight, abs tight, and your head in a neutral position.

3. Slowly bend your elbows and lower your chest toward the floor.

4. Straighten your elbows and return to the starting position. Continue for 10 push-ups.

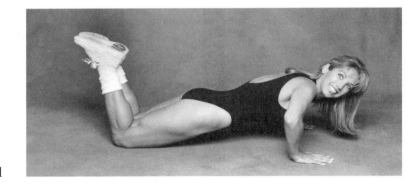

Simply the best upper body exercise!

BACK STRENGTHENER

1. Lie on your stomach with your arms folded in front of you and your chin resting on your arms.
2. Lift one leg up about 4 to 6 inches. Make sure your hips and pelvis stay planted to the floor.
3. Hold for a count of 10. Switch to the other leg and hold for a count of 10. When lifting the leg, squeeze your buttocks and don't arch your back.

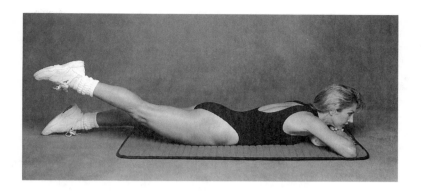

This strengthens the extensors—muscles in the back that tend to be underused and weak. Do this daily and it will help keep your back strong for life.

BACK RELAXER

1. Kneel on floor with your buttocks resting on your heels.
2. Place your hands on the floor extended in front of you with your neck and head in a natural position, resting your forehead on the floor. You should feel a stretch in your back (especially the lower back).
3. Hold for 20 to 30 seconds.

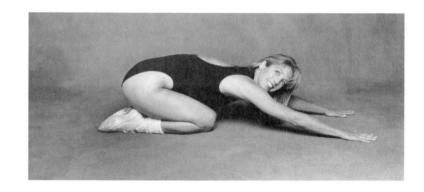

This helps to reduce pressure on your back (especially that from fatigue and emotional tension). It is also a great cool-down.

JUMPSTART

SUPER STRETCHES

FLEXIBILITY FROM HEAD TO TOE

1. Full Body Stretch

2. Runners Lunge

3 Butterfly Stretch

4. Lower Back Stretch

5. Quad Stretch

6. Reach for Toes

7. Hamstring Stretch

8. Triceps Stretch

The 5-Minute Stress Reliever

FULL BODY STRETCH

A super stretch for your whole
body, especially your arms,
shoulders, and spine, you can
do this one either sitting or
standing, and it's a great way to
rejuvenate after sitting at your
desk for long periods of time.

1. Lift your arms above your
   head and make yourself as
   tall as you can.
2. Make sure you breathe
   while holding this stretch
   for 5–15 seconds.
3. Bring your arms down in
   front of you and relax.

Variation: Side Stretch—
slowly bend slightly to the left
and then to the right.

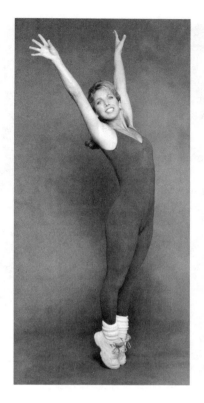 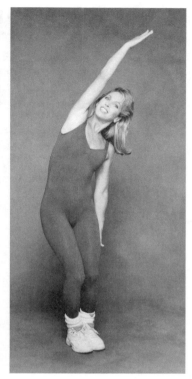

RUNNERS LUNGE

A great stretch to do after you walk, run, or after
any aerobic activity, it increases flexibility and
lengthens the muscles of the front of your hip
(hip flexors), the groin area, quadriceps, and
calf—all the muscles used in aerobic activities. If
you have time for only one stretch, do this one.

1. Stand with your feet together, take a big step
   with your left foot and place your hand on
   your thigh for balance.
2. Bend your left knee and lower yourself until
   you feel a stretch in your legs. Do not let
   your knee go past your toes.
3. Your back (right) leg should be as straight as
   possible but don't lock your knee.
4. Hold the stretch for 15–20 seconds, then
   alternate legs.

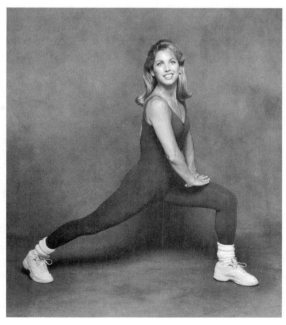

BUTTERFLY STRETCH

This stretch is designed to loosen the muscles of your inner thighs (adductors) and groin area. As with all of the stretches in your routine, make sure you take your time and *don't bounce.*

1. Sit on the floor. Put the soles of your feet together and gently bring your heels close to your groin.
2. Place your hands around your feet and slowly pull yourself forward until you feel an easy stretch in your groin.
3. Make sure you bend from the hips and not from your shoulders.
4. Hold stretch for 15–20 seconds.

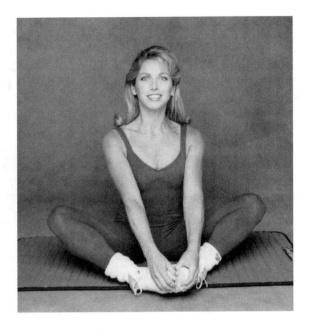

LOWER BACK STRETCH

4. Look back over your right shoulder and feel the stretch in your lower back as you twist.

5. Hold stretch for 15–20 seconds, repeat on the other side.

This lower back stretch is one of my favorites. It's easy to do and it feels great! When performing this stretch, make sure you move smoothly; you don't want this to be a "jerky" movement.

1. Sit on the floor with your legs straight out in front of you.
2. Put your *right* foot on the *outside* of your *left* knee.
3. Place your *left* elbow on the *outside* of your *right* knee while reaching back with your right hand.

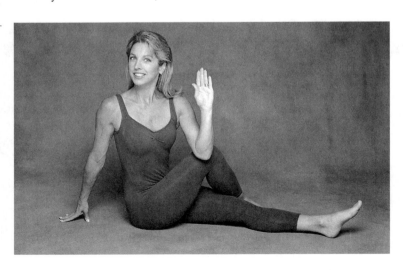

QUAD STRETCH

Your quadriceps are the four muscles in the front of your thighs. They are among the largest and strongest muscle groups in your body and are used in every activity. Jogging, biking, climbing, and even walking will be enhanced by having flexible thighs.

1. Lie on your side with your legs together.
2. Bend your right leg behind you and grasp the foot or the ankle.
3. Gently pull your foot toward your buttocks.

4. When you feel tension in the front of your thighs, hold the stretch 15–20 seconds.

5. Switch sides and repeat the movement with the left leg.

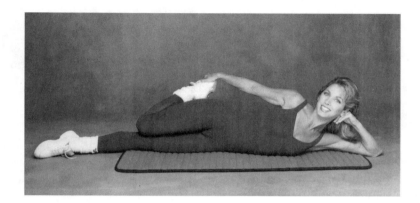

REACH FOR TOES

This is a wonderful stretch for the backs of your legs (hamstrings) and your lower back (erector spinae). Placing the towel under your buttocks will assist you in achieving proper form, making the exercise easier and more effective. The correct technique is to keep your back straight and to lengthen the space between your sternum and pelvic bone. Don't hunch shoulders forward.

1. Sit on the floor, place a towel under your buttocks and keep your legs straight out in front of you.
2. Sit up with your back straight, abs tight and your toes pointing to the ceiling.
3. Exhale as you bend forward, reaching your hands toward your toes.
4. Be sure that you keep your legs and back as straight as you possibly can.
5. Hold the stretch for 15–20 seconds, relax and repeat.

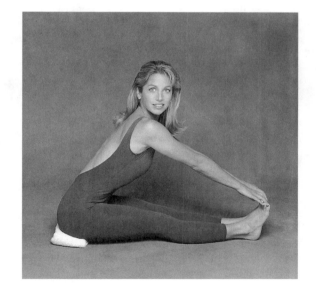

HAMSTRING STRETCH

I do this stretch all the time, whether I'm in bed, lying on the floor playing with the girls, or just watching television. It is especially useful if your lower back is bothering you. As with the rest of your stretches, be sure to Breathe, Relax, and Never Bounce!

1. Lie on your back on the floor, with your knees bent and your feet on the floor.
2. Raise your right leg up and pull it toward your chest. You can use a towel to assist you.
3. Hold the stretch for 15–20 seconds.
4. Lower the leg and repeat the stretch with the left leg.

Variation: To feel stretch more in calf muscle, wrap towel around ball of foot.

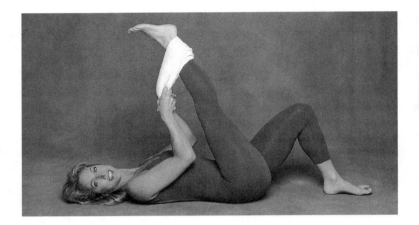

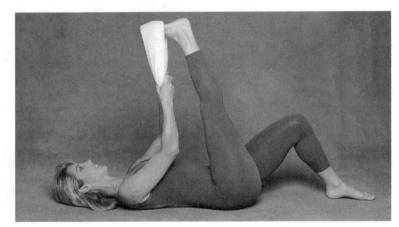

TRICEPS STRETCH

Designed to stretch the muscles of the backs of your upper arms, it can be performed either sitting or standing. In addition to doing this one at the beginning and the end of your workout, you might find it helpful to perform the stretch *in-between* exercises.

1. Raise your right arm above you and bend the elbow so your right hand is behind your neck.
2. With your left hand, grasp your right elbow and gently pull the elbow behind your head.
3. Hold stretch for 15–20 seconds.
4. You should feel a nice stretch in your right triceps.
5. Relax and repeat the stretch on the left arm.

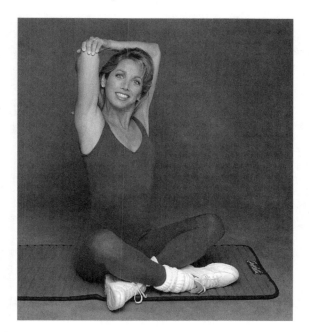

THE 5-MINUTE STRESS RELIEVER

An exercise in relaxation, it can be done at the end of all of your workouts or any time you start to feel "stressed out." It will leave you refreshed, rejuvenated, and ready to tackle the rest of your day or put you down for a good night's sleep! I suggest having someone read these instructions to you so you can close your eyes . . . and really relax.

1. Lie on your back on the floor with your feet about hips-width apart and your palms facing the ceiling.
2. Close your eyes and become aware of how your body feels. Allow your body to feel "heavy." *Breathe.*
3. Your breathing should be slow, deep, and rhythmical. With each exhale, imagine your tensions leaving your body. Slow, controlled breathing will have a calming effect on your mind.
4. Relax every part of your body, starting with all ten toes.

Relax the feet . . . the ankles . . . lower legs . . . upper legs . . . hips and buttocks . . . lower back . . . middle back . . . shoulder blades and upper back. *Breathe.* . . . Relax your shoulders . . . chest . . . rib cage . . . waist . . . pelvic and abdominal region. *Breathe.* . . . Now relax your upper arms . . . lower arms . . . hands and fingers. *Breathe.* . . . Relax your neck . . . jaw . . . lips . . . cheeks . . . nose . . . temples . . . forehead. *Breathe.* . . . Relax your eyes . . . scalp . . . ears . . . release the tension in the back of the neck and relax your entire spinal column. Feel your entire body relax and stay this way for at least 5 minutes.

JUMPSTART

TONING ROUTINES

Here are your toning routines. These exercises are designed to "spot train" specific muscles. Firming, sculpting, and toning from head to toe! Yes, you can reshape and firm up your body with these exercises, which target the arms, chest, and shoulders; the abdominals and waistline; and the hips, thighs, and buttocks.

Note: Your toning routine does not need to be done all at once. For example, in Week 3, 10 minutes in the morning and then 10 minutes in the evening is just as effective as a continuous 20 minutes.

TUESDAY: DAY 2—TONING ROUTINE

BACK ROLL-UP

1. Stand tall, feet shoulder-width apart. Place hands on thighs for support. Keep back flat.
2. As you exhale, round your back and feel a stretch in the entire back. As you do this, tighten and pull in the abdominals.
3. Relax, inhale, and return to starting position.
4. Continue in one fluid motion (flat back to round back) very slowly. This is a wonderful warm-up for the back. It elongates and stretches the muscles of the upper and lower back.

How many: 4 times.

Benefits: Lower, middle, and upper areas of the back.

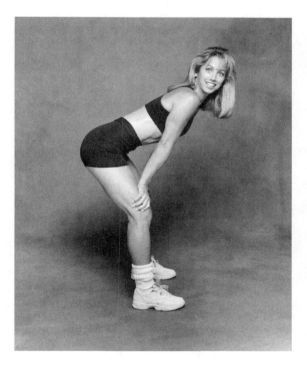 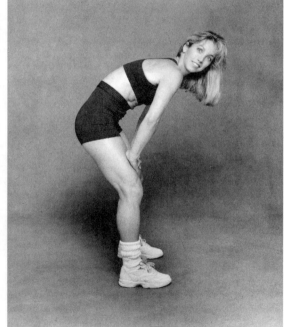

TUESDAY: DAY 2—TONING ROUTINE

BASIC PLIES

1. Stand with your feet a little wider than your hips. Your feet should be slightly turned out. Place your hand on the back of a chair for balance. Your back is straight and your abs are tight.
2. Tilt your pelvis forward and keep your hips square to the front.
3. Bend your knees and lower your hips toward the floor.
4. As you come back up, straighten your legs, exhale, and squeeze your buttocks.
5. Repeat.

How many: 2 sets of 8–12 reps each. Rest 15 seconds between sets.

Benefits: Thighs (quadriceps).

OUTER-THIGH PRESS

1. Stand with your feet together, your hands on the back of a chair for balance.
2. Your back should be straight and your abs tight.
3. With your foot flexed, slowly lift your right leg out to your side, then lower the leg. Be sure to keep your back straight. The movement should be slow and deliberate.
4. Repeat. When you have finished your 2 sets with the right leg, repeat the exercise on the left leg.

How many: 2 sets of 8–12 leg lifts each.

Benefits: Outer thigh (abductors).

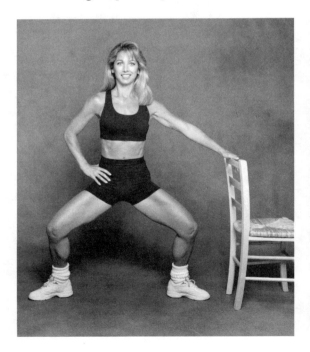

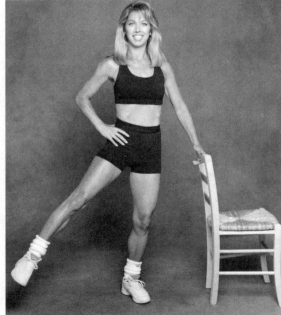

TUESDAY: DAY 2—TONING ROUTINE

INNER-THIGH PRESS

1. Stand with your feet together, your hand on the back of a chair for balance.
2. Your back should be straight and your abs tight.
3. Move your right leg in front of your left, with your right foot flexed. Squeeze your inner thigh as you move your leg. Don't let your leg just "swing" back and forth. The movement should be slow and controlled.
4. Return your leg to starting position and repeat. When you have finished 2 sets with the right leg, repeat the exercise with the left leg.

How many: 2 sets of 8–12 leg lifts each.

Benefits: Inner thigh (adductors).

STANDING LEG LIFT TO BACK

1. Stand with your feet together, your hands on the back of a chair for balance.
2. Your back should be straight and your abs tight.
3. Keeping your hips square to the chair and your right foot flexed, raise your right leg behind you. Keep the right leg straight.
4. As you complete the movement be sure that you don't arch your back at all; do really squeeze your buttocks.
5. Return your leg to the starting position and repeat. When you have finished the reps with the right leg, repeat the exercise with the left leg.

How many: 2 sets of 8–12 leg lifts each.

Benefits: Buttocks (gluteals).

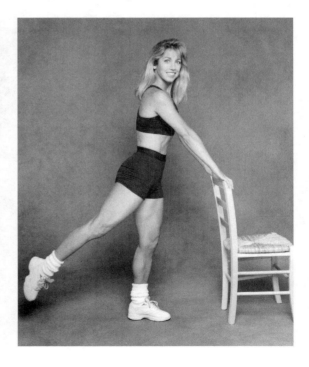

TUESDAY: DAY 2—TONING ROUTINE

BASIC STOMACH CRUNCH

1. Lie on your back with your knees bent and your feet on the floor. (If you are a beginner, or have neck problems, use a pillow under your neck and head.)

2. Press your lower back firmly into the floor. There should be no arch in your back at all.

3. Rest your head in your hands but keep your neck and shoulders relaxed.

4. Tighten your abdominals and slowly lift your shoulders up off the floor (about 6 inches).

5. Exhale as you crunch! Keep your elbows back and chin up as if you have an apple between your chin and chest.

6. Slowly lower your shoulders back to the floor and repeat.

How many: 2 sets of 8–12 crunches each. Rest 15 seconds between sets.

Benefits: Abdominals (rectus abdominis).

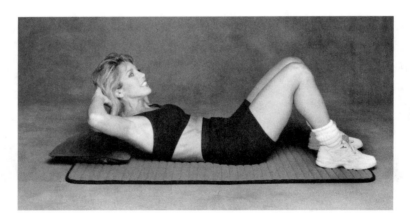

TUESDAY: DAY 2—TONING ROUTINE

REVERSE CRUNCH

1. Lie on your back on the floor, and place your hands palms down just beneath your buttocks. This allows you to keep your lower back on the floor during exercise.
2. Lift your legs off the floor and bend them slightly (cross your ankles).
3. Using the lower abdominals, lift your hips off the floor just a few inches and then release.

4. Exhale as you lift your bent knees toward your chest. Your knees should stay bent at the same angle throughout the exercise. This exercise is a very small movement. Try to control the lift using the abdominals; don't rely on momentum.

How many: 2 sets of 8–12 reps each. Rest 15 seconds between sets.

Benefits: Lower abdominals (rectus abdominus).

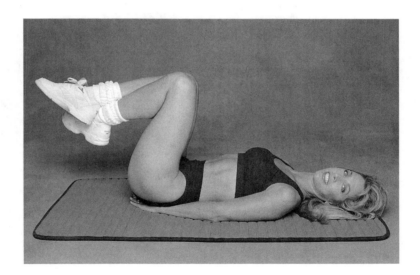

TUESDAY: DAY 2—TONING ROUTINE

PEC PRESS (WITH WEIGHTS)

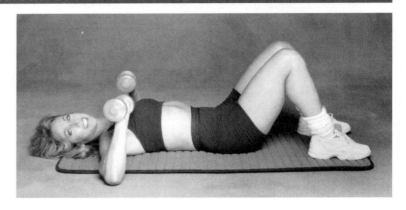

1. Lie on your back with your knees bent and your feet on the floor.
2. With the weights in your hands, slowly bend your arms so that your elbows are parallel to your shoulders.
3. Push the weights straight up so that your arms are extended directly over your chest.
4. Return to starting position.
5. Repeat the movement.

How many: 2 sets of 8–12 reps each. Rest 15 seconds between sets.

Benefits: Chest (pectorals).

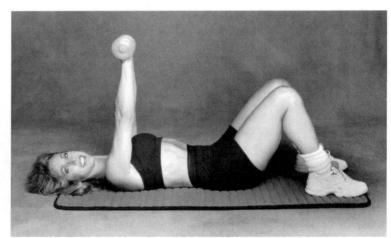

TUESDAY: DAY 2—TONING ROUTINE

CHEST FLYS (WITH WEIGHTS)

1. Lie on your back on the floor with your knees bent and your feet flat on the floor.
2. Hold the weights in your hands with your arms extended straight out at shoulder level, above your chest with palms facing inward.
3. Slowly lower your arms to your side, keeping them bent at the same angle throughout the movement.
4. Slowly return your arms to the starting position by squeezing your chest as if you're making a cleavage and repeating the movement.

How many: 2 sets of 8–12 reps each. Rest 15 seconds between sets.

Benefits: Chest (pectorals).

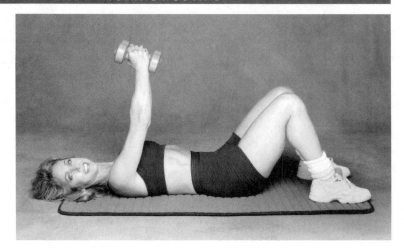

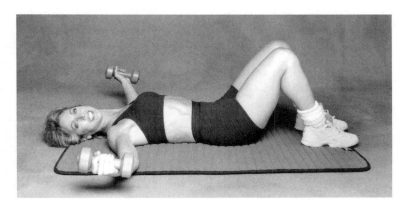

TUESDAY: DAY 2—TONING ROUTINE

FRENCH CURLS (WITH WEIGHTS)

1. Sit on the floor with your legs crossed in front of you. Sit up tall with your back straight and your abs tight.
2. Hold the weights palms in, with your arms extended straight over your head.
3. Keep your upper arms still and slowly bend your elbows so that your hands lower to shoulder level.

4. Raise the weights back up to the starting position as you squeeze your triceps.

How many: 2 sets of 8–12 reps each. Rest 15 seconds between sets.

Benefits: Back of arms (triceps).

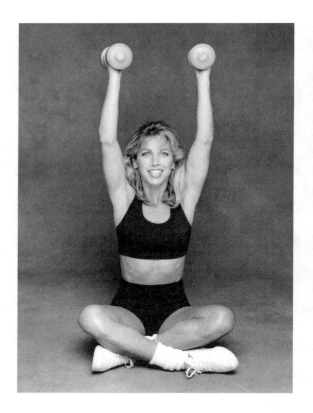
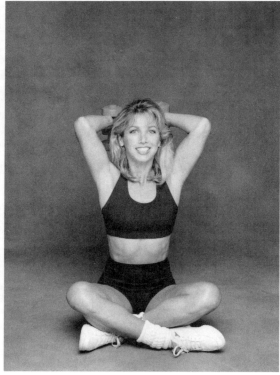

TUESDAY: DAY 2—TONING ROUTINE

BICEPS CURL (WITH WEIGHTS)

1. Sit on the floor with your legs crossed in front of you. Your back should be straight and your abs tight.
2. With an underhand grip, hold the weights at your sides with your arms extended.
3. Exhale as you slowly raise the weights toward your upper arms and shoulders, bending your elbows.
4. Hold momentarily and return your hands to the starting position. Be sure that you keep your elbows close to your body throughout the movement.

How many: 2 sets of 8–12 reps each. Rest 15 seconds between sets.

Benefits: Front of arms (biceps).

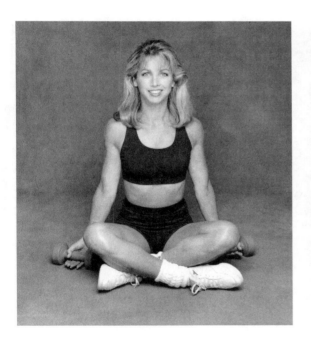 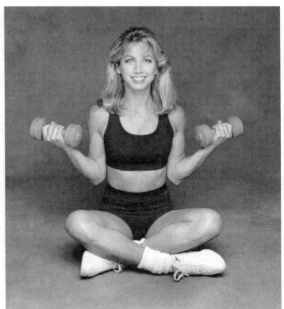

Finish with two of your favorite
"Super Stretches" on p. 188.

THURSDAY: DAY 4—TONING ROUTINE

BACK ROLL-UP

1. Stand tall, feet shoulder-width apart. Place hands on thighs for support. Keep back flat.
2. As you exhale, round your back and feel a stretch in the entire back. As you do this, tighten and pull in the abdominals.
3. Relax, inhale, and return to starting position.
4. Continue in one fluid motion (flat back to round back) very slowly. This is a wonderful warm-up for the back. It elongates and stretches the muscles of the upper and lower back.

How many: 4 times.

Benefits: Lower, middle, and upper areas of the back.

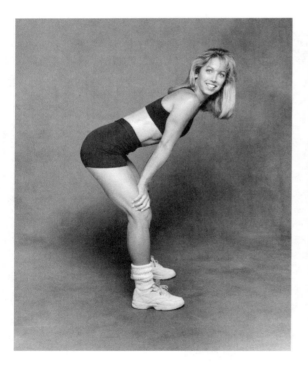 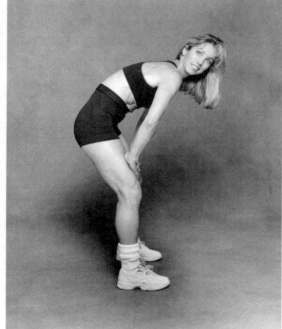

THURSDAY: DAY 4—TONING ROUTINE

BASIC SQUATS

1. Stand with your feet a little wider than your hips. Your back should be straight and your abs tight.
2. Place your hands on your hips.
3. Bend your knees and begin to squat. Feel as though you're sitting back, with your body weight through your heels. Hips should move behind your heels, like you're lowering yourself into a chair. Simultaneously, raise your hands in front of you—this will help you balance.
4. As you stand back up, exhale and squeeze your buttocks. Repeat.
5. If you have a history of knee problems, begin with a partial squat, with knees bent about 45 degrees. As you progress, you might squat to a 90-degree angle. Never go lower!

How many: 2 sets of 8–12 reps each. Rest 15 seconds between sets.

Benefits: Thighs (quadriceps), buttocks (gluteals), hamstrings.

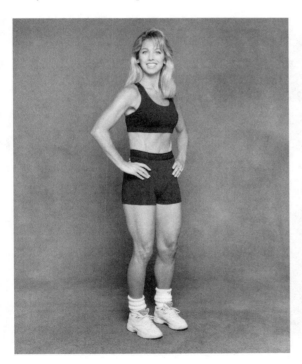
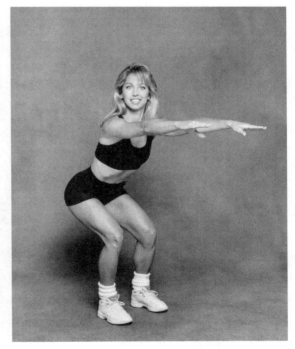

THURSDAY: DAY 4—TONING ROUTINE

PELVIC SUPER SQUEEZE

1. Stand with your feet a little wider than your shoulders. Your back should be straight, abs tight, knees slightly bent, and are turned out.
2. Tilt your pelvis slightly forward and squeeze your buttocks together.
3. Relax, then squeeze again. Repeat.

How many: 2 sets of 8–12 reps each. Rest 15 seconds between sets.

Benefits: Buttocks (gluteals).

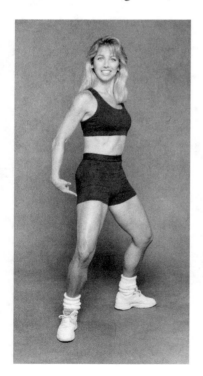

REVERSE LUNGE

1. Start with your feet about shoulder-width apart. Your back should be straight and your abs tight.
2. Take a step backward with one foot. As you step backward, bend your knees and lower your back leg toward the floor.
3. Your weight should be balanced between your back toes and your front heel (keep knees at a 90 degree angle).
4. Come back to starting position by pushing through the front heel and bringing legs together.
5. Repeat alternate lunges.

How many: 16–24 lunges each leg.

Benefits: Thighs (quadriceps), buttocks (gluteals), hamstrings.

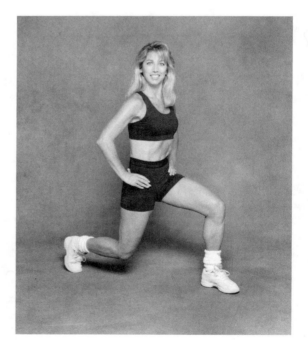

THURSDAY: DAY 4—TONING ROUTINE

BASIC OUTER-THIGH LEG LIFT (FLOOR)

1. Lie on the floor with your left side down. Your head, shoulders, and hips should all be aligned.
2. Bend your left leg, putting your right hand down in front of you for balance.
3. Keeping your right leg straight and your foot flexed, slowly raise your leg. Lower it back to the floor, then repeat. This is a very short movement, so be careful not to raise your leg too high. You should be focusing on the outer thigh of your top leg.

How many: 2 sets of 8-12 leg lifts on each leg.

Benefits: Outer thigh (abductors).

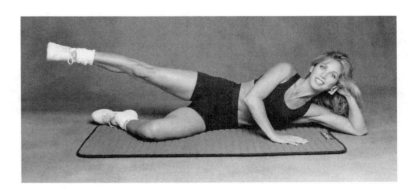

BASIC INNER-THIGH LIFT

1. Lie on the floor on your left side. Your head, shoulders, and hips should all be aligned.
2. Bend your right leg and place it on the floor in front of you.
3. Slowly raise your left leg off the floor to a comfortable height. Try to keep it straight.
4. Pause at the top of the movement, then lower the leg back to the floor. Repeat.

5. Your left foot should remain flexed and parallel to the floor throughout the movement.

How many: 2 sets of 8–12 leg lifts on each leg.

Benefits: Inner thigh (adductors).

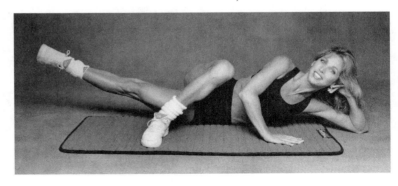

THURSDAY: DAY 4—TONING ROUTINE

BEGINNER BICYCLES

1. Lie on the floor with your legs straight.
2. Prop up on your elbows. Place your hands at your sides slightly under your buttocks, palms down. Press your back firmly into the floor. There should be no arch in your back at all.
3. Exhale as you pull your right knee toward your chest. At the same time you return your right leg to the starting position, bring your left leg to your chest.
4. Continue to alternate your legs back and forth, simulating riding a bicycle.

How many: 2 sets of 8–12 reps each. Rest 15 seconds between sets.

Benefits: Abdominals (rectus abdominis), obliques.

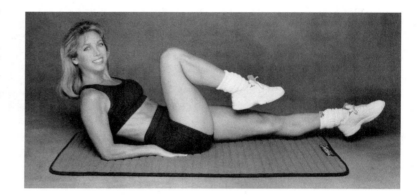

CROSSOVER CRUNCHES

1. Lie on the floor and cross your right foot over your left knee. Press your back firmly into the floor. There should be no arch in your back.
2. Place your right hand out to your side and your left hand behind your head.
3. Exhale as you lift your left shoulder blade off the floor. You're not going to actually touch your elbow to your opposite knee— just move in that direction.
4. Slowly lower back to the floor and repeat.

How many: 2 sets of 8–12 reps each per side. Rest 15 seconds between sets.

Benefits: Waistline (obliques).

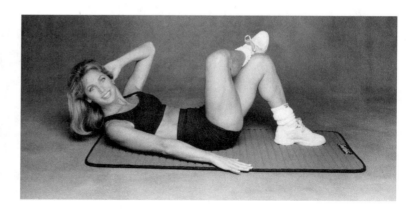

THURSDAY: DAY 4—TONING ROUTINE

LATERAL SIDE RAISES (WITH WEIGHTS)

1. Stand with your feet shoulder-width apart, abs tight, back straight, and knees slightly bent.
2. Hold weights at your side.
3. Raise the weights out to your sides. Arms should be straight and palms down. Return to the starting position.

4. Continue to complete side lateral raises up and down.

How many: 2 sets of 8–12 reps each. Rest 15 seconds between sets.

Benefits: Shoulders (deltoids).

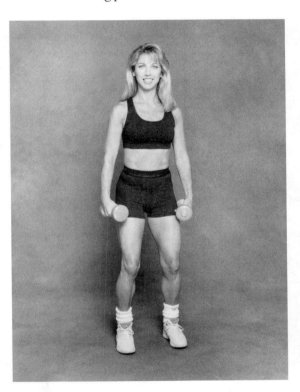 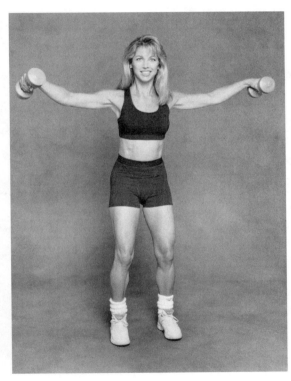

THURSDAY: DAY 4—TONING ROUTINE

TRICEPS TONER (WITH WEIGHTS)

1. Stand with your feet shoulder-width apart and knees slightly bent, with weights in your hands. Keep your abs tight, back flat, and bend slightly forward at the waist.
2. Raise your elbows so that the upper part of your arms are parallel with the floor. Keep your elbows close to your body.
3. Straighten your arms. Be sure to squeeze your triceps as you do so.

4. Return your hands to the starting position, pause, and repeat the movement.

How many: 2 sets of 8–12 reps each. Rest 15 seconds between sets.

Benefits: Back of arms (triceps).

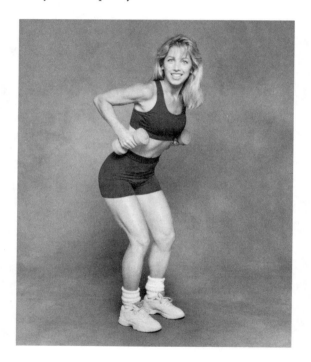 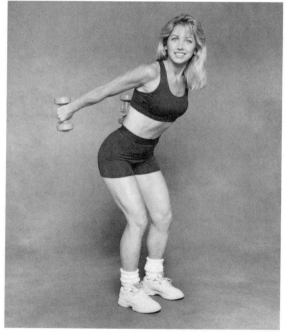

THURSDAY: DAY 4—TONING ROUTINE

UPRIGHT ROWS (WITH WEIGHTS)

1. Stand with your feet wider than your shoulders. Your abs should be tight, and your knees slightly bent.
2. Hold the weights with your palms facing in.
3. Raise the weights so your arms form the letter "V."
4. Inhale as you lift, squeezing your shoulder blades together, then return your arms to the starting position and repeat.

How many: 2 sets of 8–12 reps each. Rest 15 seconds between sets.

Benefits: Upper back (trapezius, rhomboids).

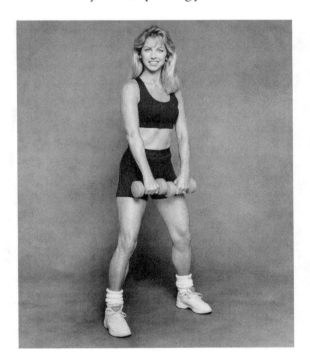 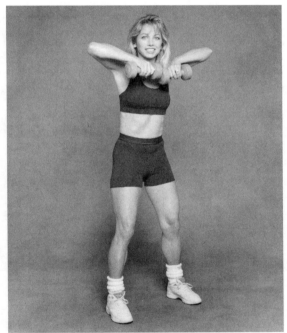

**Finish with two
Super Stretches on p. 188.**

TUESDAY: DAY 9—TONING ROUTINE

BACK ROLL-UP

1. Stand tall, feet shoulder-width apart. Place hands on thighs for support. Keep back flat.
2. As you exhale, round your back and feel a stretch in the entire back. As you do this, tighten and pull in the abdominals.
3. Relax, inhale, and return to starting position.
4. Continue in one fluid motion (flat back to round back) very slowly. This is a wonderful warm-up for the back. It elongates and stretches the muscles of the upper and lower back.

How many: 4 times.

Benefits: Lower, middle, and upper areas of the back.

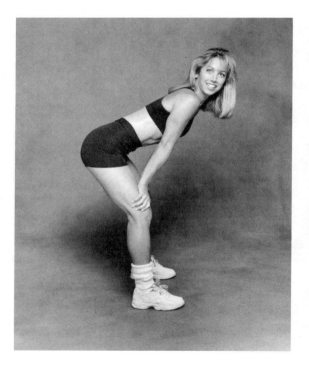 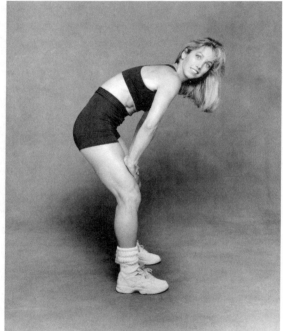

TUESDAY: DAY 9—TONING ROUTINE

BUTT TAPS

1. Stand with your feet a little wider than your hips.
2. Your back should be straight, abs tight, and your hands on your hips.
3. Bend your knees and slowly lower yourself until your butt taps the chair. Be careful not to bounce!
4. As soon as you tap the chair, straighten your legs, and return to the starting position. Repeat the movement.

How many: 2 sets of 8–12 reps each. rest 15 seconds between sets.

Benefits: Thighs (quadriceps), buttocks (gluteals, hamstrings).

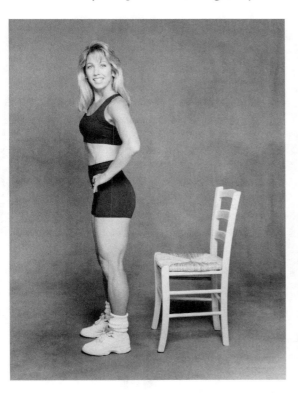
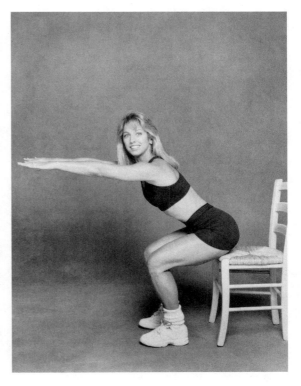

TUESDAY: DAY 9—TONING ROUTINE

BENT KNEE BUTT LIFT

1. Stand with your feet about shoulder-width apart. Hold the back of a chair for balance. Your back should be straight and your abs tight.
2. Keeping your hips square to the chair, bend your right leg, keep your foot flexed, and "squeeze" your buttocks. Heel toward buttocks.
4. Return your leg to the starting position and repeat. Bent knee—straight leg.

How many: 2 sets of 8–12 lifts per leg.

Benefits: Buttocks (gluteals).

FRONT LEG LIFTS

1. Stand with your feet together. Hold on to the back of a chair for balance. Your back should be straight and your abs tight.
2. Keeping your hips square and your right foot relaxed, raise your right leg in front of you. Keep it straight.
3. Keep supported leg (left leg) slightly bent.
4. Return your leg to the starting position and repeat.

How many: 2 sets of 8–12 lifts per leg.

Benefits: Quadriceps and all muscles surrounding your knee … a great exercise for reconditioning the knee.

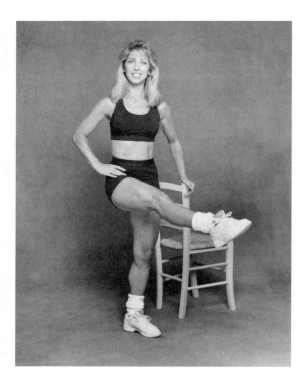

TUESDAY: DAY 9—TONING ROUTINE

STANDING CALF RAISES

1. Stand with your feet together. Place your hands on the back of a chair for balance.
2. Raise up on your toes so that you are on the balls of your feet. As you rise, be sure to really squeeze your calves.
3. Lower your heels back to the floor and repeat. This exercise can also be done one leg at a time to make it a little tougher.

How many: 2 sets of 8–12 leg raises. Rest 15 seconds between sets.

Benefits: Calves (gastrocnemius).

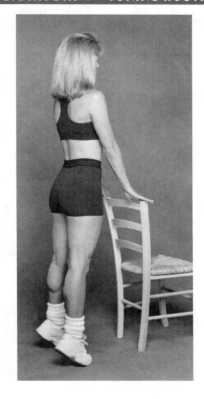

SUPER SIT-UP (WITH CHAIR)

1. Lie on your back with your knees bent and feet resting on a chair. (If you are a beginner, or if you have neck problems, use a pillow under your neck and head.)
2. Press your lower back firmly into the floor. There should be no arch in your back at all. (Propping your feet on a chair adds a slight pelvic tilt which helps keep the small of the back on the floor.)
3. Rest your head in your hands but keep your neck and shoulders relaxed.
4. Tighten your abdominals and slowly lift your shoulders from the floor (about 6 inches). Exhale.
5. Try to keep your elbows back and hold your head in a natural position. You should be able to fit your fist between your chin and chest.
6. Slowly lower your shoulders back to the floor and repeat.

How many: 2 sets of 8–12 sit-ups. Rest 15 seconds between sets.

Benefits: Abdominals (rectus abdominis).

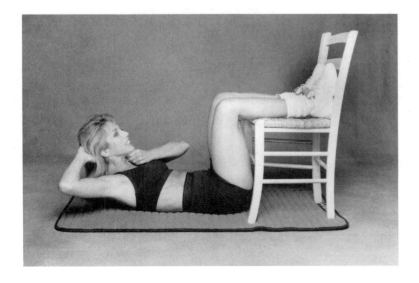

TUESDAY: DAY 9—TONING ROUTINE

DOUBLE CRUNCH

1. Lie on your back with knees bent. Legs should be lifted at a 90-degree angle with ankles crossed.
2. Place your hands behind your head for support.
3. Simultaneously lift your head and shoulders about six inches from off the floor and pull your knees toward your chest using lower and upper abdominals (it's like an abdominal compression). Exhale.
4. Return to starting position. Be careful not to let your feet drop to the floor; they should stay elevated throughout this exercise.

How many: 2 sets of 8–12 reps. Rest 15 seconds between sets.

Benefits: Lower and upper end of abdominals (rectus abdominis).

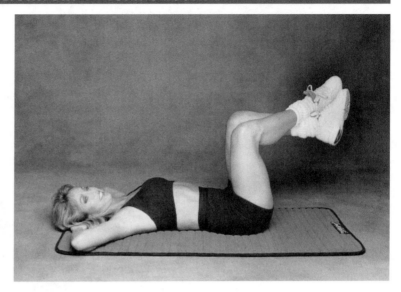

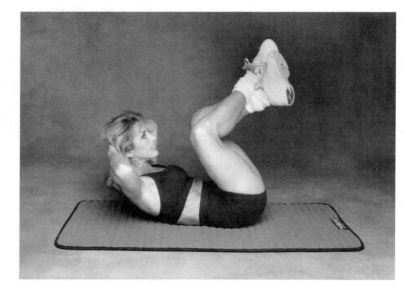

TUESDAY: DAY 9—TONING ROUTINE

OBLIQUE CRUNCH

1. Lie on your back with knees bent and feet flat on the floor. Make sure the small of the back is pressed into the floor.
2. Contract the abdominals as you lift your head and shoulders about 6 inches from the floor.
3. Twist slightly to the side, reaching your hands to the outside of your right thigh. Hold the reach . . . try to keep shoulders off the floor . . . pulsing (lifting up and down). (Those of you who need support for your neck, place your hands behind your head.) Your abdominal muscles should be contracted the entire time. Your goal is to keep the shoulder blades off the floor.
4. Hold the reach while pulsing. After completing 2 sets on right side, repeat on left side.

How many: 2 sets of 8–12 crunches each.

Benefits: Obliques.

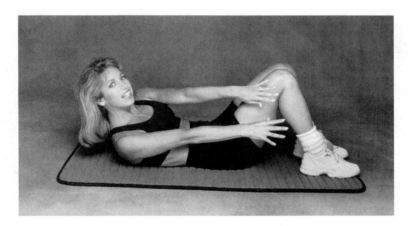

TUESDAY: DAY 9—TONING ROUTINE

OVERHEAD PRESSES (WITH WEIGHTS)

1. Sit in a chair. Keep your back straight and your abs tight.
2. Start with weights in your hands at shoulder level, palms forward.
3. Exhale as you press the weights directly over your head until your arms are straight.
4. Slowly lower the weights to the starting position and repeat.

How many: 2 sets of 8–12 reps each. Rest 15 seconds between sets.

Benefits: Shoulders (deltoids), triceps.

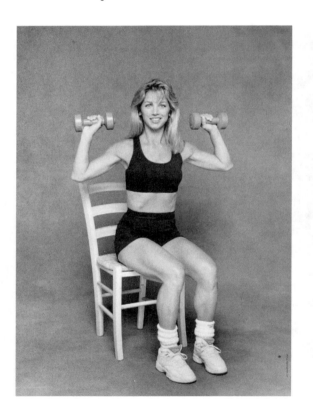
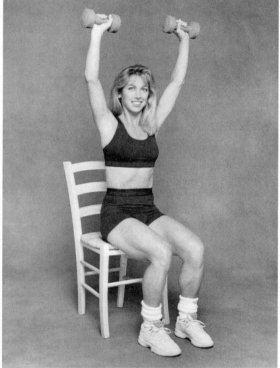

TUESDAY: DAY 9—TONING ROUTINE

UPPER-BACK FIRMER (WITH WEIGHTS)

1. Sit in a chair. Lean forward so your chest is near your thighs.
2. With weights in your hands, slowly lift your arms straight out to the sides, your pinkies up.
3. Squeeze your shoulder blades together. Return to the starting position and repeat the movement. Make sure that your movement is slow and deliberate; try not to swing the weights.

How many: 2 sets of 8–12 each.

Benefits: Shoulders (posterior deltoid), upper back (rhomboids).

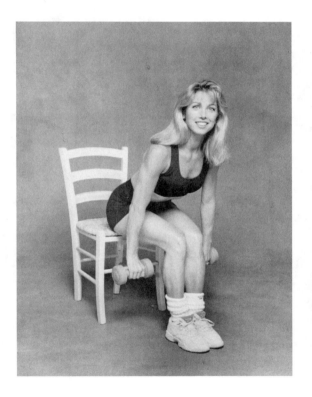 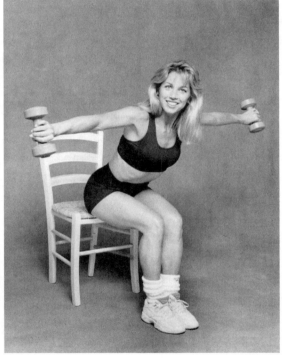

TUESDAY: DAY 9—TONING ROUTINE

UNDERARM FIRMER (WITH WEIGHTS)

1. Sit in a chair with your back straight.
2. Hold the weight in your right hand and raise it over your head.
3. Slowly bend your elbow and lower the weight behind your head. Be sure to keep your elbow close to your head.

4. Raise your hand back over your head to the starting position and squeeze your triceps.

How many: 2 sets of 8–12 each per arm. Rest 15 seconds between sets.

Benefits: Back of arms (triceps).

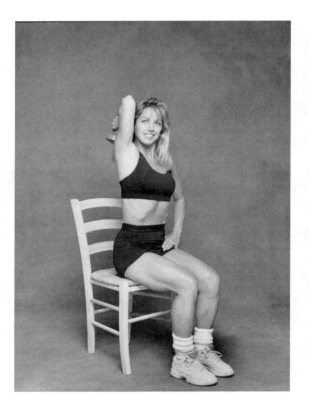 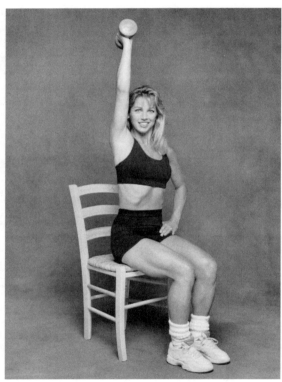

**Cool down with a few
Super Stretches on p. 188.**

THURSDAY: DAY 11—TONING ROUTINE

BACK ROLL-UP

1. Stand tall, feet shoulder-width apart. Place hands on thighs for support. Keep back flat.
2. As you exhale, round your back and feel a stretch in the entire back. As you do this, tighten and pull in the abdominals.
3. Relax, inhale, and return to starting position.
4. Continue in one fluid motion (flat back to round back) very slowly. This is a wonderful warm-up for the back. It elongates and stretches the muscles of the upper and lower back.

How many: 4 times.

Benefits: Lower, middle, and upper areas of the back.

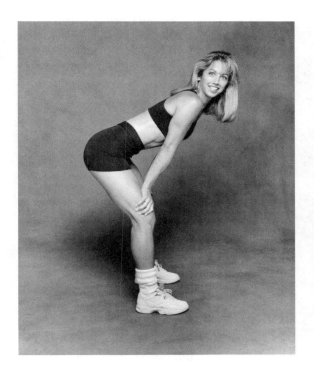 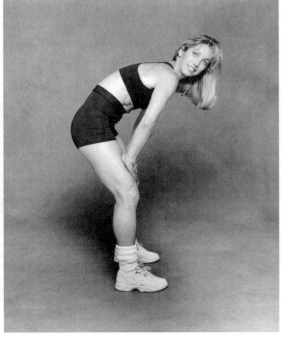

THURSDAY: DAY 11—TONING ROUTINE

WALKING LUNGES

1. Hold weights at your sides (weights optional). Start with your feet about shoulder-width apart.
2. Take a step with one foot. As you take your step, bend your back knee toward the floor. Be sure you don't bang your knee on the floor. Your body weight should be on your front heel and on your back toes.
3. Rise back up and, as you do, bring your back foot forward to return to the starting position.
4. Take giant steps forward, alternating legs. (You could do this around your house.)

How many: 2 sets of 8–12 lunges each. Rest 15 seconds between sets.

Benefits: Thighs (quadriceps), buttocks (gluteals), hamstrings.

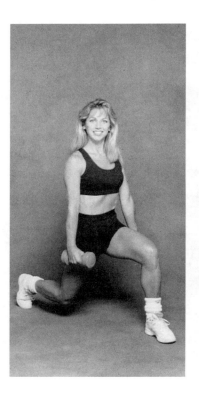 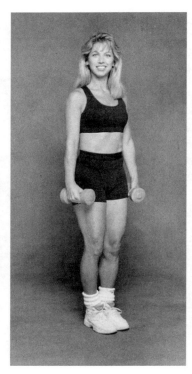 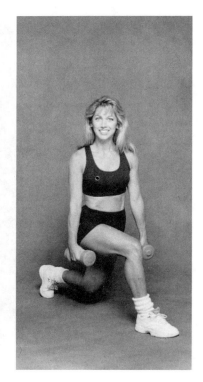

THURSDAY: DAY 11—TONING ROUTINE

PLIES WITH HEEL RAISES

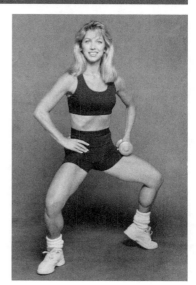

1. Hold weights in hands (weights optional). Stand with your feet wider than your hips. Your feet should be slightly turned out. Your back should be straight, and your abs tight.
2. Raise one of your heels off the ground.
3. Bend your knees and slowly lower your hips toward the floor.
4. As you return to the starting position, really squeeze your buttocks and tighten your inner thighs. The movement is a controlled lower and lift in a down-and-up motion.

How many: 2 sets of 8–12 plies each. Rest 15 seconds between sets.

Benefits: Thighs (quadriceps), buttocks (gluteals), inner thighs (adductors).

BICEPS CURL (WITH WEIGHTS)

1. Stand with your feet wider than your hips. Your abs should be tight, back straight, and knees slightly bent.
2. With an underhand grip, hold the weights at the front of your thighs.
3. Exhale as you slowly bend your arms, and raise the weights toward your upper arms and shoulders.
4. Hold momentarily and return your hands to the starting position. Be sure that you keep your elbows close to your body throughout the movement.

How many: 2 sets of 8–12 reps. Rest 15 seconds between sets.

Benefits: Biceps.

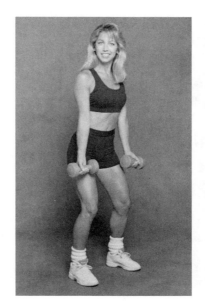
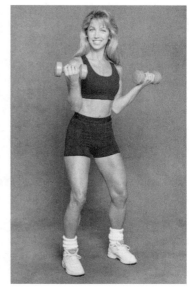

THURSDAY: DAY 11—TONING ROUTINE

FRONT LATERAL RAISES (WITH WEIGHTS)

1. Stand with your feet shoulder-width apart, abs tight, back straight, and knees slightly bent.
2. Start with your hands in front of your thighs, and with your arms slightly bent, lift the weights directly in front of you, palms down.
3. Return to starting position.

How many: 2 sets of 8–12 reps. Rest 15 seconds between sets.

Benefits: Shoulders (deltoids).

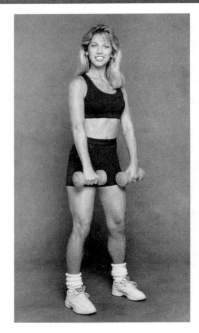 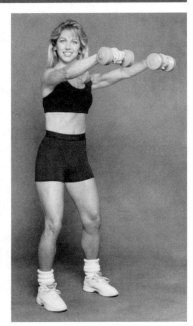

OVERHEAD PRESSES (WITH WEIGHTS)

1. Stand with your feet shoulder-width apart, abs tight, back straight, and your knees slightly bent.
2. Start with your hands at your shoulders, and exhale as you raise your hands over your head.
3. Lower your arms to your shoulders and repeat.

How many: 2 sets of 8–12 reps. Rest 15 seconds between sets.

Benefits: Shoulders (deltoids), triceps.

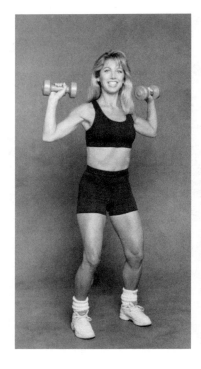 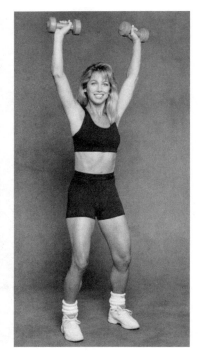

THURSDAY: DAY 11—TONING ROUTINE
ONE-ARM ROW (WITH WEIGHTS)

1. Stand with your feet apart, left foot in front of the right.
2. Bend your knees slightly and keep your abs tight.
3. Rest the palm of your left hand on your left thigh. Holding the weight in your right hand, let your arm extend to the floor.
4. Pull the weight up to your armpit, then lower it back to the starting position and repeat.

How many: 2 sets of 8–12 reps each per arm. Rest 15 seconds between sets.

Benefits: Upper back (latissiumus dorsi, rhomboid), back of shoulders (posterior deltoid).

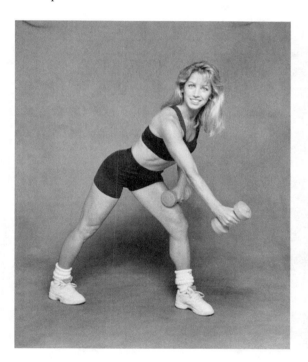

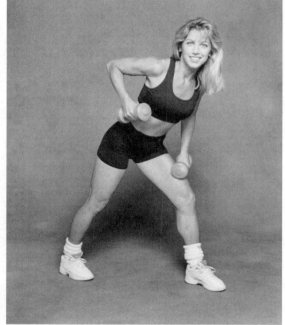

THURSDAY: DAY 11—TONING ROUTINE

PELVIC-TILT STOMACH CRUNCH

1. Lie on your back with your knees bent and your feet on the floor. Press your lower back firmly into the floor. There should be no arch in your back at all.
2. Rest your head in your hands, keeping your neck and shoulders relaxed.
3. Tighten your abdominals and slowly lift your head and shoulders about 6 inches from the floor; at the same time slightly tilt your pelvis up (buttocks are lifted about 1 inch from floor). This helps to strengthen the abdominal muscles below the navel.
4. Exhale as you crunch!
5. Slowly lower your shoulders (but not head) back to the floor and repeat.

How many: 2 sets of 8–12 reps each. Rest 15 seconds between sets.

Benefits: Abdominals (rectus abdominis).

LOWER-TUMMY TIGHTENER

1. Lie on your back with your knees bent and your feet on the floor. Press your back firmly into the floor. There should be no arch in your back at all.
2. Extend one of your legs straight out, about 1 to 2 feet from the floor (make sure the small of the back stays against the floor). Rest your head in your hands but keep your neck and shoulders relaxed. Tighten your tummy and slowly lift your shoulders from the floor. Simultaneously bend your knee toward your chest.
3. Exhale as you crunch!
4. Slowly lower your shoulders back to the floor and extend the leg. Repeat.

How many: 2 sets of 8–12 reps per leg. Rest 15 seconds between sets.

Benefits: Lower abdominals (rectus abdominus).

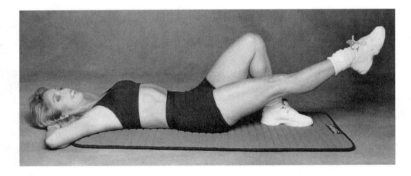

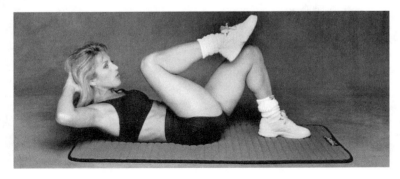

THURSDAY: DAY 11—TONING ROUTINE

REAR-VIEW SHAPER

1. Kneel on the floor with your elbows and hands on the floor.
2. Be sure to keep your back flat, abs tight, and your hips square to the floor.
3. Raise your right leg from the floor, keeping it bent at a right angle. Your upper leg and right foot should be parallel to the floor.
4. Slowly raise your knee up and down, pressing your foot toward the ceiling, squeezing your buttocks.

How many: 2 sets of 8–12 reps each per leg. Rest 15 seconds between sets.

Benefits: Buttocks (gluteals).

Ankle weights optional.

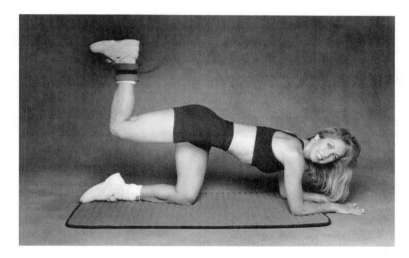

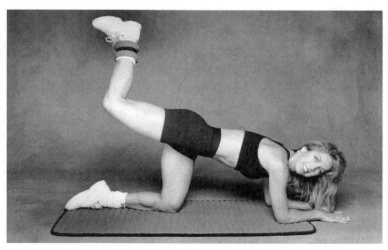

THURSDAY: DAY 11—TONING ROUTINE

BACK EXTENSION

1. Lie on your stomach with your arms and legs extended, and your feet about 6 inches apart.
2. Slowly raise your head and left arm about 4 to 6 inches from the floor. Keep neck aligned. Simultaneously lift your right leg about 4 to 8 inches from the floor, anchoring your hips to the floor.

3. Squeeze your buttocks. Concentrate on proper form—do not overarch your back. Hold for 10 seconds and relax.
4. Repeat using opposite leg and arm, and hold for 10 seconds. Then try the whole sequence again.

How many: 2 10-second holds on each side

Benefits: Back extensors (the muscles that support your back and keep your spinal column in alignment), buttocks and thighs.

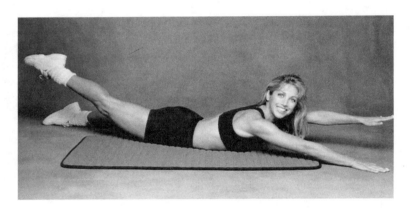

Cool down with three
of your favorite Super Stretches
on p. 188.

TUESDAY: DAY 16—TONING ROUTINE

BACK ROLL-UP

1. Stand tall, feet shoulder-width apart. Place hands on thighs for support. Keep back flat.
2. As you exhale, round your back and feel a stretch in the entire back. As you do this, tighten and pull in the abdominals.
3. Relax, inhale, and return to starting position.
4. Continue in one fluid motion (flat back to round back) very slowly. This is a wonderful warm-up for the back. It elongates and stretches the muscles of the upper and lower back.

How many: 4 times.

Benefits: Lower, middle, and upper areas of the back.

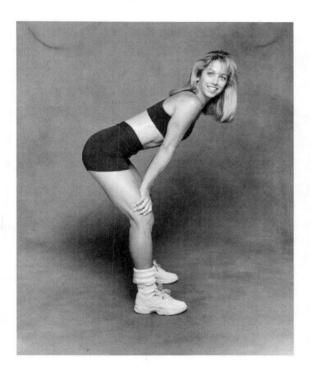
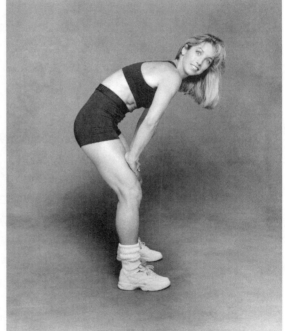

TUESDAY: DAY 16—TONING ROUTINE

THIGH AND BUN FIRMER

1. Stand with your feet a little wider than your hips. Your feet should be slightly turned out as you straddle a chair.
2. Your back should be straight, abs tight, and your hands on your hips.
3. Tilt your pelvis forward and keep your hips square to the front.
4. Bend your knees, and slowly lower your body until you "tap" the chair.
5. As you return to the starting position, exhale and squeeze your buttocks.

How many: 2 sets of 8–12 reps each. Rest 15 seconds between sets.

Benefits: Thighs (quadriceps), inner thighs (adductors), buttocks (gluteals).

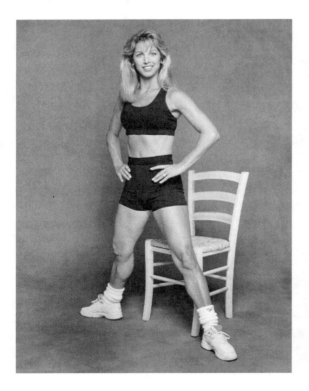 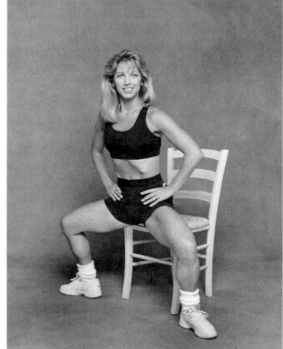

TUESDAY: DAY 16—TONING ROUTINE

LEAN LEGS

1. Stand tall, and place one hand on a chair for support and the other hand on hip. Begin in "first position" (as in ballet), with toes turned out and heels touching.
2. Your back should be straight and your abs tight.
3. Bend the knees, keeping them over the toes.
4. Lift up your heels, keeping your knees bent.

5. Push from the balls of your feet and straighten your legs, squeezing your buttocks and inner thighs.
6. Flatten heels and return to starting position. This is a 4-step exercise . . . plie down, heels lift, push up to straighten legs, heels down, and begin again in starting position.

How many: 2 sets of 8–12 reps each. Rest 15 seconds between sets.

Benefits: Quadriceps, calves, inner thighs, back of thighs, and buttock muscles.

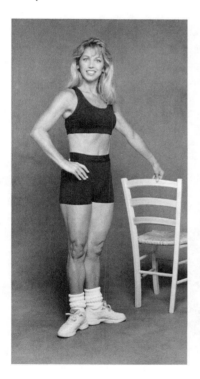
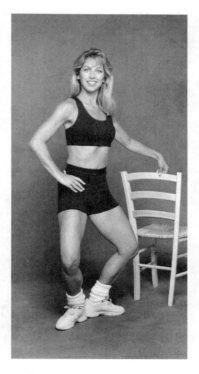
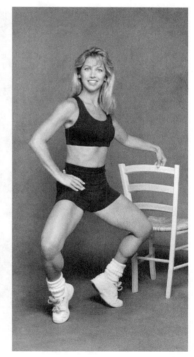

TUESDAY: DAY 16—TONING ROUTINE

LOWER BODY TONER

1. Place weights in hands at your sides (weights optional). Start with your feet about shoulder-width apart.
2. Take a step forward with one foot. As you step, bend your back knee, and lower yourself toward the floor.
3. Balancing your body weight over your front heel and your back toes, keep knees at 90 degree angles, as shown.
4. Straighten your legs and raise yourself back up.

5. Keeping your legs in the lunge position, repeat the movement up and down. After you have completed 1 set (8–12 dips, down and up), alternate legs and repeat the exercise on the other leg.

How many: 2 sets of 8–12 reps each. Rest 15 seconds between sets.

Benefits: Thighs (quadriceps), buttocks (gluteals), hamstrings.

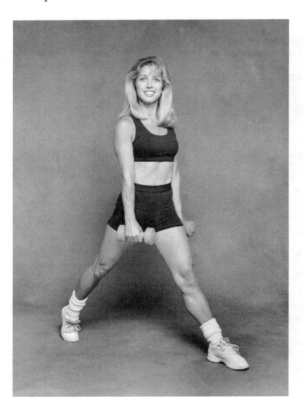
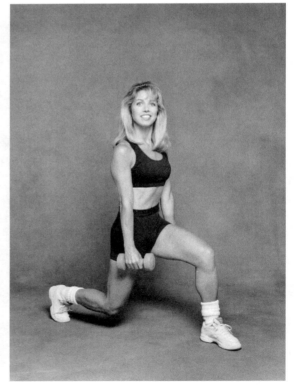

TUESDAY: DAY 16—TONING ROUTINE

KICKBACKS (WITH WEIGHTS)

1. Stand with your left leg in front of your right and slightly bend the left knee.
2. For support, you can rest your left hand on your left thigh.
3. Keep your abs tight and your back flat.
4. Raise your right elbow so the upper part of your arm is parallel with the floor. Keep your elbow close to your body.
5. Straighten your right arm. Be sure to squeeze your triceps as you straighten your arm.
6. Return your right hand to the starting position, pause, and repeat the movement.

How many: 2 sets of 8–12 reps each per arm.
Rest 15 seconds between sets.

Benefits: Back of arms (triceps).

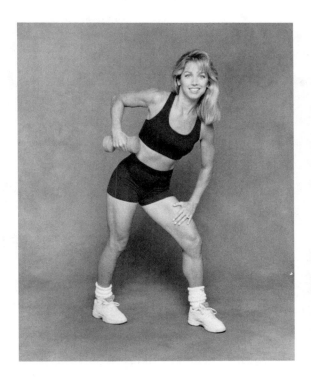
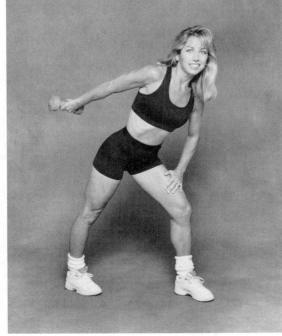

TUESDAY: DAY 16—TONING ROUTINE

SHOULDER RAISES (WITH WEIGHTS)

1. Stand with your feet shoulder-width apart, abs tight, back straight, and knees slightly bent.
2. Start with your hands at your side. With straight arms (don't lock elbows), lift the weights to the side slightly above shoulder level. Palms are down. Return to the starting position.

How many: 2 sets of 8–12 reps each. Rest 15 seconds between sets.

Benefits: Shoulders (medial deltoids).

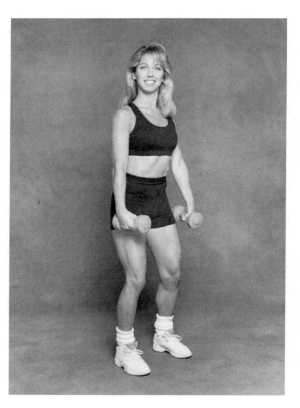
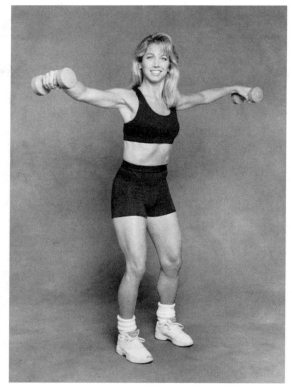

TUESDAY: DAY 16—TONING ROUTINE

PUSH-UPS

1. Kneel on the floor with your ankles crossed and your hands out in front of you on the floor.
2. Straighten your back, with abs tight and your head in a natural position.
3. Slowly bend your elbows and lower your chest to the floor.
4. Straighten your elbows and return to the starting position.

How many: 2 sets of 8–12 reps each. Rest 15 seconds between sets.

Benefits: Chest (pectorals), shoulders (anterior deltoid), triceps.

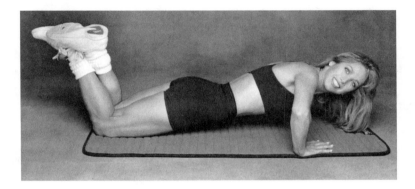

THIGH-AND-TUSH TIGHTENER

1. Kneel on the floor with both elbows directly under your shoulders, your left knee under your left hip, and hands on the floor.
2. Straighten the right leg behind you, with toes resting on the floor. Keep your back flat, abs tight, and your hips square to the floor.
3. Keeping your right leg straight, use your buttocks to lift the entire leg up. Now, lower the leg. Slowly, raise your leg up and down for two sets. Do not arch your back and squeeze the buttocks.

How many: 2 sets of 8–12 lifts each per leg. Rest 15 seconds between sets.

Benefits: Buttocks (gluteals) and back of thighs (hamstrings).

Ankle weights optional.

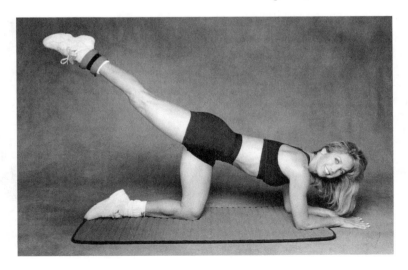

TUESDAY: DAY 16—TONING ROUTINE

BOTTOMS UP

1. Lie on your back, bend your knees, and keep feet flat on the floor. Extend your arms along your sides.
2. Lift your buttocks from the floor (3 to 6 inches) by tilting your pelvis up, squeezing your buttocks, and tightening your abdominals.
3. Hold for a few seconds and then lower your bottom down one vertebra at a time.
4. Pictured are 2 additional exercises that will increase your level of difficulty. Try these variations.

How many: 2 sets of 8–12 lifts each. Rest 15 seconds between sets.

Benefits: Buttocks (gluteals) and back of thighs (hamstrings).

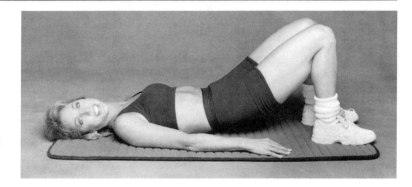

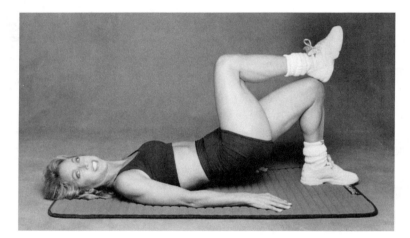

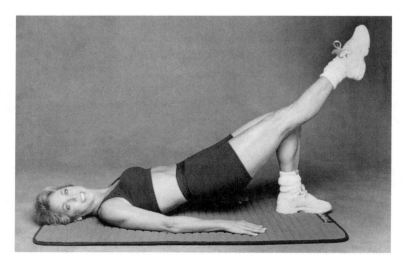

TUESDAY: DAY 16—TONING ROUTINE

WAISTLINE SLIMMER

1. Lie on your back with your knees bent and your feet on the floor. Press your lower back firmly into the floor. There should be no arch in your back at all.
2. Rest your head in your hands but keep your back and shoulders relaxed.
3. Raise just one of your shoulder blades from the floor while pressing the opposite shoulder blade into the floor.
4. As you raise up, move your elbow in the direction of the opposite knee. Slowly lower your shoulder blade to the floor and repeat.

How many: 2 sets of 8–12 reps each per side. Rest 15 seconds between sets.

Benefits: Waistline (obliques) and abdominals (rectus abdominis).

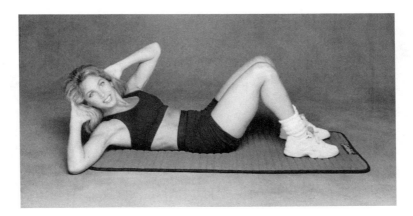

TUESDAY: DAY 16—TONING ROUTINE

ADVANCED BICYCLE

1. Lie on the floor with your legs straight. Press your back firmly into the floor; there should be no arch in your back at all.
2. Rest your head in your hands but make sure that your neck and shoulders are relaxed.
3. Pull your right knee into your chest while at the same time raising your left shoulder blade from the floor in the direction of your knee.
4. As you return your right leg and left shoulder to the starting position, bring your left knee in to your chest and meet it with your right elbow.
5. Continue to alternate side to side.

How many: 2 sets of 8–12 reps each. Rest 15 seconds between sets.

Benefits: Abdominals (rectus abdominus) and sides of waist (obliques).

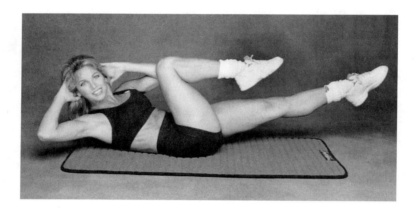

**Cool down and relax with
three of your favorite
Super Stretches on p. 188.**

THURSDAY: DAY 18—TONING ROUTINE

BACK ROLL-UP

1. Stand tall, feet shoulder-width apart. Place hands on thighs for support. Keep back flat.
2. As you exhale, round your back and feel a stretch in the entire back. As you do this, tighten and pull in the abdominals.
3. Relax, inhale, and return to starting position.
4. Continue in one fluid motion (flat back to round back) very slowly. This is a wonderful warm-up for the back. It elongates and stretches the muscles of the upper and lower back.

How many: 4 times.

Benefits: Lower, middle, and upper areas of the back.

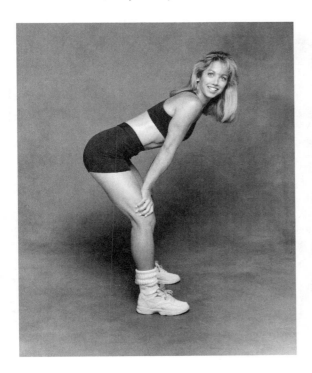
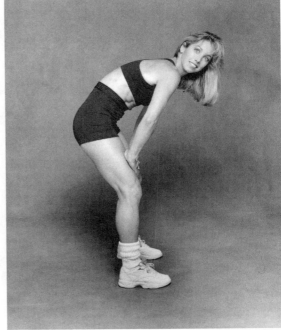

THURSDAY: DAY 18—TONING ROUTINE

POWER LUNGE

1. Start with your feet about shoulder-width apart (weights optional).
2. Take a step forward with one foot. Make sure front knee stays at a 90 degree angle. Keep your knee in line with your ankle.
3. As you step forward, bend your back knee. Be sure you don't bang it on the floor. Your weight should be balanced between your back toes and your front heel.

4. Push back to the starting position, bringing legs together and repeat, alternating your legs.

How many: 2 sets of 8–12 reps each. Rest 15 seconds between sets.

Benefits: Thighs (quadriceps), hamstrings, buttocks (gluteals).

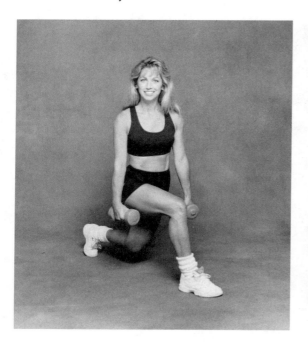
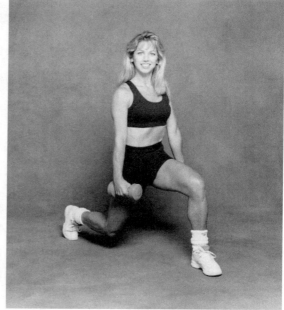

THURSDAY: DAY 18—TONING ROUTINE

BUN FIRMER

1. Stand with your feet wider than your hips. Point your toes slightly out. Place hands on buttocks with palms facing out (weights optional). Your back should be straight and your abs tight.
2. Tilt your pelvis slightly forward.
3. Bend your knees and slowly lower your hips toward the floor, as in a plié position.
4. From the plié, extend your body up. Squeeze your buttocks and tighten your inner thighs.

How many: 2 sets of 8–12 reps each. Rest 15 seconds between sets.

Benefits: Thighs (quadriceps), hamstrings, buttocks (gluteals).

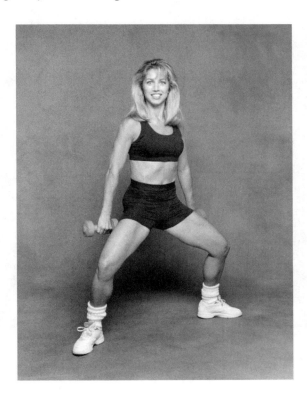

THURSDAY: DAY 18—TONING ROUTINE

UPRIGHT ROWS (WITH WEIGHTS)

1. Stand with your feet wider than your shoulders. Your abs should be tight, and your knees slightly bent.
2. Hold the weights with your palms facing in.
3. Raise the weights so your arms form the letter "V."
4. Inhale as you lift, squeezing your shoulder blades together, then return your arms to the starting position and repeat.

How many: 2 sets of 8–12 reps each. Rest 15 seconds between sets.

Benefits: Upper back (trapezius, rhomboids).

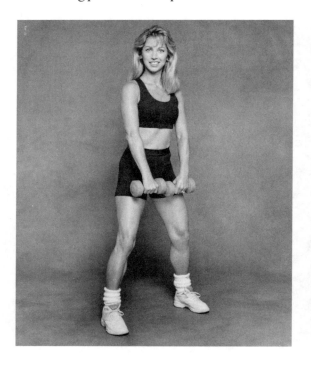
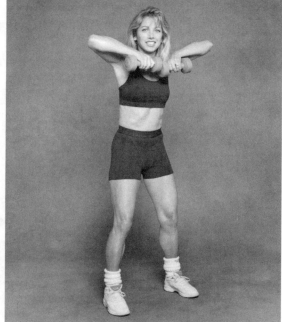

THURSDAY: DAY 18—TONING ROUTINE

BUST BUILDER (WITH WEIGHTS)

1. Stand with knees slightly bent and feet shoulder-width apart. Keep back straight and abs tight.
2. Bend your elbows out to the side at right angles.
3. By squeezing your chest, slowly bring forearms and hands together in front of your chest, initiating this movement from the pectorals (chest muscles).
4. Slowly press your arms back out to the starting position.

How many: 2 sets of 8–12 reps each. Rest 15 seconds between sets.

Benefits: Chest (pectorals).

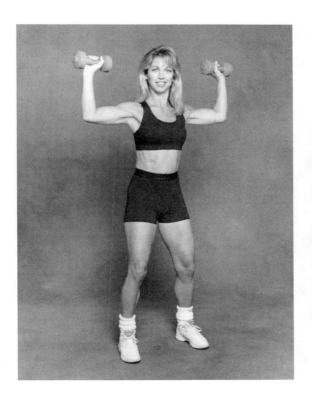
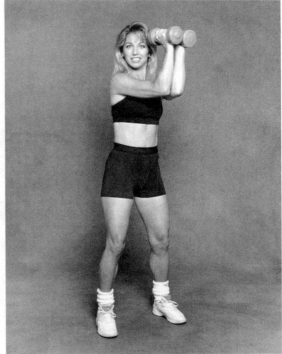

THURSDAY: DAY 18—TONING ROUTINE

UNDERARM TIGHTENER (WITH WEIGHTS)

1. Place left hand and bent left knee on seat of chair. Use right leg for balance. Keep your abs tight and your back flat.
2. Raise your right elbow so that the upper part of your arm is parallel with the floor. Keep your elbow close to your body.
3. Straighten your right arm. Be sure to squeeze your triceps as you straighten your arm. Return your right hand to the starting position, pause, and repeat the movement.

How many: 2 sets of 8–12 reps each per arm. Rest 15 seconds between sets.

Benefits: Back of arms (triceps).

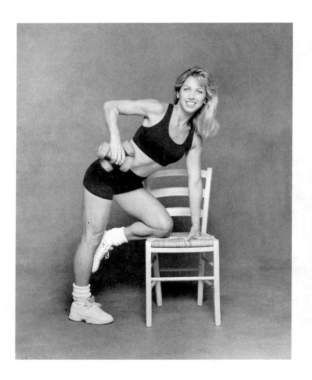
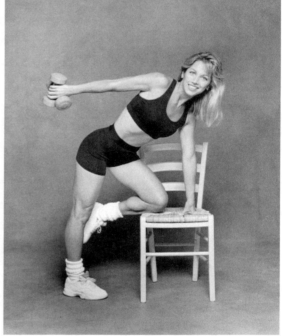

THURSDAY: DAY 18—TONING ROUTINE

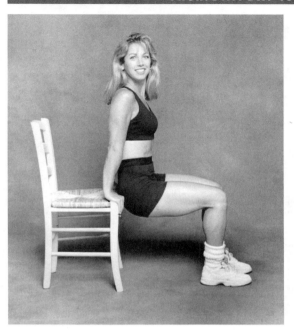

TRICEPS PRESS ON BENCH OR CHAIR

1. Sit on the edge of your bench or chair with your knees bent and feet in front of you.
2. Place your hands on the bench next to your hips and raise your body off the bench.
3. Moving your hips slightly forward, bend your elbows, and lower your body toward the floor.
4. Straighten your arms and raise your body. Repeat the movement until your reps are completed.

How many: 2 sets of 8–12 reps each. Rest 15 seconds between sets.

Benefits: Back of arms (triceps).

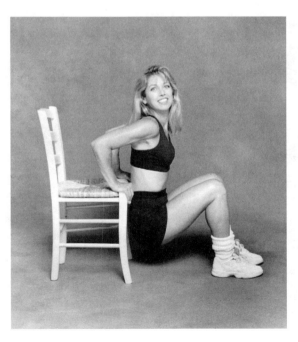

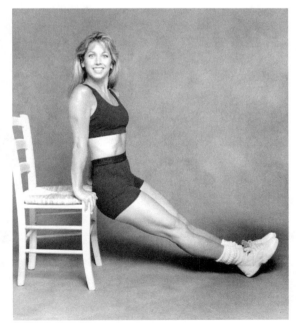

THURSDAY: DAY 18—TONING ROUTINE

SUPER CRUNCHES

1. Lie on the floor with your knees bent and your feet resting on a chair. Press your lower back firmly into the floor. There should be no arch in your back at all.
2. You may rest your head in your hands, or cross your arms in front of your chest, or extend your arms over your head, depending on your ability. Always keep your neck and shoulders relaxed.
3. Tighten your tummy and slowly lift your head and shoulders off the floor from 4 to 6 inches.
4. Exhale as you crunch!
5. Slowly lower your shoulders back to the floor and repeat.

How many: 2 sets of 8–12 reps each. Rest 15 seconds between sets.

Benefits: Abdominals (rectus abdominis).

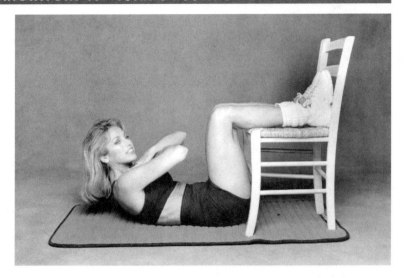

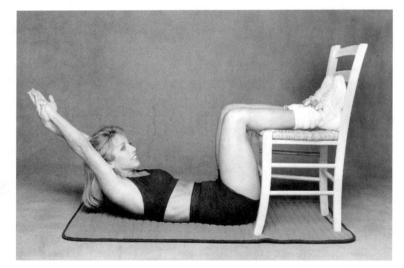

THURSDAY: DAY 18—TONING ROUTINE

ONE LEGGED V-SIT

1. Lie on the floor and place your hands behind your head with elbows extended out. Rest your head and neck in your hands. Keep your back pressed into the floor.
2. Start with one leg extended straight in front of you and the other bent with foot resting on floor.
3. Exhale and contract your abdominals as you lift your leg toward your chest. Simultaneously lifting your head and shoulders from the floor about 6 inches.
4. Lower your leg but don't let it touch the floor. This is a very slow, controlled motion. It is very important to keep back pressed to the floor the entire time. Repeat.

How many: 2 sets of 8–12 reps each. Rest 15 seconds between sets.

Benefits: Abdominals (rectus abdominus).

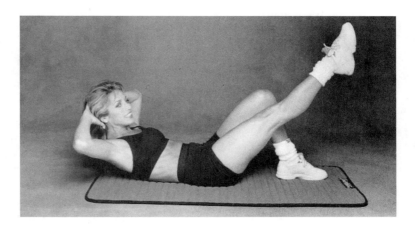

AB PRESSES

1. Lie on your back with knees bent and feet flat on floor. Press your back firmly to the floor. There should be no arch in your back at all.
2. Extend your arms to the sides. Roll your head and shoulders up from the floor about 6 inches.
3. Do an isometric hold of the abdominal muscles by adding little lifts, "pulses," keeping your shoulders off the floor. The pulses add resistance to the abdominal muscles; therefore, overloads the muscle group.
4. Stay in the crunch position for 1 set (8–12 pulses).

How many: 2 sets of 8–12 pulses. Rest 15 seconds between sets.

Benefits: Strengthens the abdominals (rectus abdominis).

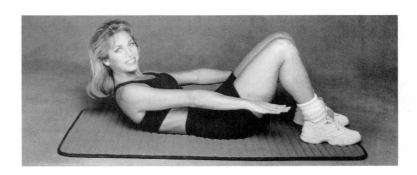

THURSDAY: DAY 18—TONING ROUTINE

BACK STRENGTHENER

1. Kneel on all fours.
2. Lift and extend your left arm and your right leg. Balance yourself by keeping your back straight, your abdominals tight, and your buttocks firm.
3. Hold for 15–20 seconds. Then relax.
4. Repeat with opposite arm and leg. Concentrate on proper form and be sure not to arch your back.

How many: 2 sets of 15–20 seconds each. Relax 15 seconds between sets.

Benefits: Strengthens your entire back (erector spinae) and firms upper back and buttock muscles.

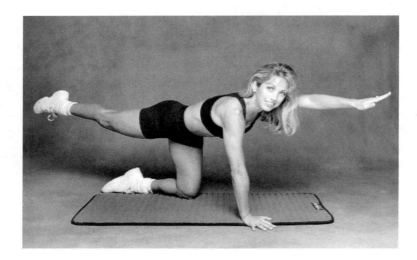

Relax and cool down with three
Super Stretches on p. 188.

PART III

KEEPING IT OFF

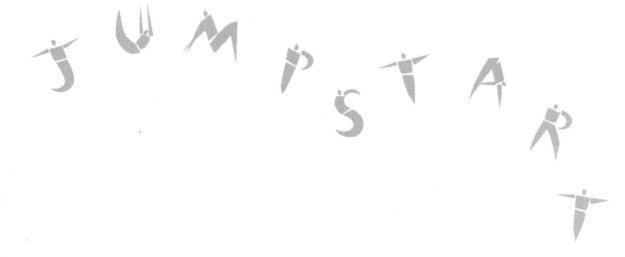

JUMPSTART

Food isn't the enemy.
Sitting still is.
—Denise Austin

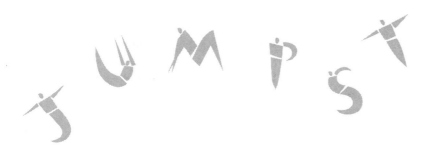

KEEP IT GOING! MAINTAINING YOUR HEALTHY HABITS

On Your Own

Dear Denise,

I want to thank you for the wonderful contribution you have made to my life. I have never felt so energetic, and have been receiving numerous compliments on my weight loss. I will continue with your health routine for the rest of my life! Many thanks.

—Helen, Coral Springs, Florida

Say hello to the good life! You will be living fit and loving it. One of the most important factors in keeping weight off is to make healthy living one of your primary goals in life. Goals help to focus our attention. Our mind will not reach toward great things until it has clear objectives, and it all starts when you set goals for yourself. It is then that the switch is turned on, the current starts to flow, and the power to accomplish anything becomes a reality. By accomplishing some intermediate and short-range goals, you will realize your long-range and ultimate goals.

Over the past three weeks you did it . . . you have met some of your goals. Great! Congratulations. Now, you must strive to commit yourself to being the best you can be.

Commitment

One of the places that we find commitment problems is in the pursuit of a healthful lifestyle. If getting in shape and living more healthily is important to you, then make it your goal to do so. Once you do so, it's important that you keep the agreement with yourself. This goes for any goal in your life. You've figured out what it is that you want, you've set goals to accomplish, and now you must commit yourself to seeing them through to the very end!

Most people when making an agreement with others—or with themselves—add a silent condition in their mind. "I'll do this . . . (if it's not too hard!)""I'll do that . . . (if it doesn't take too long!)""I'll try so-and-so . . . (if it doesn't make me uncomfortable!)" These little attachments completely negate the entire premise of commitment. Commitment is the willingness to be uncomfortable! It is the willingness to stay on track even if something is too hard or takes too long! It is the willingness that most people find so difficult. If achieving your goals and getting what you want out of life took no effort and was easy to do, these things would have no value.

Most people lack commitment because they are either lazy or they haven't yet decided what is really important to them. Focus on accomplishing your goals, understand their importance. Hold them near to you. Half-hearted efforts will get you absolutely nowhere in life. *You must have a zest, a love, a passion for what is important to you!* Without passion for what you want, it's impossible to be committed to that goal.

After 21 Days

For the past three weeks you have worked very hard to transform your negative habits into new healthy ones. Some of you might be feeling a little bit anxious, but don't be. I'm not leaving you stranded. I will stay right here as you continue the adventure we began together 21 days ago. I have more recipes for you and more great ideas to tone and firm each part of your body. Remember, the goal of the past three weeks was to find a new way of thinking, eating, and moving so that you would never have to diet again. I am bound and determined that you won't. I hope you are, too! I believe you will achieve all of your goals, including a firm, trim healthy body by continuing to think positively, eat moderate portions of healthy, high-fiber, low-fat meals and exercise regularly in a balanced program, including aerobics, toning, and flexibility.

The first three weeks were structured to introduce you to a wide variety of new meal choices and exercise alternatives along with renewing your positive attitude. Now, you should feel free to create your own menus using the recipes you enjoyed most—after all, variety is the spice of life! And, if it makes you feel better, repeat the three weeks exactly as before. There is so much variety built into the program that you won't get bored quickly. However, don't forget that it can be fun to experiment! Use some of the seasoning and preparation techniques you have learned to adapt your own family recipes to accommodate your new way of eating. Just be sure to keep that fat content around 20 percent so that those inches keep melting away. In the appendix you'll find lots more recipes, lists of ingredients, and meal suggestions.

Do not make the common mistake of deciding that "if I cut my fat intake to 5 percent, I will lose weight even faster!" Think healthy eating!

Your body needs some fat. Fat is essential to good digestion. Proper digestion leads to effective excretion. The body's ability to excrete toxins and wastes is an important component of good health and efficient weight loss. Fat also contributes to a beautiful complexion, strong nails, and shiny hair. Remember, moderation!

After you reach a comfortable weight (not skinny, comfortable!), you will need to increase your calorie allotments in order to maintain your new physique. As a general rule, the average woman should keep her daily intake under 2000 calories. (You may need to modify your daily intake based on your personal activity level—remember, calories in versus calories burned.) I wouldn't recommend increasing the fat content. Additional fat seems to creep in quite naturally, particularly in this program where we fully acknowledge the need to treat ourselves. If you maintain a daily fat intake of 20 percent, then an infrequent special snack or dessert will not be a problem. It is when our daily fat intake is already high that such indulgences cause the pounds to mount. The following chart is a general guide to daily fat allotments. Personally, I eat about 1800 calories a day and try to stay within the 20 percent allotment. Of course, there are days where I blow it. I call them my *cheat days*. I try to have only one cheat day a week and it's usually on the weekend. It's all a matter of balance.

WHAT'S YOUR FAT ALLOTMENT?

Fat in Diet	Daily Calories		
	1,200	1,500	2,000
20%	27g	33g	44g
30%	40g	50g	67g

Recently I had the opportunity to go with my husband to Spain for the wedding of one of his clients (of the famous Sanchez tennis family). While there I couldn't help but notice the beauty of the Spanish women. What I also noticed was the absence of something else . . . obesity. In fact, I didn't see much fat there, period.

I decided to do a little investigating for my book and asked some of the women their thoughts on the subject. Hearing my American accent brought an instant smile to their faces. At first I got the impression they were a little embarrassed to answer. But finally, after a bit of coaxing, one of the girls who had been a foreign exchange student in the United States spoke up. And boy, did she make her point!

Don't Let Them Scare You. . . . Food Is *Still* Fabulous!!

"I didn't understand the Americans," she said. "All the girls seemed to be obsessed with fat! Every conversation began and ended with talk about food—what they couldn't eat or wouldn't eat; what they'd like to eat or wish they hadn't eaten; how many calories were in this product, but not in that product; how this exercise burns more fat than that consumed daily."

Somehow, the American public has interpreted "no fat" and "low fat" as, "Eat as much of this as you can shove down your throat and it will make you look just like Cindy Crawford!" Now that may be a slight exaggeration, *but* only a slight one. Just the other day I was behind a women in line at the grocery. She had five packages of fat-free cookies in her basket. I wouldn't have noticed except that when she saw me, the woman smiled proudly and said, "Look, I can eat *all* these cookies without consuming *1 gram* of fat! I never would have bought cookies before. This fat-free stuff is a miracle!"

I've been thinking about her words and the excitement in her voice ever since. She spoke as though those fat-free cookies were actually going to make her *lose* weight. Without any regard for nutrition or regular calories, this woman was going to consume every single cookie in all five packages, believing she was doing the right thing. Why? Because every time she turns on the television or reads the newspaper, she sees things like, "Food doesn't make you fat, *fat* makes you fat." I wonder how many other people who have always known that a balanced diet and regular exercise is the only way to control body weight now have grocery carts filled with cookies, ice cream, cake, bread, and potatoes—and are proud as peacocks about it because they're eating "fat-free."

The information we were given that it is better to eat more food with little or no fat than it is to eat less food with high fat was never intended as a substitute for common sense or discipline. Just because there are fat-free cookies available doesn't mean you can consume five packages of them without the possibility of gaining weight. There are other variables to be considered, such as how long it took you to eat all five packages, how much and how often you had been exercising, what else you had eaten on the days you ate the cookies, and the rate of your metabolism.

That young girl in Spain was right. We think about food and the negative effects of eating way too much. Haven't you noticed? Every day there's a new report—and each one contradicts the one before. What was good for us twenty years ago will kill us today. Even worse, what was good for us *yesterday* could kill us today, according to some news releases! I'm not saying that we shouldn't pay attention to new research; a lot of it is very valuable. We now know that eating red meat every day isn't good for the arteries. And certainly what we've learned about the effects of smoking and secondhand smoke will save many lives. But let's be honest. In the big picture, haven't we always known that when it comes to eating, everything is all right in moderation? And haven't we also known that regular exercise will keep excess weight in check? Sure we have. This obsession isn't necessary. In fact, it's making us crazy!

I'm telling you to let it go. I'm going to give you the Austin Food Philosophy. If it sounds like something new, that's only because you probably haven't been spoken to about food in a rational manner for quite some time. The truth is, my philosophy of eating is an old one. But you're going to love it for two reasons. The first is that it works. If you eat the way I eat and move that body regularly, you won't get fat. The second reason you're going to love my philosophy of eating is that it will, at long last, put the fun back into food!

Don't let them scare you. . . . food is *still* fabulous. You can eat a little of anything you want—more if you exercise regularly. (Remember, a good exercise program can compensate for the lack of a healthy diet, but a healthy diet can never compensate for the lack of a good exercise program.) Don't deprive yourself. It's human nature to want what you think you can't have. That goes as far back as Adam and Eve and the forbidden fruit. Chances are, if you didn't feel guilty about enjoying certain types of food, that food wouldn't be nearly as appealing to you. Go ahead. Release the guilt. Eat, drink, and be merry . . . but only in moderation.

In-a-Hurry Thoughts

- Look for the good in people.
- Don't waste time, it's what life is made of.
- You have nothing if you don't have your health.
- Take a deep breath, get that oxygen flowing . . . you'll think better and feel better.
- Smile a lot! It's free and is beyond price.
- Don't take good health for granted.
- Keep it up.
- Never deprive someone of hope, it might be all they have.
- Fitness isn't stored, only fat is.

Weight Loss Tips

- Don't skip meals before a party; just cut back at breakfast and lunch. Enjoy the delicious food, but watch the portion size.
- If you are craving a chocolate bar, don't try to resist by replacing it with foods you don't want. Chances are you will end up eating both; instead, have the treat or just a few bites of it, and get back on track.
- Stress causes many people to overeat, so learn how to relax.

Some good options are yoga, meditation, and walking.

- Try eating slowly to avoid overindulging.
- Did you know that fitness walking is the number one outdoor fitness activity for adults in the United States today? Fitness walkers walk an average of 2.86 miles per walk, 110 days per year and 315 miles per year.
- To keep your blood sugar and energy level up, try eating small meals throughout the day. By eating small meals, you won't overwork the digestive system by making it digest three big meals, leaving the body with little energy to complete other necessary tasks.
- If you must, eat small samples of the foods you are craving. If you deprive yourself of food you like, you will be more likely to gorge yourself later.
- For dessert, choose low-fat dishes like sorbet, fruit, or angel food cake.
- Challenge breakfast foods to the paper-towel test. If foods like muffins or croissants exude oil onto a paper towel, they are high in fat and should be eaten in moderation.
- Never think you are going on a diet because it implies you will be going off it at some point in the future.
- To escape that sluggish feeling after eating, avoid fat. Fat causes our digestive systems to work overtime, because fat is the hardest nutrient to digest.
- Eat larger amounts of food earlier in the day, so you will burn off those calories. Eat breakfast like a king, lunch like a queen, and dinner like a pauper.
- Put a curfew on your eating. Do not eat anything for three hours prior to your bedtime.
- Eat small meals throughout the day instead of three large meals. Smaller meals provide the energy needed for immediate demands, while large meals have excess calories not needed for current tasks, which leads the body to store these extra calories as fat.
- Avoid alcohol! It stimulates hunger and causes you to forget the importance of nutritional eating. Drinking alcohol reduces the rate at which the body burns fat. So, not only is the body receiving empty calories from the alcohol, it is also not burning off calories from other foods as rapidly. Remember your health and your waistline the next time you're about to grab a drink, and choose sparkling water.
- Always use 95 percent lean ground beef instead of regular ground beef (165 calories versus 225 calories per 3-ounce serving).

- Women: Do your Kegels! Tighten up the vaginal wall by squeezing the muscles in the pelvic area. To learn where these muscles are located in the pelvis, next time you are going pee, stop the flow. Those are the muscles you use during a Kegel exercise.

- Don't smoke and if you do, *quit!* Nicotine is a drug; it artificially induces a high, which means you'll crash. Smokers lack the stamina needed to live active, healthy lives. And as we all know, cigarettes are extremely harmful to our health.

- When you feel overwhelmed by your career and/or your family, take a minute to prioritize your tasks for the day. Consider what is really important and what might be put off until tomorrow.

- Losing weight with good eating habits and activity offers many health benefits . . . unlike liposuction.

- No magical cream has been proven totally effective for combatting cellulite and in many cases liposuction has made the cellulite on women's legs look worse; however, you are likely to see improvement by reducing the fat in your diet and increasing exercise.

- Exercise isn't an isolated part of your life. How you eat, drink, and rest is essential to your overall health.

- To avoid hurting your back when lifting heavy objects, bring the load as close to you as possible, separate your feet, putting one slightly in front of the other, bend your knees so you use your leg muscles and not your back, don't jerk the load—lift slowly, and don't twist your body while carrying a heavy load.

- Every 10 years your metabolism slows by 7 percent, so you have to either increase your exercise or decrease your food intake to maintain your normal weight.

- Did you know that shoveling snow burns 710 calories per hour?

- You would have to eat nearly 2 quarts of plain, unbuttered popcorn to get the calories found in 1 ounce of potato chips (about 15 chips).

- Prioritize your tasks for the day. What are the major and what are the minor tasks for the day?

- Write out a list of your objectives for the day, from the most important to the least important.

- Schedule and plan your day. It helps. With two small children in our lives, Jeff and I have to schedule a time to be alone.

- If you have a sweet tooth and feel like eating an entire cake (you know, PMS time), try eating a graham cracker with low-fat vanilla frosting spread lightly on top.

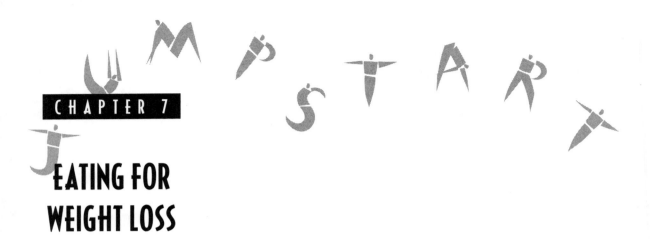

CHAPTER 7

EATING FOR WEIGHT LOSS

f you have decided that it's time to lose weight, I'm here for you. I will show you how to do it safely and make the experience as fun for you as possible. I just want you to look at the reasons that you want to lose the weight and evaluate your motives. Do you want to lose weight for a certain occasion such as a party, your wedding, swimsuit season, and so on? If so, understand that these occasions are one-time goals and therefore, your weight loss is likely to be temporary. You can do it, of course, as I'm sure you already know. Most people who need to lose weight have lost it a dozen times throughout their lives.

Wanting to lose weight for a certain occasion is normal. And, in fact, an occasion can be a great motivator, the thing that gets you started. But, unless you want to have to lose the weight over and over again, your reasoning for doing so has to be bigger than that. I've said it before and I'll say it again, anything you do temporarily will only last temporarily.

Losing weight for your health, however, would be an ongoing commitment, just as losing weight in order to be able to do more in life or to keep up with your children would be ongoing commitments. See the difference? These reasons might not seem to have the urgency of a wedding or swimsuit season but, believe me, their impact is far more powerful because they are much more likely to promote lifestyle changes. When you've committed to a lifestyle change, one that you know will last for the rest of your life, you won't ever have to worry about going back to the "fat" you. That person will no longer exist in your mind. And if she doesn't exist in your mind, she won't exist in your body. You'll be able to eat something sweet or fatty now and then without guilt, fear, or disgust.

You now know that the key to healthy eating is a low-fat food plan. With a diet high in complex carbohydrates, a moderate amount of protein, and a little fat, along with regular exercise, you won't gain weight. In fact, your body will naturally be able to find the weight that suits it best if you feed it properly and move it consistently. You'll have strength, energy, and much less sickness and stress in your life.

If you need to lose a significant amount of weight, you'll probably want to jump-start the process. This doesn't mean you'll have to eat different foods than you'd eat on a normal healthy eating plan, but you may want to eat them a little bit differently. When I talk about eating to lose weight, I'll sometimes refer to it as "the royal eating plan." Eat breakfast like a king, lunch like a queen, and dinner like a pauper. It's a simple matter of mathematics. If you burn more calories than your body uses, you'll lose weight. That's why you should eat the bulk of your calories early in the day, while you're active. After you've incorporated regular exercise into your life and your body develops some muscle, you'll burn calories even as you sleep. But until then, you don't want your stomach filled with food late in the evening, because unless your job keeps you up and moving at night, you won't have as much opportunity to burn the calories your body doesn't need.

While there is no doubt that calories from fat are the real culprits in weight gain, it is wise to consider all calories when trying to lose weight. I don't mean to go crazy and count every calorie that you put in your mouth, but you should know that starches are high in regular calories. For someone who wants to maintain her weight or for someone who is already active, it won't be a problem. You can and should have them in your diet. It's only the creamy sauces, butter, and sour cream that will make you fat. Still, don't fill up on bread, pasta, potatoes, or rice and then go straight to bed. If you do, your weight loss won't happen as fast as you'd like. As a general rule, remain up and somewhat active for at least 3 hours after you've eaten your dinner. Try to eat most of your starches at breakfast and lunch, cutting back on them at dinner. You can have some starch at night, but keep it to one serving.

When you're trying to lose weight, avoid alcohol. Generally, there is nothing wrong with a glass of wine but alcohol, for the most part, just provides empty calories. And, more important, alcohol can enhance your appetite, making you think you're hungry when you're not. One study found that just 4 ounces of alcohol slow down your metabolism, making it harder to burn fat.

By far the worst thing you can do when trying to lose weight is to starve yourself. Skipping meals will not support your efforts, only hurt them. If you've ever lost weight and then gained even more back in its place, it is likely due to what you didn't eat rather than what you did. You see, when your body is accustomed to being fed regularly, the shock of not eating sends it into survival mode. This is not something you have control over, it just is. The body wants to live and will fight to keep itself alive. When you stop eating, the body thinks it might starve. To avoid that, it will slow down its metabolism in order to save energy. It will not burn fat, but keep the fat in place in order to protect itself. People always have a difficult time believing this, yet they continue to wonder why their diets never produce lasting results.

The best way to lose weight once and for all is to eat three healthy meals a day and exercise regularly. The meals should consist of foods you enjoy and that satisfy you. If you are used to eating too much of the kind of food that promotes weight gain (food high in fats and/or sugar), you will have to train yourself to crave different types of food. Believe it or not, this will be *easier* than it was to train yourself to crave the food you eat now.

Your body wants you to eat well. Eating healthy foods makes you feel better and have more energy, as well as reducing stomach and digestion problems and mood swings. Healthy eating doesn't mean a lettuce leaf and a bowl of consommé for dinner. As you've seen, you can prepare wonderful dishes that are low in fat and calories but high in taste.

Eating for Energy

There are reasons for changing your eating habits other than to lose weight. Your doctor may prescribe a new food plan in order to adjust your cholesterol level, blood sugar level, or blood pressure. It's possible that a person can look slender—even thin—but have a high percentage of body fat. Being thin and feeling fit are not the same thing at all. Fitness requires not only eating well, but having strength and stamina to do the things in life that make you happy.

Do you ever notice that some people seem to be able to fit so much into their day? They can get up, work out, go to work, take care of the kids, keep a clean house, have a hobby, and still have time for a relationship? You, on the other hand, often find yourself exhausted before half your list of things to do is completed. If the thought of doing anything that requires more effort than finding your way to the couch at the end of the day is too much, and you don't know why, the first place I'd look is at the way you eat. You'd be surprised at how much more energy you'd gain with a new food plan, like my JumpStart.

Although a lack of food can make you weak, lightheaded, and irritable, too much food will always make you sleepy. Rich, heavy foods will leave you lethargic and in no mood to do anything but rest. The longer you remain in that state, the longer the things in your life will remain undone. Pretty soon the to-do list will get so big that it really will become impossible to complete, and your chronic tiredness could turn into depression.

Before this happens to you, take control and make up your mind to do something about it. The 21 Day JumpStart Plan is a perfect place to begin or rebegin. If you need more energy, try to follow this eating plan as closely as possible. It will take a little while for your body to realize the change. You can help it along with a little extra light exercise. Take a walk after dinner or as soon as you get home from work—no matter how tired you are—even if it's just for a short ten minutes. You will find that just 10 minutes will give you an energy boost . . . rev you up.

You may think sugar is a good way to get a quick burst of energy. But the rush from sugar is so fleeting that it won't do you much good unless you're feeling faint. The problem with eating sugar, other than the harm it does to your teeth and the unnecessary calories it adds, is that sugar brings your energy level up quickly and then drops it quickly, usually 20 minutes after you eat it. If you're not in a position to take advantage of that quick burst, sugar just makes you more tired. Don't kid yourself into thinking that a candy bar at three in the afternoon is going to give you the strength or put you in the mood to get things done after work. It won't.

At no other time should you avoid alcohol more than if you have a lot to do or you need a clear head. Regardless of how happy you become after a couple of drinks, alcohol is a depressant, make no mistake about *that*. It will make you tired and groggy but won't necessarily enhance your ability to sleep. A few drinks may have you drifting off sooner rather than later, but unfortunately, you could wake up feeling extra tired, queasy, and even more guilty for not accomplishing what you needed to get done.

Eating for energy means eating clean, eating regularly, and eating light. Forget alcohol, stay away from late-night snacking, and move, move, move! Within a short period of time, your days and nights will not only be filled but *fulfilled,* and your to-do list will be done!

Be Knowledgeable About Nutrition

In spite of the opposition lodged by food manufacturers, one of the greatest boons to the nutrition industry was the passage of the Food Labeling Law. Due to the diligent efforts of nutritionists and some consumer advocacy groups, all food products are now required to bear a standardized label entitled *Nutrition Facts.* The Nutrition Facts label lists the quantity of a serving, as well as the calorie content, the fat content in grams, and the percentage of total fat to total calories. It also clearly lists similar important information for those who must monitor cholesterol, sodium, carbohydrates, fiber, protein, and sugar, in addition to a general overview of vitamins and nutrients contained in the product. Another thing to consider is that the ingredients are listed in order on labels and that list is more accurate than the pictures companies might use that deceive the consumer.

The new labels make healthy eating much easier than it used to be! However, should you ever need to determine the percentage of fat within a food item yourself, the formula is quite simple. Each gram of fat has 9 calories. Multiply the number of fat grams by nine. Divide the total number of calories by the number of fat calories to get the total percentage of fat. Here is a quick example:

- 1 cup of Uncle Ben's Boil-In-Bag Rice contains 170 calories and .5 grams of fat.
- Multiply $.5 \times 9$ to get the fat calories, 4.5 (round it up to 5 if that is easier).
- 5 divided by 170 is equal to .0209 or 2 percent fat.

Obviously, the rice is well below 20 percent, so we can consider it a healthy low-fat food. Make your selection brown rice and you will not only get low-fat food, but one that is high in fiber as well.

Of your total caloric intake, 50 to 70 percent should come from complex carbohydrates (high-fiber cereals, vegetables, pasta and grains), and 15 to 20 percent from protein (preferably lean, such as skinless chicken, fish,

FOOD GUIDE PYRAMID
A Guide to Daily Food Choices

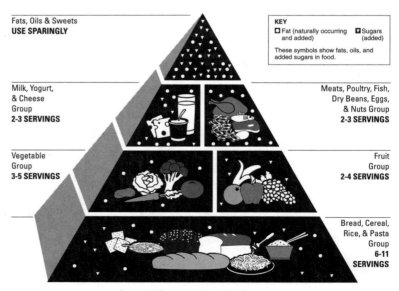

Fats, Oils & Sweets
USE SPARINGLY

KEY
□ Fat (naturally occurring and added)   ■ Sugars (added)
These symbols show fats, oils, and added sugars in food.

Milk, Yogurt, & Cheese Group
2-3 SERVINGS

Meats, Poultry, Fish, Dry Beans, Eggs, & Nuts Group
2-3 SERVINGS

Vegetable Group
3-5 SERVINGS

Fruit Group
2-4 SERVINGS

Bread, Cereal, Rice, & Pasta Group
6-11 SERVINGS

Source: U.S. Department of Agriculture &
U.S. Department of Health and Human Services

beef, and beans). I prefer not to calculate anything! These are just general figures to help you get a mental image of how to proportion your meals. A famous method of depicting a balanced diet is the Food and Drug Administration's Food Guide Pyramid. The pyramid is shaped like a triangle with all the complex carbohydrates located in the wide bottom. Right above complex carbohydrates are fruits and vegetables. Next highest are the meats and dairy products, with oils, fats, and sweets at the very narrow top. Notice that there is no food left off the pyramid. The FDA agrees that there is room in a healthy diet for all foods, it is simply a matter of proportion.

Good Health 101

"So complex carbohydrates, fruits and vegetables, proteins, fats are all important. But why?" Good question! Nutrition is one of those topics that we all should know more about. Knowledge is power, so I want to give you a general understanding of how your body uses these essential components for energy and good health.

Complex carbohydrates provide energy. They also have the secondary benefit of filling you up and curbing your appetite for fats and sweets. Complex carbs are high in fiber (which is good for your colon) and they take a while to digest. The two best types of carbohydrates to eat are: starchy (such as brown rice, oatmeal, beans, and legumes) and fibrous (such as broccoli, cauliflower, and spinach).

Protein is probably the single most important nutrient because it is a component of every cell in your body. Since our bodies are in essence just one mass of cells . . . I think you get the point. Protein is essential to the overall maintenance of a healthy body. It contributes to strong bones, teeth, hair, fingernails, cartilage, muscles, ligaments, tendons, skin, and other tissue, cells. . . . you name it! Protein helps you stay healthy because it is a source of antibodies which keep infections and viruses at bay. Protein is also the nutrient that the body uses to repair and rebuild muscle, a process that never stops. Your body requires more fuel to sustain a muscle. You need protein in order to build muscle, so protein becomes an essential component to burning fat.

Did you know that a new study has confirmed that patients who regularly consumed protein from soy products had significantly lower blood-cholesterol levels than patients who ate animal products? Try some tofu!

The Strive for Five campaign sponsored by the National Institutes of Health introduced the general public to the concept that eating healthily can also mean avoiding disease. Their research shows that the consumption of five servings of fruit and vegetables each day can actually prevent cancer. The key here is five servings. The average nutritionist's definition of *serving* is really much smaller than the quantities of food generally scooped onto a plate. One serving of broccoli (approximately ½ cup) is the equivalent of two fresh spears. I easily eat three times that at any one meal! Half a banana, a small apple, or a cup of salad also equals one serving. And broccoli is power-packed with anticancer nutrients: beta carotene, vitamin C, nitrogen compounds, and sulforaphane (this chemical raises the activity of enzymes which counters the effect of carcinogens.) Other vegetables containing sulforaphane include cauliflower, carrots, green onions, and brussels sprouts.

Celery has a nutrient called 3-n-butylphthalide which can help lower cholesterol and blood pressure. And, don't forget about garlic and onions (found in a multitude of my recipes). They have been found to have some beneficial effects in individuals with high blood pressure and cholesterol. As a matter of fact, some homeopaths consider garlic an effective preventative and treatment for a wide variety of ailments, possibly including slowing the growth of tumors. Strawberries and other fruits, which contain pectin (fruit fiber), have been proven to contribute to reduced cholesterol levels, as well as the prevention of colon cancer. And do not discount the value of fresh fruits and vegetables as a dietary source of fiber. A diet high in fiber seems to lower the health risk of colon, prostate, and breast cancer, too. So, strive for five servings every day.

The Bottom Line on Sodium

Cutting back on salt can help lower your blood pressure. However, avoiding salt can be tough because you can't always taste the sodium in the prepared foods we eat. So, to lower your salt intake, check labels for the lowest sodium contents. Try to avoid foods that have more than 480 mg of sodium per serving. Cut sodium to 2400 mg a day, and set a goal of 1800 mg a day.

One dill pickle spear can have as much as 440 mg of sodium. Check your labels!

Water Works!

Do not make the common mistake of waiting until you are thirsty to drink water. When you become aware that you are thirsty, your body has already gone into survival mode and is warning you of pending dehydration. By the time you become thirsty, your body has depleted its healthy fluid reserve level. And, on days when you are exercising and traveling (particularly on planes and/or when you go to a dryer climate), not to mention when you are sick, pregnant, or nursing, you lower your body's water level even more. If you are vomiting, running a fever, or suffering with diarrhea, you should particularly think water! Not only will you assist your body in flushing out impurities, but you will also be replenishing the liquids being lost at a pace more rapid than normal. Did you know water was your best defense against jet lag? I'm serious! Try drinking water instead of sodas or alcoholic beverages next time you fly. For every hour you fly, you should drink at least 1 glass of water. So, if you're on a 3-hour flight, you should have at least 3 glasses of water. See if you don't feel less tired and have a better ability to concentrate when you land.

The body uses fluid to flush itself of toxins. Toxins are literally poisonous byproducts derived from our body's digestive processes. Toxins are always present and, in a limited quantity, quite normal. However, when we go for long periods without adequate hydration, particularly when combined with eating less, the body is unable to expel toxic chemicals fast enough. Our organs become *polluted* (for lack of a better term) with poisons, and cannot perform efficiently. When your organs—the kidney, liver, and colon—become sluggish, so do you! One possible short-term side effect is constipation. Boy, will that one slow you down, in energy and in weight loss! Did you know that your colon can store 8 to 10 pounds of fecal matter? Your digestive tract needs fluid to help everything flow smoothly and function properly. In the most extreme cases, your body's inability to excrete toxins properly can lead to kidney stones and other serious illnesses.

Always drink a couple of glasses of water before you begin exercising. Consume another glass or so every 15 to 20 minutes during your workout. If you want to know why this is so important, just try your routine without replenishing your water reserves. You will notice that the routine feels harder, you are more lethargic, less motivated, and your mouth is distinctly dry. I promise you it will not be fun at all! When you exercise, you perspire. Even if you are not the type who completes a workout dripping wet, you are still sweating. Sometimes you may not be aware of the wetness because the wind or the lack of humidity causes it to evaporate very quickly. Perspiration is the component of your body's temperature control system that cools you down.

A recent trend has been to carry a bottle of water with you wherever you go. I think that's great because I have done that for years! Fill up a sport bottle, or some other plastic container that is convenient in size. Don't feel that you have to spend a fortune on bottled water either. Refill empty "designer" water bottles (whatever the brand) from the tap. Now, most tap water is carefully regulated and is very safe to drink. Keep a few cold bottles in the fridge so you'll always have some to take with you. I know that you will need to visit the rest room more frequently than normal. But that's okay, it will keep you moving more. So drink water! It'll give you energy!

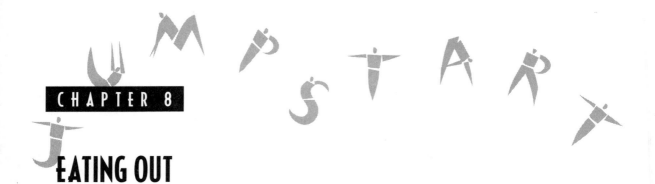

CHAPTER 8

EATING OUT

Dining Healthily in Restaurants

Dining out in a restaurant is, and should be, fun! But it does not mean that your new eating habits have to go out the window. Maintenance of your healthy standards can be achieved with a bit of initiative and wise choices from the menu. As a matter of fact, in response to consumer demand, many restaurants have added special icons to help their patrons identify low-fat, healthy entrees. If not, be sure to specify to your server how you want your food prepared. Do not allow yourself to be intimidated! Do not forget that these establishments are in business to serve *you*. They want you to be happy with your dining experience, satisfied with your food, and ready to return! Remember, take action to overcome obstacles!

Sometimes it helps to be *menu savvy*. A little advice can help you to avoid some unintended high-fat choices. For instance:

- Any type of grilled dish is great, but if your selection is chicken, request the skin be removed prior to cooking for the lowest fat possible. If you did not know the dish came with chicken in skin, go ahead and remove it at the table. You will still save yourself a lot of fat and calories.
- When a dish includes toppings of nuts, cheese, olives, bacon, or other items you know to be high-fat, ask that they be left off.
- If the entree you choose is in a sauce, you may wish to avoid some fat by asking that the chef "go lightly," or better yet request it be served on the side. That way you can control the amount of sauce on your meal.
- Always request salad dressing on the side. Try sticking only your fork tips into the dressing, then picking up the salad. You get the benefit of the taste at a fraction of the fat grams.

- Choose dry toast, plain or multi-grain rolls, or breadsticks instead of butter-drenched garlic toast and rich croissant dinner rolls.
- Order an appetizer, a broth-based soup, and a salad as opposed to a full meal. I assure you that you will not be hungry, and these items tend to have fewer hidden fats than many entrees.

Ethnic foods of all kinds are very popular and scrumptious to eat, but it can be confusing to identify ingredients with foreign names. Here is a brief list to help you navigate those international delicacies!

ITALIAN

What to Look for	What to Avoid
Lightly sautéed	Alfredo
Light red or white wine sauce	Parmigiana
Primavera	Stuffed or topped with cheese
Herbs and spices	Cream sauce
Lemon sauce	Fried

- Ask your server if you can have the appetizer-sized serving as your entree.
- Ask for salad dressing on the side.
- Have plain, dry bread with dinner rather than garlic bread or toast.

CHINESE

What to Look for	What to Avoid
Simmered	Fried or deep fried
Steamed	Crispy
Fresh fish fillets	Egg foo yong or egg noodles
Lobster sauce	Cashews or peanuts
Light wine sauce	Sweet-and-sour sauce

- Ask the chef not to use MSG.
- Try to skip the soy sauce if the low-sodium kind is not available.
- Substitute another entree for any stir-fry prepared with vegetable or peanut oil.
- No crispy fried noodles, please!

MEXICAN

What to Look for	What to Avoid
Grilled	Served/topped with sour cream
Marinated	Served/topped with guacamole
Picante sauce	Fried or deep fried
Shredded chicken	Stuffed/topped with cheese
Wrapped in or served on top of a tortilla	Black olives
Shredded lettuce, diced tomato, and onion	Layered with refried beans

- Have shredded chicken instead of shredded beef to avoid excess fat and calories.
- Ask the server to hold the sour cream and/or guacamole.
- Order soft corn tortillas on the side, and the salad without the fried tortilla shell.

CONTINENTAL OR AMERICAN

What to Look for	What to Avoid
Grilled	Fried or deep fried
Poached	Cream or creamy
Red sauce	Butter or buttery
Light wine sauce	Sour cream
Steamed vegetables	Sautéed vegetables

- Ask for fish that is grilled or poached: It is rich in flavor without the added fat or calories.
- Make a habit of asking for baked or roasted potatoes or rice, instead of french fries.
- Ask the chef to prepare the dish with a minimum amount of oil and salt.
- Try to choose natural ingredients.

Good Fast Food?!

Fast food has become a staple of the American diet. Our hectic schedules and the speed of modern life have made such quickie meals a matter of survival. (Not to mention that they serve the one thing that even the most finicky child will eat. . . . hamburgers and french fries!) I have been known to frequent McDonald's, Hardees, Burger King, you name it. Who doesn't in a family with children? And with my on-the-run lifestyle, sometimes a fast-food meal is the only meal available. It is not unheard of for me to ask the limousine driver who drives me back and forth from my appearances on QVC in Philadelphia to cruise past a drive-through window! With menus that for years have been full of fat and virtually fiber free, these restaurants seem to have finally recognized the need for at least one or two options which register on the good health meter. All it takes is knowing what to ask for in this fat-filled minefield, and you can enjoy a relatively low-fat meal.

- Many restaurants now offer grilled chicken sandwiches. Make sure the chicken on the sandwich is skinless, and order the sandwich minus any special sauce or mayonnaise. You can add your own zip with mustard, ketchup, relish, or barbecue sauce for one-quarter the fat and calories.
- Avoid batter-dipped or deep-fried chicken sandwiches. A regular hamburger has less fat and fewer calories. (I am talking about a regular hamburger here, not a Quarter Pounder!)
- Ask for a whole-wheat bun if there is a choice. It contains more fiber than white bread.
- Order a dry baked potato topped with low-calorie dressing, salsa, or other salad-bar ingredients.
- If they are available, pretzels are a good alternative to french fries.
- Salad bars are great, but stick to the fresh veggies and low-calorie dressing. The pasta and potato salad may look delicious, but they are laden with high-fat mayonnaise.
- Many fast-food restaurants now offer soup. Choose only those soups that are broth based, like chicken noodle and beef vegetable. Cream-based soups are tasty, but they are also fattening.
- When chicken is available, choose baked or roasted instead of fried. And always, always remove all skin, which contains three-quarters of the fat.
- When ordering pizza, consider trying it without the cheese. Pizza sauce, green peppers, onions, mushrooms (and any other veggie toppings) with a sprinkle of Parmesan has a great deal of flavor with a lot less fat.

Here are menus from some of my frequent fast-food haunts:

McDonald's	Chef salad with fat-free dressing and vanilla shake
	(460 calories, 10g fat)
	Single hamburger
	(255 calories, 9g fat)

	Chunky chicken salad (140 calories, 3g fat)
Burger King	BK broiler chicken sandwich (550 calories, 10g fat) BK broiler chicken garden salad (reduced-fat Italian dressing) (200 calories, 10g fat)
Wendy's	Small chili (370 calories, 6g fat) Grilled chicken sandwich (290 calories, 7g fat)
Roy Rogers	Roast beef sandwich with lettuce, tomato, pickles, onions, and mustard. Seven-ounce orange juice. (416 calories, 10g fat.)
Hardee's	Ham sub, side salad, fat-free dressing (390 calories, 7g fat) Apple (bring your own) Chicken 'n' pasta salad (1 tablespoon low-cal dressing) (239 calories, 4g fat)
Taco Bell	Light taco supreme (160 calories, 5g fat) Light chicken soft taco (180 calories, 5g fat) Light burrito supreme (350 calories, 8g fat) Light taco salad (without chips) (330 calories, 9g fat)
Arby's	Light roast chicken deluxe (276 calories, 7g fat) Light roast turkey deluxe (260 calories, 6g fat)
Subway	Turkey (6-inch) (308 calories, 9g fat) Ham and cheese (6-inch) (if you hold the cheese, it will be a lot less fattening) (322 calories, 9g fat)

Veggies and cheese (6-inch)
(272 calories, 9g fat)

Jack in the Box / Jack's   Chicken fajita pita
(292 calories, 8g fat)

Carl's Jr.   Barbecue chicken sandwich
(310 calories, 6g fat)
Junior hamburger
(200 calories, 8g fat)
Grilled chicken salad
(260 calories, 9g fat)

Domino's   12-inch cheese pizza (2 slices)
(360 calories, 10g fat)

Chick-Fil-A   Chargrilled chicken salad (lite Italian dressing)
(148 calories, 3.1g fat)

Boston Market   Turkey sandwich
(312 calories, 2g fat)
Chicken breast sandwich
(422 calories, 4g fat)
New potatoes
(129 calories, 3.5g fat)
Zucchini marinara
(89 calories, 3.9g fat)

Long John Silver's   Ocean chef salad with fat-free ranch dressing
(160 calories, 1g fat)

Popeye's   Spicy and mild tenders
(110 calories, 7g fat)
Mashed potatoes (no gravy)
(100 calories, 6g fat)

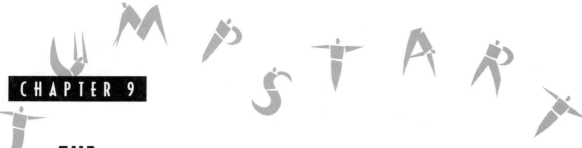

CHAPTER 9

THE PHYSICAL FACTS—GET MOVING!

Dear Denise,

For me, exercise was a four-letter word. I couldn't stand to be part of the conversation when my friends would bring it up. All they ever talked about was this video or that aerobics class. I thought it was such a bore, but that wasn't really it. I was ashamed because I had never tried exercise and I knew they knew it. I always thought they were trying to give me a hint, or something. Now I know what no one would ever think to hear me say, Exercise is fun!!! My friends weren't just saying that for my benefit. Thanks Denise, for all the giggles and inspiration.

—Darlene, Detroit, Michigan

wish that I could tell you that exercising and getting fit were easy. But you and I know that would be a lie. It isn't easy. To my knowledge, there are no miracle cures, but it isn't overwhelmingly difficult or complicated either. I can promise you that getting up and getting moving is the most important decision you can make to improve your overall health and quality of life!

First and foremost, exercise increases your metabolic rate and your body's ability to burn fat, which means that you will lose weight. Even more than that, exercise is the single best antidote to the stress of everyday life. It is known to stimulate the release of *endorphins,* a chemical in the brain that could be considered a natural antidepressant. All forms of exercise prompt you to use muscles in a different way from sedentary activity, which forces oxygen-rich blood to flow throughout the body, increasing alertness. The stretching and contracting of muscles and tendons which are normally held in the same positions for extended periods of time relieves stiffness and tension. Let's take a moment to understand why.

Total fitness requires dedication, fortitude, and planning. It also takes reliable information to be incorporated into your life as a regular habit. As you have started following the JumpStart Plan, many of you have added aerobic activity, toning and resistance exercises, and stretching to your weekly routine for the first time. I'll bet you are feeling firmer, stronger, and more energetic every day! I am confident that if you haven't already seen the beautiful things that are happening to your body, you will very soon!

Fitness Know-How

The 21 Day JumpStart Plan completely mapped out the basics of a sound fitness regimen so that you did not have to worry about any details initially. I supplied the structure needed in order to help you adapt to a new lifestyle. I am sure that as you began the 21 Days you barely had time to work exercise into your daily schedule, much less plan every single activity so that it was balanced and safe. But as the plan progressed, you became more knowledgeable and more confident about what felt right. Now we need to investigate the components of a balanced fitness program, why all this fitness stuff makes you feel better, and what is happening inside your body. This will not only help keep you dedicated to pursuing a healthy body, and motivate you when you feel frustrated or bored by results that seem too slow, but it will also free you to vary your plan and seek alternative forms of exercise.

Building a Fitness Plan

There are three basic components of a good fitness plan:

1. Aerobic exercise
2. Toning/resistance training
3. Flexibility

Each area is equally important to your overall goals for very different reasons. As a matter of fact, each component is so important that the next three chapters will be dedicated to explaining each of them thoroughly. In addition, I will include the answers to the five questions I get asked most frequently by my viewers.

A solid exercise program requires approximately 30 minutes a day. That is about the minimum amount of time it takes to complete even the most streamlined routine. You should do some form of aerobic exercise at least three times a week. The other two days should include some muscle conditioning and stretching. It's also great to incorporate an aerobic activity and toning in the same day. If you have only 30 minutes here is a perfect routine breakdown: 20 minutes of an aerobic activity, 9 minutes of toning, and 1 minute for stretching. Can this vary? Absolutely! Your program is whatever you can fit into your life consistently! Consistency is probably the most critical goal as you continue to pursue a fit body.

If your schedule is particularly hectic and you can spare only 10 minutes to walk around the block, 4 minutes for toning, and 1 minute to stretch, so be it! It is better to have done something than nothing. Then, on a day when you have more time, take more time. Walk for 30 minutes, use 10 minutes to tone, and 2 minutes to complete the Super Stretches Routine. It is more important to make it a regular part of your day than to beat yourself up over how long you spend at it.

Remember, this program is to make you feel better—don't allow your new eating-and-exercise program to increase your stress level, particularly during a hectic time. If that is the case, exercise will make you feel unhappy and burdened instead of better. It is better to do what you feel you *can* do, instead of persecuting yourself for not fitting another thing into an already overburdened schedule.

We all have time to exercise. The only difference is that some of us have to work harder to find the time than others. There are 168 total hours available in every week. Your week, my week, it doesn't matter. The same 168 hours are available to all of us. If you were to commit to a minimum of 20 minutes of exercise 3 days per week, the total time you would have exercised would be 1 hour! One hour is only one-half of one percent of your entire week! Commit to 30 minutes 3 days per week and you would have exercised one-and-one-half hours, which is still less than one percent of the time available to you. See? We are not talking about a major time commitment. Even if you exercised seven days per week, it would only add up to just over 10 percent of your time!

Number of Minutes	Days per Week	Total Hours	Percentage of Week
20	3	1	.5%
20	4	1.2	.7%
20	5	1.6	.9%
20	6	2	1.1%
20	7	2.3	1.3%

Just to be healthy and lose up to 1 pound per week	3 times a week of a 30-minute aerobic workout	
To look great in clothes and lose up to 2 pounds per week	4 times a week of a 30-minute aerobic workout. 2 times a week of a 15-minute muscle-toning workout.	
To be in perfect bikini shape	5 times a week of a 30–45-minute aerobic workout. 3 times a week of a 30-minute muscle-toning workout.	

Pick the Shape You

Want to Be In—

3 Fitness Categories

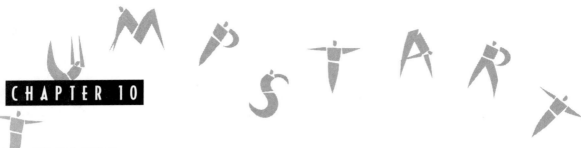

CHAPTER 10

IT TAKES HEART TO BURN FAT

Dear Denise,

My daughter and I have recently started to work out with you, and we enjoy your program a lot. We have ordered Tone-Up 1-2-3, many of your tapes, and some of your workout equipment. I have been recording your program every day. In just a short time, we have noticed an improvement in our body tone! We admire you and feel inspired by your enthusiasm. We have been working out with you since December 1994. You have changed our lives completely! At times, we do not feel like exercising but when you say, "Get up and exercise," we feel guilty if we stay seated. After exercising with you, we feel revived!! Your exercise program is the only one we follow. You are the greatest!!

—Steluta, Dania, Florida

To "Air" Is Human

Let's talk about the heart of the matter. Do you want to burn fat? Do you want to shed pounds? Of course you do! We all know how—regular exercise and a healthy low-fat diet. Let's explore why it works.

The benefits of regular aerobic exercise have been well documented. Aerobics is any activity maintained at a moderate intensity for at least 15 to 20 minutes, like walking, slow jogging, easy cycling or swimming. No one will argue the fact that some form of even the mildest exercise several times a week is a good idea for any relatively healthy individual. In addition to waking up that sleepy metabolism, which increases weight loss and fat burning, putting your body in motion results in improved circulation and a strengthened heart (and is one of the best preventatives against heart disease) and lungs. Exercise contributes to lower blood pressure, and raises HDL levels ("good" cholesterol).

Aerobic exercise contributes to your total fitness far beyond the benefits of weight loss, as it maximizes the spread of oxygen-rich blood throughout the body. When you move around for a period of time, your muscles demand more and more oxygenated blood from the heart and lungs. The heart and lungs have to work even harder than normal to keep pace with your activity. That is why your first walks, or other aerobic activities you engaged in initially, seemed so hard and left you exhausted! Your body was forced into overdrive to supply a requirement of oxygen and energy it was not accustomed to. Over time, however, being active became more comfortable. Now that you are capable of exercising for longer periods more frequently and with ease, I'll bet you even feel, dare I suggest, invigorated after a workout.

The brightness you experience following an aerobic activity comes from the inflow of oxygen throughout your system. That is why we call it *aerobics*—receiving *life* from *air*.

If there is an answer to any one question I would like to have taped to my forehead it would be "What is the minimum amount of time that I have to spend exercising to get benefits and burn fat?" The answer is 20 minutes! What has changed in recent times is that we used to think that you had to exercise aerobically for at least 20 *consecutive* minutes to realize any cardiovascular and fat-burning benefits. New research from the American College of Sports Medicine, however, seems to indicate that you can derive equal benefit from two ten-minute sessions in a 24-hour period as from one 20-minute workout. What does this mean to you? Fitting an effective aerobic routine into your hectic schedule is even easier. It is sometimes much easier to find 10 minutes here and there than 20!

All in all, I personally recommend you strive for 20 consecutive minutes at least three times per week, mostly because once you are in gear, you might as well just go for it. It is too easy to lose track of that second 10-minute workout in the rush of everyday activity. But keep the 10-minutes twice-a-day theory as a resource to use when life is simply too busy to enable you to afford that large a block of time.

Faster Is Not Better!

Now let's talk about anaerobic activity. Anaerobic activity is what many people mistakenly understand aerobics to be. You are anaerobic when you engage in sudden bursts of motion like sprinting as fast as you can, cycling at high speed, or doing rapid jumping jacks. These activities are performed at high speed and with a great deal of intensity. Usually an anaerobic activity will leave you breathless and unable to talk without gasping for air.

Why is this distinction important? Because when you try to use an anaerobic activity in place of an aerobic exercise, you are being counterproductive to your goal of improving the body's ability to burn fat. When you demand that your body perform at high intensity, your heart and lungs begin to work furiously to keep up with the need for oxygen. In addition, the overall priority in your system becomes utilizing the most readily available sources of fuel to keep you going.

Your body burns simple carbohydrates (sugars) first, since it can convert sugar into energy most quickly, then it takes the complex carbohydrates, the proteins, and, last of all, the fat. To be honest, you would be dead before you could keep up an anaerobic activity long enough to get to the fat-burning stage. It takes so much work for the body to convert fat to energy that when it is taxed by intense exercise, it will access every other resource first. When you exercise moderately, the body is not asked to perform at its maximum capacities and it takes an approach that will provide you with energy over an unknown length of time. Hence, exercising more slowly allows your body to tap into fat stores that can keep you going over the long haul.

The good news here is that we don't have to kill ourselves by engaging in high-intensity workouts. Slower is better for fat burning! When I go to the local gym, I never cease to be amazed at the intensity with which people ride exercise bikes and stair-climbing machines. They are literally dripping in sweat, and practically collapsed over the machines! The poor beginners watch these fools for torture and think that they should strive to be so fit and dedicated. Phooey! I know I get some surprised glances when I set my machine on levels one to three. But my goal is to burn fat (and not to be miserable while doing it). I choose to work out at a lower level of intensity, within my target heart range, over an extended period of time. Those high-intensity people may feel superior but, take my word for it, those of us who stay aerobic versus anaerobic will be more successful at the fat-burning game!

Confused? Read the Signs!

There are a couple of methods to test whether you are exercising anaerobically or aerobically. The first and easiest I call the *talk test*. The talk test is very simple. Can you talk while you are exercising? If you are with a friend, could you conduct a reasonable conversation without gasping for air? Now I don't mean slightly winded, since you should be taxing your cardiovascular system to some extent. I mean gasping or struggling to breathe. Any physical activity when sustained for any length of time will leave you a little winded! (For that matter, if you can talk without even being winded, it is time to push yourself a little harder.) Aerobic exercise, like managing your diet and your life, is all about balance and moderation.

A second, slightly more technical, way to determine if you are exercising aerobically or anaerobically is to check your heart rate by taking your pulse. As an added benefit, your heart rate can be a great tool to monitor your physical improvement beyond your measurements. Your heart rate indicates the intensity of your exercise by the number of times your heart beats per minute. The higher your heart rate, the more intense the activity. In order to determine the best intensity level for your body to maximize its ability to burn fat, you need to know how to find and count your pulse and how to calculate your *target zone*.

The target zone is 60 to 85 percent of your maximum heart rate (that is the greatest number of times your heart could possibly beat in one minute without you keeling over). The closer your heart rate is to the 60 to 65 percent range, the more fat you are burning. As the intensity increases to the 75 and 85 percent range, the fat burned begins to lessen, even though you are still exercising at a safe level for your heart.

Together, let's calculate your personal target zone:

1. Subtract your age from 220. The number you get is your estimated maximum heart rate.

   $220 - \text{age} = \text{maximum heart rate}$

2. Now, determine your aerobic training zone:

   Maximum heart rate $\times .60 = $ best for fat burning

   Maximum heart rate $\times .85 = $ less fat burned

   For example, since I am 38 years old, my formula would look like this: $220 - 38 = 182$.

   I would burn the most fat when my heart rate was closer to 100 beats per minute ($182 \times .60 = 109.2$ or 109).

   I would be getting closer and closer to anaerobic as I approached 155 beats per minute ($182 \times .85 = 154.7$ or 155).

Since my principal goal is burning fat, I would want to stay somewhere between 109 and 135 beats per minute. This may seem like a lot of work, but once it is done it's done. Your fat burning range does not change from day to day, only once a year—on your birthday!

In order to use this information, you need to know how to take your pulse. Two easy-to-find pulse points are at the side of your neck right below the jaw and on the underside of your wrist. Use your index and middle fingers, placing them in the position pictured.

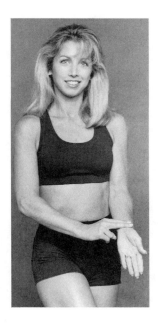

You should feel a slight thumping. That is your pulse. Your arteries thump every time the heart pumps. Get a watch with a second hand to keep with you when you work out. Count the beats of your pulse for 6 seconds. Add a zero to that number. For instance, when I am sitting still I can count 6 beats in 6 seconds. My resting heart rate is 60 (the average is about 75). Obviously, I am at rest and my body is functioning at a normal pace. If

I were exercising, however, it could easily double to 12 beats in 6 seconds—then I would be burning the maximum fat possible at a heart rate of 120. If I counted 13, 14, 15 or more beats per minute, I would slow down my routine by moving less quickly or reducing my arm motions.

The third and probably the best way to judge how hard your body is working is how you feel, or *rate of perceived exertion*. Can you breathe freely and without struggling? Are you experiencing any pain or cramping? Do you feel dizzy or faint? If so, slow down and then stop. Our goal is to enjoy the benefits of exercise, not endure misery. Listen to your body. If you are not feeling well on a particular day, do not force yourself. There is always tomorrow, and the next day, and the next.

The rate of perceived exertion can also be registered on a scale between 0 and 10, where 0 indicates no effort, and 10 the greatest effort without blacking out. To remain in the best fat-burning range, I recommend you stay somewhere between 3 and 5.

Rate of Perceived Exertion

0	No effort
1	Very little effort
2	A little effort
3	Moderate effort
4	Somewhat strong effort
5	Concentrated strong effort
6	Transition level into high intensity/anaerobic range
7	Very strong effort
8	Transition level out of safe target zone
9	Nearing maximum effort
10	Near exhaustion and collapse

Think F.I.T.

Thinking F.I.T. is the best rule of thumb I know to understanding and enjoying a trim healthy body for the rest of your life! F.I.T. stands for *F*requency + *I*ntensity + *T*ime. These three elements comprise the principal elements of an effective fat-burning aerobic program. Let me explain.

1. *Frequency* indicates the number of days per week you engage in an aerobic activity for some sustained period of time. The percentage of benefit to the metabolic rate, ability to burn fat, appearance of the body, and cardiovascular system is significantly increased by each additional day you exercise per week. Think of it this way: If one day of aerobic exercise per week is good, two is better, three terrific, and four

stupendous!! Just imagine how much you will accelerate the results in your measurements, your attitude, and your energy level every time you choose aerobic exercise!

2. *Intensity* refers to your heart rate during exercise. The intensity of aerobic exercise directly impacts whether or not your aerobic workouts are consistent with your overall fitness goals. We have already discussed how effective your heart rate can be as a monitor of whether your aerobic activity is burning fat or not. Exercising at too high an intensity level becomes, in essence, simply spinning your wheels if your goals are weight loss and fat reduction. Low intensity and slower workouts are what burn fat. I cannot emphasize this point enough. Please do not allow yourself to become frustrated by dedicating yourself to an exercise intensity level that will never allow you to be successful! Remember, slow and steady wins the race!

3. *Time* refers to the duration of each occasion you engage in an aerobic activity. Strive for a minimum of 20 minutes several times per week. If your schedule will not permit a workout of 20 consecutive minutes, break it down into two 10 minute sessions; maybe one in the morning and a second before or a little while after dinner. Every minute you engage in an aerobic activity burns calories, and the longer you pursue the activity at any given time, the more opportunity your body has to delve into your fat stores! So exercising longer means ridding your body of unwanted fat faster!!

Keep Moving the Whole Year Through

Varying your activity is very important. Selecting from a variety of aerobic activities not only alleviates boredom, it also creates options when for one reason or another you cannot participate in a particular activity. Personally, I work out differently depending upon the time of year. I think of my routines as seasonal. I choose my activities so I can take advantage of good weather when possible, and avoid the more inclement weather by staying indoors. There certainly is a wide variety to choose from.

Walking	Stair climbing (on a machine or the stairs at home)
Jogging	Stationary bike
Jogging in place	
Swimming	Cross-country skiing or simulated machines
Bike riding	Ice skating/sliding and similar winter activities
Hiking	Jumping rope
Rowing	Aerobic dancing (low or high impact aerobics)
Step aerobics	Roller skating/roller blading
	Aerobic riders

And that only scratches the surface!

Like many of you, I find too much of the same kind of exercise boring. I use all sorts of tricks to keep my mind occupied. As a matter of fact, it is not unusual to see me on my stationary bike with the phone in my hand! Often, I use my exercise time to solve problems. I will focus all my attention on a particular issue that is on my mind or bothering me, like upcoming negotiations with ESPN, some aspect of my career, or something as mundane as what I'm going to make for dinner. By the time 20 minutes have passed, I have usually reached a decision, conclusion, or plan of action. So I feel better physically *and* emotionally!

All About Walking

I'm going to talk a little about walking because I believe it was the best and fastest way I lost weight after both babies were born.

My cute little mom, who is seventy years old, walks for fitness. Walking has become America's favorite form of exercise. In fact, last year alone over 72 million people walked for fitness! Walking is one of the easiest ways for you to start exercising. After all, walking is a natural movement, and we do it without even thinking. Even if you haven't exercised in a long time, you can easily get started just by going for a walk. What's great is that there is no expensive equipment to buy, club to join or dues to pay. All you have to do is tie up those shoes (it helps if they are comfortable to begin with), and put one foot in front of the other. There is a difference, however, between walking for exercise and taking a stroll around the garden.

When we walk for exercise, there are several things to keep in mind. We must think about our posture, our legs, and our arms. In order to lose weight and inches in the most effective way, we must also consider how often, how fast, and how far. On average you burn about 100 calories per mile whether you walk or run.

Walking Form

When walking for exercise, keeping proper form is essential. Good form will allow you to walk longer and more comfortably, enabling you to *burn more calories.* Let's go through a quick check for proper body alignment. First, make sure that you are standing up nice and tall. Your head, shoulders, and hips should all be in line. By keeping your body up as straight as you can, you will enhance your body's ability to take in oxygen. Imagine how difficult it would be to breathe if your shoulders were hunched over! Second, pull in that tummy and make a conscientious effort to keep it tucked in—almost like you're being tickled. Third, as you walk, occasionally "squeeze" your buttocks for that extra benefit.

In walking for exercise, it is very important for you to use your arms.

Your arms should be bent at a 90-degree angle and your hands should be relaxed in a soft, fistlike position. When walking, you should swing your arm from the shoulder, keeping your elbow bent at the same angle the entire time. Always be sure to swing your arms from front to back, *not* across your body. Pumping your arms helps you build and maintain speed while at the same time burning more calories! The more muscles you use, the more calories you burn.

Finally, let's talk about your feet. They are, after all, the most important part of the walking picture. When you take a stride, your front heel should be the first thing to hit the ground. As your heel strikes and your momentum takes you forward, you roll forward, transferring your weight from your heel to your toes.

Walking Intensity

Now that we've talked about proper form, let's discuss intensity. *Intensity* can be defined as how fast, how long, and how often you should walk. Not everyone burns the same amount of calories performing the same exercise. This being the case, not everyone will walk at the same level of intensity. There are four major factors that determine the safest and most effective intensity level for you! They are: your age, your weight, your health, and your level of fitness.

One of the nicest things about walking for exercise is that you can adjust the intensity on your own. You can walk faster for speed, farther for distance, and longer for time.

You have a lot of flexibility in adjusting your walking program to fit your individual fitness needs. The one area, however, that is not flexible is that you *must* walk at least three days a week for the exercise to be most effective. I don't expect anyone to be able to just jump right into this or any other kind of exercise program so it's okay if you start gradually. Walk as often as you can at first, with the goal of working up to at least three days a week.

Research shows that the recommended speed for walking for the most effective results is 4 miles per hour. This means that you would walk 1 mile in 15 minutes at the rate of about 110–120 steps in a minute.

This may be a little quick for some people just starting a walking program so I recommend the following pace to begin with:

Starter Speed

3–3.5 miles per hour
1 mile in 18–20 minutes
90–100 steps per minute

When starting out, your minimum goal should be to walk for 20 minutes. Your ideal goal should be to walk 2 to 3 miles, 4 to 5 times a week.

Walking Tips

There are some things that you can do to make your walking program more effective from start to finish. I suggest you begin by finding a track to walk on. Most junior-high and high schools have tracks you can use. Walk on the track until you are comfortable with the feeling of walking a mile (usually 4 times around a standard-size track). When you begin your walking program, it's important to set a specific walking schedule. If you don't schedule it into your day, and assume that you'll do it at some point, chances are that you won't get it done. Schedule it into your daily list of things to do, just as you would an appointment. The third thing you can do to make your walking program easier to adjust to is wear comfortable walking shoes. Most companies make shoes specifically designed for walking that have great arch support and cushioned soles. You don't necessarily need special shoes but I suggest you wear something that is comfortable and gives you good support. Also, if you walk 3 days per week, your shoes will break down, so every 6 months you should buy a new pair for good shock absorption. Last, I suggest you take water with you when you walk. Water is vital in replacing essential fluids lost during exercise.

Healthy Parents, Healthy Kids

While you are building good habits, try to include your spouse and your children. Along with family outings and activities, Jeff and I encourage Katie and Kelly to share our more traditional workouts as well. We don't ask the girls to pump iron or anything like that! We just try to live the example that exercise can and should be an important part of everyday life.

My favorite aerobic activities are those I can do with my family and friends. Sometimes our only workout is going to the local park or a nearby pool to play with the girls. There are times you will see Jeff and I playing hopscotch, jumping rope, or hula-hooping with the girls. I'm sure some of the other parents probably think we are a bit crazy, but I think it is important for the girls to see that adults can run around, and laugh, too! Jeff and I often play tennis, while the girls go after the extra balls. And since Jeff is a far better tennis player, there is often a ball or two to chase on my side of the court! When I am in town, several of my girlfriends and I get together to walk and talk. Sometimes that is our only opportunity to get together.

I feel it is important that my children, and all children for that matter, learn to be active. Studies indicate that excess weight in young girls seems to accelerate the onset of puberty. Preliminary research shows that an early menstrual cycle seems to have some correlation with the incidence of breast cancer in later life. It seems that the percentage of fat cells being carried within the female body triggers the onset of the menstrual cycle. This makes sense because fat is a part of the maturing process, and is how flat and straight little girls achieve the curves of womanhood.

When very young girls are overweight, the body thinks that the extra weight means maturity, hence the reproductive cycle begins. The modern thinking is that we should help young children, and particularly preadolescents, keep body fat percentages to a healthy level in order to delay menstruation. Regular exercise, through play, dance classes, and sports is ideal for this purpose.

JUMPSTART

BOOST YOUR BURNING ABILITY: TONING, SCULPTING, SHAPING, FIRMING, AND A LITTLE BIT OF WEIGHTS

Muscle Burns Calories Even When You Sleep!

Dear Denise,

I always thought that since I wasn't fat, I was in shape. But I've learned, from having to go on disability for a bad back, that it isn't true at all. Being skinny and being fit aren't the same. My chiropractor recommended working out with you to help build up my strength. A lifetime without exercise had left me tired and weak. He said you were the best in your field. And he was right! When I heard that cheerful little girl with the sweet smile telling me (I assume it was me you were speaking to because I was just laying around on the couch at the time) to "get off my butt!" I had to laugh, but I did get off my butt. Now, I know what fun is! Keep up the good work.

—Cheryl, Cincinnati, Ohio

Who burns more calories in 24 hours? An aerobiciser or a weight lifter? If you guessed the weight lifter, you are absolutely correct! Weight lifters burn more calories in 24 hours because their bodies contain so much muscle that the metabolism works to burn fat and calories 24 hours a day. The bottom line is this: the more muscle you have, the more food you can eat!

You do not have to join a gym and become Ms. Universe to experience the same metabolic results. The exercises we began on the 21 Day Plan have started you well on your way. The key is consistency. Aerobics and challenging toning exercises must become a part of your weekly routine. I promise they will work. You have to promise to do them! Two little phrases I like to use are: If you don't use them, you will lose them! Or, if you rest, you rust!

During the early eighties, when I lectured to groups of women, I could feel the room recoil when I mentioned building muscle. Thank heaven some of the fear of weight-bearing exercise has been dispelled as fitness has increased in popularity. Weight-bearing exercise is truly the secret to burning the maximum fat day and night! Now, women realize that they cannot possibly amass the bulk of a man. Women's bodies just achieve firmness and definition.

Steady muscular exercise, whether from a sit-up or using a dumbbell, strengthens and firms the muscles, giving them a flatter, longer appearance. As the muscle strengthens, it becomes more compact, which demands that your metabolism produce more energy reserves. People find this hard to believe, but it really does take more calories for the body to maintain developed muscles. Your body struggles to keep up fuel supplies, which forces your metabolism to work at a faster pace. Not just when you exercise, but all the time—even in your sleep! Think about it: By building more muscle, or increasing your *lean mass,* as they say in the fitness world, you will require your metabolism to work for you 24 hours a day.

I often hear individuals complaining that they have lost a significant amount of weight, but their bodies still look the same—just a bit smaller. "I thought if I lost 20 pounds I would get rid of my . . . thunder thighs . . . pot belly . . . huge backside!" I am sure you can fill in the blank with your own problem area. Let me give you the answer to changing your body. Use some form of resistance-bearing exercise in order to strengthen and firm your muscles. Yes, weight lifting! I'm not talking about super-heavy weights or about hours in a gym. I'm referring to leg lifts, sit-ups, and biceps curls, using a soup can as resistance if that is all you happen to have. Just use those muscles! Work them! That is why I incorporated these types of exercises into the weekly plan.

When muscles are not used, they become a storage site for fat. As a matter of fact, they become "marbled" like cuts of beef. The more marbled your muscle, the shorter and rounder its shape. All of your other fat deposits (you know, the ones you can pinch around your waist and thighs) rest on top of the muscle. So now you have a short, round, soft muscle padded by another layer of mushy, jiggly fat. Ick! Dieting helps you to reduce the fatty padding, but does nothing to eliminate the marble in your muscle or change its soft, round shape.

Muscular, or toning, exercises increase the muscle mass while reducing the marbled fat. As a result your muscle becomes denser, or hard. That is why we use the term *firming up* in reference to isometric or stationary muscular exercises. The elimination of the marbled fat within the muscle causes the muscle to become leaner, providing a longer, sleeker appearance. Increased muscle mass combined with the flattening that comes

The only way you will ever change your shape is by developing muscle.

from fat reduction will eventually give you contours and curves that you never dreamed were possible.

Aside from just doing toning or resistance exercise, you need to do the exercises correctly. Proper form is as important to work the muscle most effectively as it is to avoid injury. Completing a set of exercises incorrectly can prevent you from isolating the right muscle group, and significantly reduce the benefits to your body. So, concentrate while you complete an exercise. Think about that muscle you are toning and imagine it getting firmer and sleeker with every repetition. Envision the contoured, fat-burning machine you are creating with every set. Really work it, in both directions! Concentrate as you tighten and slowly release for maximum benefit. If you are standing, do not ignore the rest of your body, which may not be directly involved in the exercise. Stand up straight, pull your tummy in, and maintain a solid stance with your shoulders down and your feet shoulder-width apart. And never lock your knees! Keep them slightly bent for added balance and blood flow. Remember, you are the architect. Create a physical structure that is balanced and strong.

Weighs More, But Looks Smaller

Please bear in mind that muscle weighs more than fat. But in the same vein, muscle development can do more to change your shape that any weight-loss program alone. That is why I emphasize using measurements to evaluate your progress over the bathroom scale. No matter what your scale is reading, just keep repeating to yourself that you are increasing your fat-burning potential while reshaping your body!

I see my friend Karen on a fairly regular basis. Karen had an extensive history as a yo-yo dieter, and overcame that problem by teaching herself good eating and exercise habits. She had been following a low-fat diet and regular aerobic program for over two years. During the first year, she lost some weight (she really did not have that much to lose—about 15 to 20 pounds—like most Americans) and during the second year was maintaining her weight quite effortlessly. But she was still dissatisfied.

Karen hated the doughy look of her physique, and was sure that 10 more pounds would make all the difference. But it would not come off. The reality was that at its present composition of lean muscle to fat, her body had found a set point at which it felt comfortable and it was refusing to give up another pound. I convinced her to try adding a weight program to her regular regimen. Not being one to do anything halfway, Karen joined a local gym. She chose to invest in a couple of sessions with a personal trainer to set up a routine. It cost about thirty-five dollars per hour, but as she explained to me, "It is worth the price of what I would spend on one dinner out to know that I am doing this correctly." She committed herself to three times per week, sometimes getting there as early as 6:00 A.M. to fit it into her busy schedule.

The results were dramatic. Not only did she lose that last bit of fat, but she transformed her appearance. (And the numbers on the scale barely changed!) I cannot emphasize the difference it made in Karen's mental attitude. As she says, "I am a new person. The body I thought I was cursed with is totally different. Not only that, I can eat like a normal person. I feel great about myself. I used to think that I was incapable of being attractive." Of course, that last comment is untrue. She was always attractive to the rest of us—the difference now is that she believes it too!

How Often Should I Do Muscle-Toning Exercises?

I recommend that you engage in some type of muscle toning exercises at least twice a week. In a perfect world, and to get a great body, do it 3 times per week. You can add these exercises on the same days that you exercise aerobically, or alternate muscle toning and aerobics.

How Much Weight Should I Use?

You should be able to complete a set of particular exercises without torturing your body, and yet it should feel difficult. Sometimes the weight of our bodies and the resistance of gravity make toning exercises difficult enough without added resistance! If your exercises become *too* easy it may be time to increase the intensity through weight. For instance, if you can complete a set of eight squats two times (or 16 total squats) without too much trouble, try the exercise the next time using soup cans or three-pound hand weights. Toning exercises should never be something you cruise through, but they should not be overwhelmingly painful either.

When Should I Increase the Amount of Weight I Use?

When you are able to complete all of the exercises in the program twice, with relative ease, it is time to think about increasing the intensity of the exercise. Gradual increases in weights are best. Suddenly adding a 10-pound dumbbell in each hand could surely injure you if you are not prepared for it. Go slowly. Start with soup cans if that is all you have. When you feel ready, purchase a set of hand-held weights. They are relatively inexpensive, but worth their weight in gold in results for you!

The Top Five Questions I Get Asked About Toning

How Many Repetitions Should I Do?

You should start by trying to complete 8 to 12 repetitions of every exercise. In the beginning, if you can only do five correctly, then five repetitions are fine. Gradually begin to increase the number as the exercise gets easier. If you can accomplish 20 in a row, twice, think about adding some weight next time. For abdominal, I recommend starting with 15 to 20 repetitions if you can. Once again, however, listen to your body. Do what you can, and increase from there. The most important thing to remember is that this is your program, so make it something you can stick with!!

What Is the Difference Between Muscular Strength and Muscular Endurance?

Muscular strength is the ability to lift a heavy weight one time, whereas muscular endurance is the ability to sustain activity in a muscle or muscles over a period of time. The exercises in this program are designed to help you develop muscular endurance while realizing some increase in strength.

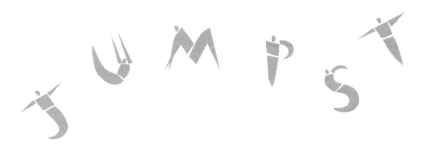

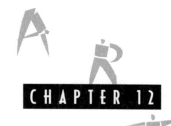

CHAPTER 12

HIT
THE SPOT!

Abdominals

Dear Denise,

I just wanted to thank you for your great stomach exercises. I have been doing them faithfully since the birth of my baby girl 1½ years ago. My stomach is flat and hard. I never thought I'd reach that goal again. You've been a great inspiration to me.

—Deborah, South Salem, New York

or every inch your waistline exceeds the size of your chest, you can deduct two years from your life expectancy.

Keep those abs fit . . . no other body part indicates a person's level of fitness as precisely as the centerpiece of the torso—the abs!

Your abdominals are an area of your body that you can and should try to work on every day. I start with abdominals because they are "the core"—the center of your body. These muscles are responsible for maintaining good posture and they protect most of your vital organs. Furthermore, the more fat around your middle, closest to your heart, the greater the chances of heart disease. The risk of colon cancer is twice as high in men who don't exercise, and having a large waist (more than 43 inches) also doubles the risk. Strong abdominals are a must! Don't be discouraged if you can only do a couple of reps the first few times you try these exercises. Most people find abdominal work very difficult for a couple of reasons. First, their abdominals and lower backs are in terrible shape. Second, the only movement that remotely mimics the ab crunch is getting out of bed. Most of us get out of bed only once a day so our muscles aren't trained to repeat that motion several times in a row.

> I spend only 3 to 4 minutes a day on my abdominals.
> —Denise Austin

291

Here are a few very important things you should know about doing abdominal exercises to make them as safe and effective as possible:

1. It is critical that you keep your lower back pressed firmly to the floor throughout the movement. Feel as though you are pressing your navel directly into your spine.
2. Never pull on your head during the movement. This can put unnecessary strain on your neck and upper back. Always *rest* your head in your hands and keep your chin up. I like to tell people to imagine an apple or orange under their chins. If you look too far up, it will fall out; look too far down and you'll squeeze the juice out of the orange.
3. I can't tell you how many times over the years people have confessed to me that they do tons of crunches but they still have tummies that stick out. Here's a little secret to guarantee that you get the greatest flattening effect from your crunches. When you are in the crunching phase of the exercise, it is *imperative* that you exhale! If you do your ab work with a diaphragm full of air, you'll build a hard tummy that actually sticks out. No kidding. Just making sure that you exhale as you come up with each rep that you do means the difference between a hard round tummy and a flat sexy tummy.
    1. Practice proper breathing during a sit-up right now.
    2. Lie on your back, bend your knees, and place your hands on your tummy.
    3. Inhale and slowly fill your diaphragm with air—your hands should be lifting as if your tummy is inflating a balloon.
    4. Now, slowly raise your head and shoulders (crunching) and exhale all the air—deflating, flattening your tummy—letting all the air out of that balloon . . . navel to spine, hollow . . . that's how you breathe during each sit-up (crunch).
    5. Slower is better when doing sit-ups—using the muscle, not momentum.
    6. Come only halfway up—once you go past a 45-degree angle you are no longer using your abs but perhaps straining your back.

You will want to work on the entire rectus abdominus—the muscle that runs vertically from the chest bone (sternum) all the way down to the pelvic bone. You should also zero in on the internal and external oblique muscles—the sides and front of your waistline.

Now you can choose to do all of the abdominal exercises that I showed you in the 21 Day Plan—from the basic crunch on Day 2 to the advanced bicycle on Day 16. This takes me only a few minutes a day for my "rock hard" tummy.

The most important part of doing abs is proper alignment. Don't cheat! When doing sit-ups, slower is always better.

When to see results: Do three of the ab exercises at least 4 days a week and you will see a noticeable improvement in 3 weeks.

Laugh, laugh hard—you're toning your tummy!

Hips and Thighs

Dear Denise,

I work out with you every day. In the past 3 months I have lost 20 pounds. I firmly believe that my weight loss is because of your low-fat diet and exercises. I am so excited about the inches I have lost around my hips and thighs. Thank you for being a great motivator and encourager.

—Tanya, Ft. Benning, Georgia

The hips and thighs are crucial areas for all women. It seems that we are more critical of these areas of our bodies than of any other. I don't know anyone who doesn't want shapely legs that are free of cellulite—and yes, all cellulite is plain old fat that dimples from lack of muscle tone! Of course, genetics play a role in the shape of this region (about 50 percent) but you can tighten, tone, and shape your legs, and in particular your inner and outer thighs, to achieve a great-looking lower body!

Keep in mind that your legs are the largest muscle group in your body so it will take a little more work to see results. This doesn't mean you have to knock yourself out—a nice, concentrated effort is all you need to get lean legs!

I recommend that you look through the Tuesday and Thursday pages of the 21 Day Plan for great hip and thigh exercises. Try to complete 4 thigh exercises, at least 4 times a week, and you'll see results in a matter of 3 weeks. I like to do at least 1 exercise for the outer thighs, 1 for the inner thighs, and then a couple that really target the hips and the entire thigh, like the lunge or squat. It takes only a few minutes. . . . Go for it! You'll have "hot legs."

Buns

Dear Denise,

I have really enjoyed your exercises for the hips, thighs, and buttocks. I have found they truly work. I used to spend many days seeing the doctor for lower back pain, but your exercises have strengthened my back, keeping me out of the doctor's office. You have been a lifesaver for my back as well as for my well-being, and I look better in pants. Thank you! Thank you!

—Myra, Perris, California

"Squeeze your buttocks—anywhere, anytime—turn that idle time into exercise time."

Get a great "rear view" with these easy exercises that give your buttock muscles—your glutes—a lift! No more sagging rears, because if your muscles are out of shape, gravity will make them droop.

Do you want to look great from behind and feel sexy in jeans? Then try a few of the effective exercises for the best BUN workout ever. . . . Make the most of your bottom!

I recommend the toning routines on pp. 213, 214, 222, 227, 228, 230, 231, 232, 235, 236, and 241. To see results, pick at least three of your favorite bun exercises, do them 4 days a week and you'll see a noticeable improvement in just 3 weeks. It will take you only a few minutes and you will have a fabulous derriere. . . . A tight tush!

Upper Body

Dear Denise,

I have always been a physically active person. My favorite exercise is running. My problem, though, has always been my upper body. Even though my legs and hips are quite toned, I tend to have the most flab on my arms and back. Your upper body toning excercises have been a lifesaver! Now that I spend about 15 minutes on them after my runs, I have a whole new body. No more flabby underarms or rolls on my back! Now I don't hesitate to wear a backless sundress. Thanks a million!

—Schuyler, Louisville, Kentucky

Do you want to get rid of saggy arms and bra overhang? Do you want to develop and firm your chest muscles to achieve an uplifted breast and sexy shoulders? All it takes is a few of these upper body exercises to have a firmer, younger, more feminine figure, regardless of age.

Beautiful Back

A well-developed back makes an incredible difference in your overall appearance. The development of your back determines the posture of your body, and a stronger back will keep your shoulders from slumping.

As you work out your back, and it begins to take shape, you will notice that your waist will look smaller, and so will your hips and buttocks! Because your back supports your shoulders, you will see that you look better in all of your clothes.

Try One-Arm Rows and Upright Rows on pp. 211, 225, and 242, and the Upper-Back Firmer on p. 219.

Great Arms

You can wear baggy pants to hide your fanny and thighs and even wear black all the time to look thinner, but one of the most visible parts of your body every day is your arms. All the upper body exercises I have shown you also benefit your arms a little. It is important, however, that you do some exercises specifically for your arms. I'm sure that we all had a teacher in elementary school who had flabby arms that would jiggle every time she wrote on the chalkboard. Yuk! Granted, you'll have to do some cardio to get rid of the majority of fat on your arms, but by doing these few simple exercises, you can make a *huge* difference in the look and shape of your arms. These exercises can be performed *anywhere*. I sometimes do my arm exercises while I dry my hair in the morning and when I make lunch for Kelly and Katie. And you can do your arm exercises using *anything!* You don't necessarily need to use hand weights. You can use your hairdryer, a can of soup, your briefcase, or even your kids. With all of these options, you really have no excuse not to do these exercises!

Try the Biceps Curl on Day 2 (p. 203) and the Triceps Toner on Day 4 (p. 210).

Sexy Shoulders

Weak and sloping shoulders can make you look tired. By developing these muscles you can create a wonderful appearance of youth, energy, and self-confidence.

Your shoulders are a very important part of your body. Think about all the clothes that you own that have shoulder pads. By doing these exercises you won't have to depend on shoulder pads any longer! By developing strong, sexy shoulders, you will have that shapely look no matter what you wear.

You should aim for 8 to 12 reps of each exercise. As soon as you complete this with relative ease, add a second set of each exercise.

Let's try this quick lesson to understand exactly how your shoulder girdle moves and works. Try rounding your shoulders forward and then squeeze them back; next, lift them up toward the ears, and then press them back down.

Try Overhead Presses from Day 9 (p.218) and Lateral Side Raises from Day 4 (p. 209).

Chest

Your chest is an important part of your body to exercise because it generally receives so much attention. The muscles of your chest lift and give shape to your breasts, and a properly developed chest will enhance your firm and feminine figure.

Women always ask me if working out the muscles of the chest will make their breasts disappear. *No way!* When you work these muscles, you will develop an attractive line of cleavage regardless of the size of your breasts. Furthermore, firm muscles underneath your breasts will help to counter the downward pull of gravity and help to form firm, uplifted breasts that might otherwise start to sag as time and age take their toll.

Aim for 8 to 12 repetitions of the exercises every time you do them. As soon as you can do this relatively easily, add a second set of each exercise.

Try the Chest Flys and Pec Presses on Day 2 of the 21 Day Plan (pp. 200 and 201).

How Often?

I recommend you do at least 4 different exercises 3 days a week . . . it will take only 5 minutes. To get the best contours, incorporate a variety into your routine: include an exercise for the upper back, one for the arms, one for the shoulders, and one for the chest.

About Weights

Dumbbells are great tools for training the upper body; they're convenient and effective and they let you work through a complete range of motion. To see results you should do all these exercises with weights (except tricep dips on chair). It is the quickest way to see true definition in the muscles. Begin using soup cans or 3-pound hand weights . . . dumbbells.

When Do I Increase the Amount of Weight?

Toning exercises should never be something you cruise through, but they should not be overwhelmingly painful either. When you are able to complete all of the exercises in the program twice, with relative ease, it is time to think about increasing the intensity of the exercise. Gradual increases in weights are best. Suddenly adding a 10-pound dumbbell in each hand could surely injure you if you are not prepared for it. Go slowly. Start with soup cans if that is all you have. When you feel ready, purchase a set of hand-held weights. They are relatively inexpensive, but worth their weight in gold as far as results for you!

How Many Reps?

You should aim for 8 to 12 repetitions of each exercise. As soon as you can complete this with relative ease, add a second set of each exercise. I personally use 5-pound weights in each hand and do 2 sets (16 to 24 reps).

Almost 80 percent of all Americans will, at some point in their lives, suffer from debilitating back pain. In fact, estimates indicate that approximately six-and-a-half-million people are incapacitated on any given day. The United States Health Service estimates that back impairment is the most frequent cause of activity limitation in Americans under the age of forty, as well as the third most prevalent disabling condition in over-forty Americans. Back pain, however, is a malady mostly within our control. In other words, back pain is often preventable.

Back pain is a disorder that reflects our living habits, mostly a muscular response to overload. Realizing and understanding this will put you in control and allow *you* to help your back. Although experts theorize that 80 percent of back problems are degenerative in nature, stemming from misuse (poor lifting technique) or lack of use, a number of factors can also contribute to back pain.

1. *Weak Abdominal Muscles*—Weak abdominal muscles are the result of improper exercise. Without strong "tummy" muscles, the muscles of your lower back have to work double duty to keep your body upright.
2. *Tight Hamstring Muscles*—Tight hamstrings, the muscles in the backs of the thighs, can trigger back pain by pulling on the pelvis, which in turn pulls on the lower spine.
3. *Weak Back Muscles*—Muscles not exercised will deteriorate; therefore, weak and unexercised back muscles will provide inferior support of the spine.
4. *Emotional Stress/Chronic Fatigue*—Many experts believe that stress is the single most important factor contributing to back pain. The spinal musculature is overstressed by chronic emotional fatigue. Relaxation techniques and proper coping mechanisms can be implemented when fatigue is the cause of back pain.
5. *Overweight*—Poor nutrition and lack of exercise contribute to excessive abdominal weight. The more weight you have in your stomach, the more stress it puts on your back.

Try to do a few exercises every day to prevent any back problems in the future. Do 1 minute's worth of sit-ups (Day 2, pp. 202 and 203), the Back Extension on Day 11 (p. 228), and the Hamstring Stretch from Super Stretches on p. 192.

Too often, in our zeal for a leaner fit body we overlook the component of fitness that provides our best insurance against injury. No, it is not

Your Spine Is Your Life Line: Keep It Strong!

Flexibility: Too Important to Forget

sitting still! It is *flexibility training!* Understanding of the importance of flexibility training, or stretching, has greatly increased over the past twenty years in the fitness industry.

Every fitness expert used to encourage you to begin your routine with "static stretching." You know, the whole "Can you touch your toes?" thing. It was called warming up! Today we know better. A warm-up should involve the entire body in slow movements. Warming up means exactly that. You should literally feel slightly warmer as the oxygen and blood flow freely to all your extremities, whether you walk slowly before you jog or you march in place before you jump on your bike and ride off.

Stretching is wise only following exercise. After exercise our muscles are very warm and more pliable. To understand this concept, think of a rubber band, which is very elastic when it is warm. You can stretch it to double or triple its size before it will break. A cold rubber band, on the other hand, is quite stiff and can easily snap in two when it is stretched.

Now imagine your muscles. After exercise they are very warm and prepared for slow, steady, and gentle pressure (forget bouncing!) which will expand and lengthen the muscle group. Try the same stretch on a cold muscle group and you risk damaging a tendon, ligament, or the muscle itself. A cold muscle will "snap" like the cold rubber band much more readily than the warm one. Believe me, that will not only hurt when you do it, but also for several weeks afterward. An injured muscle can really put a damper on your entire fitness plan.

After exercise, stretching can feel great, particularly if exercise is new to you and causing some stiffness. Use the stretching exercises I have taught you as part of the 21 Day Plan after every workout. I promise that a good stretch following exercise will help you feel a lot less achy! Stretching restores the free flow of blood and oxygen to the muscle following tension, whether that tension comes from activity like toning exercises or stress at your desk. Stretching can help release the aches that come from "uptight" muscles.

If You Don't Use It, You Will Lose It!

Flexibility increases in importance as we age. Remember my saying "If you don't use it, you will lose it?" It is never more true than when in reference to regular stretching. One of my friends is a personal trainer at a local country club in our area. She trains several mature adults whose ages range between sixty-five and eighty-five. (You are never too old to become fit!) She confided in me one day that for all of her education regarding the importance of stretching and flexibility to overall fitness, she had never truly known why until she began training older clients.

To illustrate what she meant, she related to me the story of a gentleman who had spent his entire career as a dentist. Dentists do most of their work hunched over a patient with their arms in front of their bodies. As a result, over the course of his lifetime, he rarely had a need to raise his arms above his head. The bottom line was that now, as a senior citizen, he was unable to lift his arms higher than his cheeks! Due to lost flexibility in his shoulders he could no longer reach above his head to change a light bulb. The good news is that you can always reestablish flexibility if you work at it regularly. Fairly soon after starting his program, to his wife's delight, he changed his first light bulb in fifteen years! See how important this is?

I mentioned earlier that flexibility is important in preventing injury. And it is. Flexibility training will not only help you avoid injury while you are exercising, but also when you are not. For instance, the winter of 1994 in Washington, D.C., was unusually cold. We were experiencing sub-zero temperatures in the minus teens combined with a great deal of precipitation. Those of you from way up north know what that means . . . *ice!* And being a region of the country unused to the harshness of winter, the D.C. area was hardly prepared! There was simply not enough sand and salt to melt the quantities that fell. It was treacherous!

I cannot tell you how many times I slipped trying to get to my car, the grocery store, or even just up our driveway. You know what? I did not get seriously injured (except for a few bruises—and a bit of embarrassment) in any of my spills. Some people said I was lucky. But I know that it was because my body was flexible enough to handle my legs sliding out from under me in two directions. Fortunately, I stretch as a regular part of my workout routine. My muscles were long and loose. Had I ignored this component of my overall program, I could have easily snapped a tendon or torn a ligament in any one of my mishaps.

Could I have injured myself in spite of my flexibility? Sure. Some accidents are too violent, or pull too hard on a muscle, and it has no choice but to tear. But at least I have a little assurance that my muscles will give me the maximum leeway, whatever the instance.

Invest in your own insurance against injury—STRETCH THOSE MUSCLES! Unless you are already flexible, stretching isn't going to be an easy task. In some cases it will be downright painful. Don't you worry, with continual stretching you will notice a marked improvement . . . and much less pain!

When you initiate a stretch, it's important that you stretch the muscle to the point of slight discomfort. As you hold the stretch for a couple of seconds, this initial feeling of discomfort will dissipate and it will become easier to do it the second time. (Yes, you'll have to do this more than once.) I recommend that you hold each stretch for a minimum of 6 seconds. This allows sufficient time for the "stretch reflex" to take effect, an involuntary muscle contraction that prevents you from overstretching. After about 6 seconds, an "inverse stretch reflex" occurs, and it is at this point that the muscle actually starts to lengthen. So don't cut your stretch short because it is uncomfortable or you won't realize the full benefit of the movement.

There are two other crucial pointers I want to share with you. First, you should *never* stretch a cold muscle. Get up and move around a bit and warm up your muscles *before* you start to stretch. This will increase the blood flow to your muscles and raise the core temperature of your body, making it much easier to stretch. The easiest way to warm up is simply to walk around a little, or march in place, or climb steps, all of these for at least 3 minutes.

Second, be careful when you do any type of stretching that you don't bounce or have a jerky movement. Bouncing while you stretch (also called ballistic stretching) can actually damage the very muscle you are trying to improve by causing microscopic tears. When you stretch you should be very relaxed as you ease into the movement (also known as "static" stretching).

For some stretches to incorporate into a daily routine, see p. 188. If you are going to do your other exercises on the same day, perform these stretches after you have completed your workout. It really doesn't take very long to stretch your muscles and become more flexible. If you spend only 5 minutes a day going through these stretches, you will become more limber, you will move better, and you will be less prone to injury. Always wear comfortable clothes while stretching. It doesn't matter whether you have shoes on or off . . . whatever is most comfortable for you.

How Often Should I Stretch?

I personally believe that 5 minutes of stretching every day is insurance against the likelihood of injury and aches and pains from stored tension in the muscles. If this is impossible, make sure that you stretch at least for 1 minute following your workout. It is important to re-lengthen all muscles that were working so hard to contract.

Will Stretching Improve My Flexibility?

Absolutely! When you stretch, as I have demonstrated, you will notice substantial increases in your flexibility. It is never too late, and you are never too old. Stretching will keep your body supple and ready for movement.

Why Is Stretching So Important?

When you increase your flexibility you also boost joint lubrication, which makes it easier to move your limbs through their full range of motion. There is the added bonus of releasing tension and making your body less prone to injury.

Should It Hurt When I Stretch?

No! Stretch to where you feel the "pull," but not to the point of pain. Good common sense is the best rule to follow: If something is very painful . . . stop. But do take the time to stretch properly. Never bounce. Instead, apply steady pressure for at least 20 seconds. And this may sound silly, but don't forget to breathe. Holding your breath contributes to nothing but unconsciousness.

If I Don't Have Time to Go Through All of the Stretches You Show, What are the Best One or Two to Do?

This answer really depends upon the individual. If you had to pick only two or three stretches, choose the ones that concentrate on your least flexible body parts. I always like to do one stretch for my thighs, like the Quad Stretch on p. 191 or Hamstring Stretch on p. 192; one for the back, like the Lower Back Stretch on p. 191; and also one for the upper body, like the Triceps Stretch on p. 193.

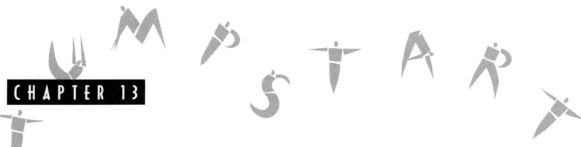

CHAPTER 13

A DAY WITH DENISE: IN-A-HURRY EXERCISES YOU ALWAYS HAVE TIME FOR!

Turn idle time into exercise time!

This chapter will solve your number-one problem. Right here and now, I am going to debunk every excuse you have ever come up with to avoid fitting exercise into your day! I am here to tell you that I have heard them all: from pets pooping in shoes to "I can't afford it." I firmly believe that there is time to exercise in a day that appears to have not a second to spare. You simply cannot tell me that you do not even have time to stretch in the morning. Yes, stretch. Elongate your spine and swing your arms over your head. Reach for the ceiling while you inhale deeply. This is a marvelous way to wake up and get that circulation going. And how many of you are so busy that you cannot at least take a moment to wash your face and brush your teeth? Not many, I am sure. Why not add a few hamstring curls and rear leg lifts to that wash-up, brush-up time? And what about a squat or two while blowing and styling your hair? See what I mean? Before you even leave the house on a day with no time you have completed four or five exercises. And that is only the beginning!

I am going to walk you through my own busy day to illustrate how I often incorporate 20 minutes of exercise without ever putting on my workout clothes! As we discussed in chapter 9, the American College of Sports Medicine notes that individuals can significantly improve the strength and tone of their muscles by simply working out 20 minutes per day. (We'll sneak some aerobic activity in there too!) The 20 minutes does not have to be consecutive. So, why not spread your workout over 16 hours! The truth is that you really can improve your overall fitness, increase energy, tone your muscles, and flatten your stomach throughout even the busiest day while on the telephone, in line at the bank, driving, cooking, and doing the dishes.

Once again, if you can manage to complete a 30-minute workout that includes 20 minutes of aerobic exercise a couple of times per week, that is the fastest and most effective method. But since we do not live in a perfect world, use this routine to supplement those days when even the most organized schedule goes awry!

JUMPSTART

IN-A-HURRY EXERCISES

All exercise is preventative medicine. These common sense, do-it-yourself, anytime, anywhere exercises are like getting extra interest on your savings. They set off a chain reaction that revs up circulation and stimulates your energy levels! The instantaneous benefit is release of tension.

You can do these exercises throughout your day. They each take only one minute to perform. You don't have to change your clothes and don't worry, you won't break out in a sweat—these in-a-hurry exercises are designed to stretch and tone your muscles. (As I am writing this, I'm tucking in my tummy.)

These exercises will become a part of your life: You'll start stretching your hamstrings. You'll start toning your thighs—automatically, easily—while you're doing something else.

IN THE BATHROOM

TUSH AND THIGH TONER

Did you know you should brush your teeth for at least 2 minutes? Here's a great exercise to tone and tighten your buttocks and the backs of your upper thighs! You'll have white shiny teeth and nice buns!

1. Extend your leg out behind you.
2. Bend your knee with your heel lifting toward your buttocks.
3. Continue for one full minute.
4. Switch legs and repeat.

Benefits: Firms the back of the thighs.

LEG SQUATS

This is one of my favorites. The squat is the best thigh exercise you can do. It is the fastest way to firm up your thighs.

1. Slowly bend your knees halfway down and back up.
2. Continue doing them until your hair is done!

Benefits: Tones thighs.

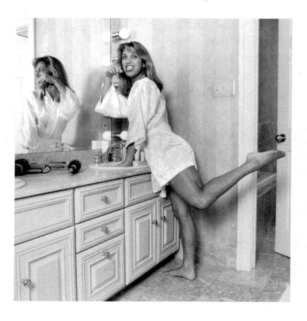
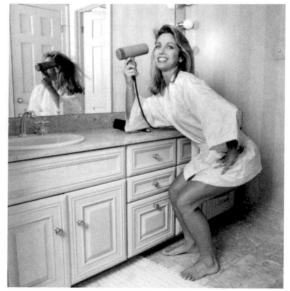

IN THE BATHROOM

TOWEL STRETCH

You can use your towel for more than just drying off. . . . Why not improve your posture, rejuvenate your spine, and work your waistline . . . all before hopping into the shower.

1. Grasp a towel and extend arms overhead.
2. Bend and stretch side to side.

Benefits: Stretches arms, chest, shoulders, and sides of waistline.

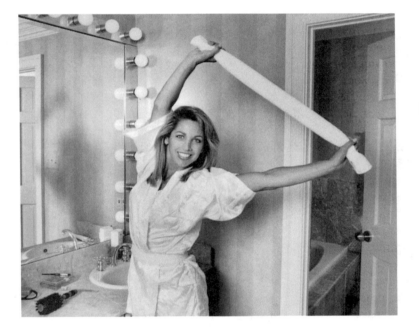

BUN FIRMER

If you spend 1 minute or 15 minutes putting on your make-up, then you have time to firm your buns! This is an easy exercise that "lifts" your derriere, preventing your rear from drooping. Look great from behind. . . .

1. Slowly lift and extend your leg straight behind you.
2. Squeeze your buttocks; hold 10 seconds.
3. Switch legs and repeat.

Benefits: Lifts and firms the buttocks.

IN THE KITCHEN

SADDLEBAG SLIMMER

Even if you're slender everywhere else, those curves in the outer thighs can collect fat. Fortunately, those saddlebags can be unpacked.

One of the best ways of trimming them is the side leg lift. You can do it standing just about anyplace—behind a counter, at a desk, while pumping gas, waiting in a grocery checkout line, diapering the baby.

1. Stand up tall, lift your right leg out to the side a few feet, and pull it back in.
2. Complete 15 repetitions of lift and lower with right leg.
3. Repeat with left leg.

Benefits: Toning your outer thighs.

INNER THIGH FIRMER

To get rid of bumps, lumps, and bulges and to develop sexy and shapely thighs, try this inner-thigh tightener. No more jiggly inner thighs! Firm it up while making dinner.

1. Stand up tall, pull your right leg in front and cross over the front of your left leg, gently squeezing your inner thighs.
2. Return to starting position. Do 15 repetitions.
3. Switch legs and repeat.

Benefits: Firming your inner thighs.

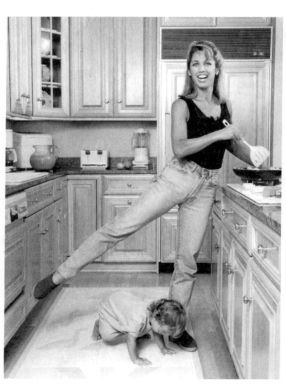 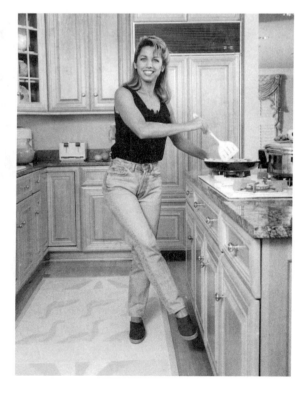

IN THE KITCHEN

BUN BLASTER

Many women complain that their bodies are pear shaped. That's because women tend to store fat in their buttocks and upper legs. You can give your derriere a pick-me-up even while you're cooking, ironing, or loading the dishwasher.

1. Stand straight.
2. Lift your right leg straight out behind you, only a couple of inches off the floor. Point your toes.
3. Squeeze your buttocks tight and feel the muscles tense and work. Keep your hips facing straight ahead; don't slouch.
4. Return your foot to the floor.
5. Lift and squeeze and lower 20 times.
6. Relax.
7. Switch legs and repeat.

Benefits: Tones and tightens the back of your thighs and your buttocks.

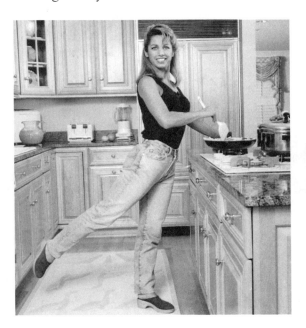

LEG STRETCH

I've been known to do this stretch in the most unusual places—my legs parallel to the floor of the plane when I travel, my feet propped one at a time on the bathroom sink while drying my hair. I've even plopped them on the kitchen counter while rinsing dishes. Remember what I said . . . any time and anywhere! Stretching your hamstrings will alleviate lower back pain and stiffness.

1. Stand in front of a stable, waist-high fixture such as a table.
2. Raise your left heel slowly and brace it on the edge.
3. Keeping both legs as straight as possible, hold the stretch for 10–15 seconds.
4. Lower your leg and repeat the stretch with your right leg.

Benefits: Increases flexibility in back of thighs (hamstrings).

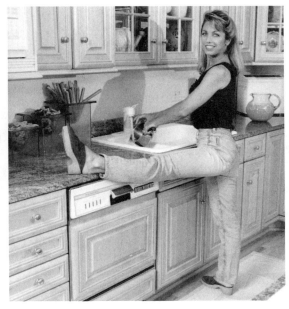

TENSION TAMERS FOR THE OFFICE

Did you know the average person sits for over seven-and-a-half hours a day? One of the toughest physical challenges our bodies can face is sitting all day. Standing is a more natural posture; sitting increases the pressure on your lower back by 40 percent and if you hunch over while sitting, the pressure is increased by about 80 percent. Plus, sitting disrupts the circulation between the upper and the lower body. That's the reason why people in desk jobs often experience neck and back pain. The best tip I can give you is to take breaks by standing up, walking around, and doing some of the following stretches. You'll get more energy from stretching tight muscles than from gulping coffee!

NECK RELAXER

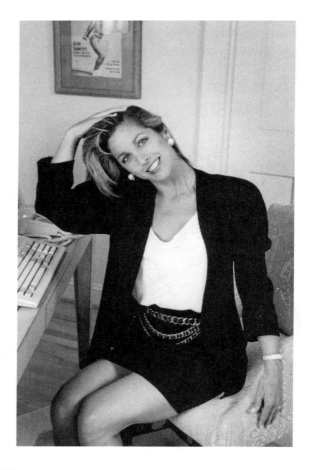

To ward off fatigue and release built-up tension in your neck, here's a great stretch to do whenever you feel a knot in your neck.

1. Sit up straight, with your shoulders relaxed and your neck extended.
2. Lower your left ear slowly to your left shoulder. Hold for 15 seconds.
3. Roll your head to the right and hold your right ear to your right shoulder for 15 seconds.
4. Roll your head to the center. Touch your chin to your chest for 15 seconds.
5. Keeping your chin to your chest, rock your head slowly to the left, then to the right, semicircle continuously for 15 seconds. Be sure to keep your neck long throughout the entire exercise. Relax.

Note: Never jerk your head or roll it backward or in a full circle. Such movements can compress the top two vertebrae and cause injury.

Benefits: Keeps your neck from getting stiff, relaxes a stiff neck and aching head.

TENSION TAMERS FOR THE OFFICE

SHOULDER ROLLS

A few hours of inactivity can make your shoulders ache. Tension collects behind your neck and at the points your arms join the trunk of your body. You can feel like Atlas carrying the world on your shoulders. The best relief is an exercise that decreases muscle tension.

1. Lift your shoulders to your ears. Inhale. Lower your shoulders and exhale. Repeat.
2. Roll your shoulders up and back 5 times.
3. Roll your shoulders up and forward 5 times.
4. Execute 3 sets of shoulder rolls, backward and forward.

Benefits: Releases tension and reduces stiffness in your neck and shoulders.

NO MORE SLOUCHING

Bad posture habits are the culprit behind tense-tight shoulders and neck. To relieve stress, you've got to relax those muscles. Here's a great stretch to open up the chest to improve your posture. About 60 percent of women slouch, a problem that can cause neck and shoulder pain and even reduce your energy level.

1. Clasp your fingers behind your neck.
2. Pull your elbows back as far as you can. Hold for 10 seconds. Keeping your fingers clasped, try to bring your elbows together in front of you. Hold for 5 seconds.
3. Release your hands and relax for five seconds.
4. Repeat the sequence three times.

Benefits: Keeps you from slouching, stretches your pecs, eases you into a positive posture.

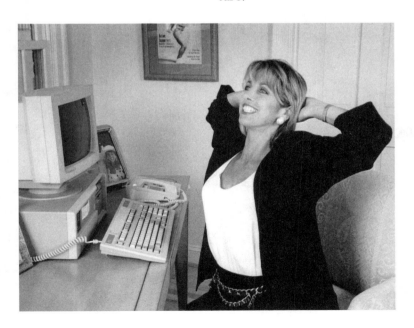

TENSION TAMERS FOR THE OFFICE

SIDE STRETCH

Stay fit at work by elongating and stretching your spine. When you sit for long periods of time, the muscles around your vertabrae tighten, which can lead to back pain and stiffness. This side stretch is a great way to give a lift through the spine and improve circulation.

1. Interlace your fingers and lift your arms up over your head.
2. Press your arms back as far as you can.
3. Slowly lean to the left and then to the right.

Benefits: Stretches the muscles along the side of your body from your arm to your hips.

REACH BEHIND

This stretch is effective for stretching the muscles of your chest, shoulders, and arms and is another great way to rev up if you're getting tired at work. This is perfect when you find yourself slouching. It can be done sitting or standing.

1. Sit or stand up straight and interlace your fingers behind you.
2. Bring your arms up beind you until you feel the stretch. Try to keep your back and arms straight.
3. Hold stretch for 5 to 15 seconds and relax. Repeat.

Benefits: Stretches chest, arms and shoulders.

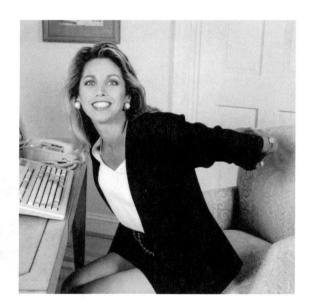

TENSION TAMERS FOR THE OFFICE

TUMMY TUCK

Why not get a great tummy workout right in your chair? You can do this anywhere. I even do this tummy tuck on my couch while watching television. I've also been known to do it while on an airplane (with long pants on). Turn idle time into toning time and get that rock-hard tummy!

1. Sit upright and grasp a chair's arms or a point underneath the chair.
2. With feet together and knees bent, lift your knees toward your chest while contracting your abdominal muscles.
3. Hold for 3 to 5 seconds. Relax and repeat.

Benefits: Tones and tightens abdominal muscles.

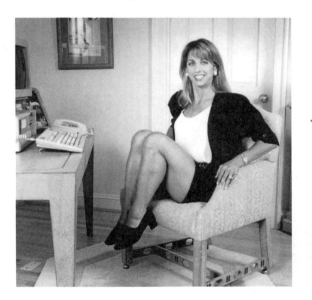

THIGH FIRMER

Anyone who knows me knows I talk on the telephone a lot. My business depends on the phone. I'm really very busy, rushing here, flying there, so the phone has become the best way to keep up with my friends and to check on the progress of my professional activities. But as you might guess, I never, never just sit there when I'm on the phone. It'd be a waste of perfectly good exercise time.

1. Lean back lightly against a wall.
2. Flatten your spine against the wall.
3. Lower your body along the wall until your knees are bent to at least a 45-degree and no more than a 90-degree angle. Pretend you are sitting in a chair.
4. Hold for as long as you can, up to 60 seconds.

Benefits: Tones and strengthens your quadriceps; especially great for skiers.

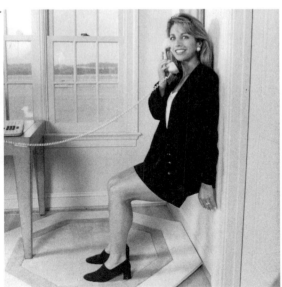

TENSION TAMERS FOR THE OFFICE

LEG SHAPER

Eighty percent of American women wear high heels at least twice a week. Even though high heels make your legs look great, they can cause your muscles to tighten from heel to calf and can lead, in turn, to tired, aching legs, ankles, and feet. I usually wear high heels only for dressy social functions. When my feet begin to hurt, I get relief by slipping away from the crowd and doing this exercise. I don't even have to take off my shoes.

1. Place the ball of your right foot at the edge of a step.
2. Press your right heel downward until you feel a stretch in your lower right leg. Hold for 30 seconds.
3. Release.
4. Switch legs and repeat.

Benefits: Increases flexibility in your calf muscles and stretches your Achilles tendons.

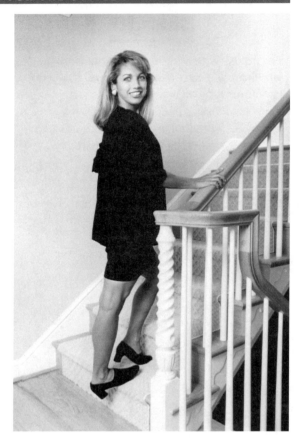

IN THE CAR

All these exercises are called *isometric* exercises, and are designed to firm and tone the body. If you are ever stuck in traffic, why let those muscles just hang out? Contract those muscles. Do these exercises at the next stop light. Make it a stop-light habit.

In your stopped car:

Tighten Your Tummy: Press the small of your back into your car seat, tightening and contracting your abdominal muscles. Hold for 10 seconds and relax. *Try to do 10 seconds.* There—you did a sit-up without ever getting out of your car!

Benefit: Strengthens the abdominal muscles. Practices the tummy to tuck in!

Mini Chin Lift: Lift your chin just a bit—keeping your eyes on the road, of course. Raise your lower teeth over your upper lip, then lower them quickly. Repeat as many times as you can in 1 minute.

Benefit: A marvelous way to head off a double chin.

1-Arm Ceiling Press: Place one palm on the ceiling of your car and press upward. Hold for ten seconds and relax. Now try it with the other arm.

Benefit: Firms the arm muscles. No more underarm sag.

WAIST TWIST

Most of us spend an awful lot of time in automobiles. I've heard of people who won't walk even half a block for a quart of milk. And even when we're not being lazy, a lot of us end up spending hours waiting around in parked cars for one reason or another. The next time you're sitting in a parked car, turn waiting time into trim-your-waistline time.

1. Sit comfortably, with your back straight.
2. Twist your torso toward the right, far enough that you can grab the back of the seat with both hands. Feel the stretch through your waistline, upper arm and back.
3. Hold for 15 seconds and relax.
4. Twist toward the left.

Benefits: Tones and stretches the muscles on your sides (the internal and external obliques).

After a Long Day

Your poor, aching feet! Think about them for a while. You walk on them all the time. You stuff them into shoes that are too tight. You stub them, you get them wet. They get no respect. When was the last time you soaked them in warm, sudsy water, and sprinkled them with talcum power? Maybe, just maybe, you rub them at night, but that's not enough. Feet need massaging before they reach the point of exhaustion. All you need is a minute—let's say while you're on hold—and a tennis ball.

1. Take off your shoes and socks
2. Place a tennis ball under one foot
3. Roll the ball back and forth under the foot for 30 seconds.
4. Switch feet and repeat.

Benefits: Loosens up your feet, and your whole body follows suit.

Commercial
Break

Next time you're watching your favorite TV show, each time a commercial comes on, get up and exercise: march in place, do arm circles, anything that moves your body. Then when your show resumes you can get back on that couch. Did you know there are approximately 6 minutes of commercial time in a 30-minute show during which you can exercise? And you're not missing anything (except some inches around your waist)! Do sit-ups and push-ups during every commercial. You'll soon get a flat tummy and firmer arms!

Reeducate Those Muscles

Here is a pop quiz. Which do you think would be more effective? Pulling your tummy in all day long, or 5 minutes of sit-ups and then forgetting about your abdominal muscles. Pulling in your tummy all day, of course. Think of it as 16 hours versus 5 minutes of exercise.

I challenge you to try this. Make an effort to keep your posture erect for the rest of the day. Put a reminder in places you cannot help but see several times throughout the day. I like to use those little self-stick dots sold at office-supply stores. Put them on your phone, in your wallet, on your dashboard, on the refrigerator—wherever you will see them often! When you see that dot, straighten up and pull it in! Boy, will you feel those muscles by tonight. After awhile, standing and sitting straighter should become automatic as your muscles adapt and become strong and firm.

Muscles are like inanimate clay. Left alone they form soft, round blobs. Those blobs, however, can be shaped by deciding to tighten or pull them in. Of course, you are reshaping them through the toning and aerobic exercise. But think of how much faster your body will change when you tax those muscles consistently during every waking hour, instead of just for 5 or 10 minutes 6 days a week! All activity has the potential to work your muscles. It just takes some awareness and some concentration from you.

Now, before I go any further, I want to clarify that what I am about to tell you should not be used as a replacement for the toning exercises, at least not if you can help it. This bit of advice is best used in addition to the resistance training routine. The toning exercises provide an opportunity for you to focus on a muscle group and achieve maximum results in the shortest time frame. But, and it happens to all of us, if you are truly pressed for time or simply cannot stick to the routine, there are ways to work your muscles throughout the normal course of your day.

Sounds great, right? Then let's begin! The first step toward becoming your own architect is to think about your posture. It really is as important as your mother told you it is. Posture is as critical to how you feel as it is to how you look. And believe me, good posture demands strong muscles. Holding your skeletal structure erect, pulling in that tummy, and straightening the spine by tightening and pulling in that rear end all take a great deal of muscle and concentration.

For example, how are you sitting right this minute? Don't move, just observe. Is your spine curved in a C shape? Is your middle region scrunched together? Is your tummy a lump in your lap? Are your shoulders rounded over your chest? If so, sit up straight right now. Pull in that abdomen, spread those shoulders back, straighten that spine, open up that middle region. Now look at yourself again. In two seconds you have tremendously improved your appearance. I'll bet you look thinner, not to mention more alert, just because you have asked your muscles to do their jobs. Would you like to know a secret way to look like you have lost at least 10 pounds instantly? Stand up straight! Sit up straight! Hold that body erect and with pride!

Are you beginning to feel tired and uncomfortable in this position? I'll bet you are, because your muscles are not accustomed to working as they were meant to. They have become lazy. You are feeling them now, just like during your daily exercise routine, because they are really working.

Now take a minute to make sure your posture is correct. Stand sideways in front of a mirror with your feet shoulder-width apart. Imagine a taut string running from your earlobe, through your shoulder, into your hipbone, and down to your ankle on both sides of your body. When all of these parts of your body are in proper alignment you are standing properly. While it may feel strange at first, you should feel very relaxed when standing and sitting properly. As a matter of fact, locking up muscles, particularly around our shoulders and neck, is one of the leading causes of back pain, neck pain, and headaches. Sitting and standing improperly disproportionately distributes the weight that any one muscle, vertebra, or tendon must support. When a muscle is forced to carry more weight than intended, it becomes stressed and begins to ache.

I know this from personal experience. In my Catholic school, if a classroom was getting unruly the sisters would punish the entire class. My second-grade teacher, Sister Sharon Ann, had a unique way of getting our attention. She would make the entire class stand with their arms extended perpendicular to their sides. Then, after a moment or two, she would begin selecting individuals and allow them to put down their arms and be seated. Needless to say, the sister usually had a pretty good idea who the culprits instigating any trouble were, so the usually well-behaved children got to sit down first.

Let me tell you, we waited anxiously for her to call our names. Try holding your arms out like that for even a short time. It really begins to hurt, because our small shoulder muscles were simply not designed to carry the weight of our arms that way. The same principle applies to the neck when we hold our head too far forward, our lower back when we slump and curve the spine, and our upper back when we hold our shoulders tightly hunched up around our ears. Those muscles start to ache as well as tighten in an attempt to hold this unnatural position. So, the next time you feel an ache or pain, particularly in the neck or back, check your posture. Stretch all those muscles to release the constricted blood flow and then sit or stand properly. I'll bet you will feel some immediate relief.

Exercise Wherever You Are!

The great thing about the exercises that accompany the 21 Day JumpStart Plan is that they do not require a lot of special equipment. This will make it much easier for you to keep up with your exercise routines while you are traveling. Just throw your walking shoes and some workout clothes into your travel bag and you are off!

Walking is the most transportable exercise I know! You can walk almost anywhere. Think of it as an adventure as you take the time to wander through every location you visit! If business travel or a vacation takes you to a hotel or motel, just be sure to check with the front desk regarding the surrounding area. Is it safe to walk in any direction? Should I avoid a particular area? Is it safe to walk alone after dark? Personally, I subscribe to the buddy system. I think it is best to go walking or jogging in pairs. Consistent exercise is important, but it is not worth risking your safety.

Also, many hotels have added workout facilities for their guests, including everything from stationary bikes to free weights. However, always check to see if the facility is staffed. I never use a hotel facility by myself. It is just not safe to be in an isolated, unmonitored area. If your location does not, ask if the establishment has a cooperative relationship with a local gym or aerobic studio nearby. Often the front desk will have passes that enable their guests to use a local facility at little or no charge for the duration of their stay. Some local gyms and studios allow a nonmember one free visit. Subsequent days may be subject to a day rate. Do not be afraid to ask around! It can be a lot of fun to experience new places and different forms of exercise.

If you normally incorporate weights into your toning routine, do not try to take them with you unless you are prepared to pay for baggage assistance. (If you are driving, go ahead and throw them in the car. That is, if, as in my case, they can fit after the port-a-crib, stroller, car seats, and toys! I am lucky that Jeff and I get to bring clothes!) The good old standbys: sit-ups, push-ups and standing squats will still be effective. Instead of weights, challenge your muscles by testing their endurance levels. Double the amount of times you repeat the exercise if you can. For instance, if you have been doing 2 sets of 8 standing squats holding 5-pound weights, try doing 2 sets of 16 in a row. Don't worry, you will feel like you have worked out!

If you are on vacation, and there simply is not time to complete your regular routine, then forget it! Yes, I said forget it. Not exercising completely, just your regular routine. Find other ways to be aerobic. Play Frisbee or volleyball on the beach with your children. Go on a hike if you find yourself near a national park. Swim in a hotel pool as a relaxing way to end a hard day of sightseeing. Or race your children to the next ride at the amusement park. Wherever you are there is some kind activity available to help you keep that fat burning going strong—even on vacation!

CHAPTER 14

BABIES, BUSINESS, AND BICEPS: HAVING IT ALL . . . IT'S ABOUT BALANCE

If Life Is a Tightrope, Where Is My Net?

Dear Denise,

I have been working out with you for 6 months. After having a baby a year ago, I needed the firming and energy to keep up with being a working mother. I have a long way to go, though I have regained my energy and started to firm. I tape your show so that I can do it when I get home from work. It allows me to get the necessary exercise while being able to stay at home with baby and family, and each day is a different workout so I never get burned out. Your program has been incredible for me and my lifestyle. You are fun, motivating, and challenging. Thanks!!

—Beth, Lawrenceville, Georgia

I am not, nor do I want to be, a superwoman. I just want to be a happy person who determines her success in life by how well she cares for her family and maintains her values and principles. I never want professional achievement to deter me from ensuring that Jeff and the children remain my top priority. I am seeing this shift in my friends as well. There seems to be a renewal of the commitment to parenting and family life over professional status. Does that mean I am ready to give up all that I have worked for in my career? No way! Does that mean I should not have friends and hobbies, or take a moment or two for myself now and then? Absolutely not. But there are many times I feel stretched beyond belief, like I am walking on a tightrope without a net or safety harness. And, I think, is this the way I want to live? Is this the environment that will allow Katie and Kelly to grow up to be strong, confident women? Is this the person Jeff looks forward to seeing when he comes home? Is all this rushing worth it?

In my mind, life is a delicate balance of the personal and professional things that are the most important to me. For instance, I made the distinct decision to work at home and be as much of a full-time mom as I could. Jeff and I firmly believe that the only way to convey our values and heritage to the girls is by being a traditional family. On the positive side, I was there to share many of my girls' firsts: first teeth, first steps, first words. I love picking up Kelly, and sometimes one or two of her friends, after school. It tickles me to hear of the day's adventures and to see the joy on Katie's face as her big sister jumps in the car. I am thankful that I am home on days when the children are not feeling well. I know that for many working mothers it is impossible to remain home unless their child is seriously ill. Even then, some employers are not very understanding. On the down side, it is difficult to keep myself from running downstairs every time I hear a cry to see if the girls are all right. And sometimes, babysitter or not, Kelly and Katie get pretty determined to be with Mommy. I laugh when I hear that recording of President Kennedy telling John, Jr. to behave in his office during a live radio address. I have had a few situations like that myself!

"No": It's Not A Dirty Word!

I believe that the positive habits you have acquired through the 21 Day JumpStart Plan are the key to balancing all of life's demands. But there is one critical factor to balancing it all that I have yet to discuss: the ability to say *no*. I know, I know, it sounds simple enough. However, one of the most difficult problems women face is saying no to others. When you overload yourself and run yourself ragged because of an inability to turn others down, those you care about the most end up with the leftover crumbs of your time and energy. In 1995, the *Washington Post* reported a study from the American Journal of Psychiatry that stated that women with degrees in the corporate world are paying a high price—they were suffering from more stress, depression, and feelings of being on the verge of a nervous breakdown than were their male counterparts. The price you pay for life in the fast lane can be high.

I try to balance professional obligations and personal relationships with appropriate healthy limits. I am now unwilling to sacrifice my personal values and priorities. It's all in balance and planning ahead.

Prioritizing

The number-one step in prioritizing is to focus your energies on what's most important to you. It is important to focus on the big picture and where you want to go in life. It helps to establish short-term and long-term goals, and a vision of where you want to be. We all have dreams and aspirations, we all have goals, we all want to achieve something in this life.

What are they for you? I want you to write down three things you want to get out of your life. This can really help you bring the big picture into focus. From there, you will be able to set your priorities as to how you want to achieve these goals.

In my life, the race is on from the moment I wake up in the morning until I go to bed. Between getting up, working out, getting the kids up and out the door to school, running errands, cleaning house, doing chores, work, spending time with the kids, and making dinner, it is sometimes hard to see what is the most important. I try to realize that some days certain things just aren't going to get done. For me, it's hard to have a neat house with children, but I'd rather spend the time with them than cleaning up. Always focus on the big picture.

Balance

One of my goals is to have a happy, healthy family life. This requires balancing time among my husband, my children, my friends and family, and my career. I believe that to make all of these pieces fit together, you have to believe in each other, encourage each other, and support each other. Within my home, I have made a little pact with myself to create a positive environment. I feel, as a mother and wife, a responsibility to be the heart of the home. My attitude determines the environment of my family. A smile goes a long way, and a cheerful atmosphere will affect your whole family and those around you. I have a girlfriend whose seven-year-old always says "Watch out, my mom is in a bad mood," or asks, "Do you know what mood my mom is in today?" Well, this shows you do have the power in your home to set the mood. Remember that slogan, never underestimate the power of a woman. How true that is!

This places a lot more pressures on women—and especially on mothers—since our moods and levels of happiness set the atmosphere in each home and make it a happy one for our children. I have found that the best way to alleviate this pressure is through regular exercise. Exercise is a proven way to reduce stress and anxiety, and it's a natural tranquilizer. Exercise also helps you to sleep better, which will give you a much needed good night's rest and allow you to wake up and feel refreshed. I feel exercise is my mental filter, flushing out all my grouchiness and crabbiness. So, it's only fair to me and my family that I stick to a regular fitness schedule as a part of my balanced day.

My husband does just fine when I'm away for a day or two. But I try not to travel and be away for more than three days in a row. It's too hard on Jeff and the two girls. I need my family as much as they need me. I'm a mother now and my priorities have changed. Before children, I was a lot more competitive, and would spend weekends giving lectures, seminars, everything I could to get ahead. But now I come home from a long day in New York and Kelly runs up to me and hugs me and says "I love you!" That means more to me, and is more precious than anything else I have achieved.

We waited seven years before beginning a family. It was a wonderful time to establish our marriage first, before having children. Once I had my baby, things did change, and it's all worth it. Some days I wonder if the pace of motherhood keeps me from getting enough done, or if life is passing me by. But then Kelly will get on the phone while I'm away on business and say to me "I love you bigger than the whole sky!" and I'll just cry. My girls help me with my career by giving me perspective and helping me to get some distance from work frustrations. I don't get bogged down because when I'm with them and see their little faces, everything falls into place. It's all about balance.

Plan Ahead!

Have you ever wondered why your neighbor seems to get so much more done than you do? Her home seems immune from dust and stray toys. Her family raves about her home-cooked meals. And to top it all off, she seems to exercise regularly and always look pulled together. How does she do it? Is she a Stepford wife? No, of course not, but she is prepared and she is organized. These are the two essential factors to maximizing the time you have available every day.

I must confess, I am not the woman I just described. But each of us knows someone like her. She is the envy of every woman who ever got married and gave birth. But, I have learned a few tricks from the most incredibly efficient and productive woman in my life, my mother. My mother was divorced when I was eight and left on her own to raise five children. I cannot remember a time while I was growing up that she was not working at least two jobs. But I never look back on those years and think that we kids lacked her time and attention. Somehow, in spite of her responsibilities, she always seemed to be there for us. Our meals were always hot and nutritious, and her warm hugs and cheerful words were constant.

As an adult, and mother of my own children, I have become even more aware of the great job my mother did. I only have two children, and work at home when I am not traveling, and it is a major challenge to keep up. Before Jeff and I had children it was fairly easy to skimp in the cooking department, as we could always pick something up or grab a quick sandwich or salad. If the laundry didn't get done that day, no big deal. And so on.

Then we had Kelly. All of a sudden little laundry piles became mammoth mountains. As Kelly grew and stopped nursing, my kitchen became the source of what seemed like an unending food fest. It seemed that as soon as I would clean up from breakfast, it was time for lunch. After lunch, it was snacks, and then dinner! The meal preparation never ended.

I asked my mom to explain how she managed all those years with five children. "Denise," she said, "it's all a matter of thinking ahead and getting as much done in advance as possible." Boy, is she right!

I quickly realized that some organization was needed, and fast. Jeff and I began to use Sundays as planning days. It was not as formal as a meeting, we just agreed to cross-check our schedules to make sure neither of us had double-booked the other by accident. Also, with my travel schedule, we needed to confirm that Kelly's (and now Katie's) schedule was covered either by Jeff or our frequent babysitter. I also had our new house built so that my kitchen and family room were all in one. That way, on Sunday afternoons I try to prepare as much in advance as possible for the meals that week, Jeff plays with Kelly and Katie, or works at the kitchen table while they watch videos. I wash and precut vegetables and meats, and put them into plastic bags for easy access. I also take a quick glance at any recipes I will be using. How many times will I need sliced green or red pepper, carrot or celery? I try to get as many of my ingredients ready as well so that in the evenings when time is short it is more a matter of assembly.

Here are five tricks I use to keep my busy schedule in order:

1. Use Sunday to plan for the week ahead.
2. Keep a calendar.
3. Try to exercise in the morning, before the day's activity begins.
4. Don't be afraid to ask for help if you need it. Delegate.
5. Prepare meals in advance and freeze them.

A few tips for working mothers:

Try to make your time with your children. Have the babysitter run errands for you, like getting the milk, picking up the dry cleaning, and stopping at the pharmacy. Stay with your kids—they need you—and have others run to do the chores. It is important to me to spend at least one hour a day with my children, giving them my undivided attention.

A few tips for at-home mothers:

Even if you don't have any help, call relatives and friends and pool your resources. Sometimes you might want to just get out of the house. (I know, I've been there!) After my second baby was born, I just couldn't wait to go to the grocery store—it was a joy and a relief. So I asked a friend to come over and she watched the girls while I ran out and, when I came back, she did her errands and I watched her kids and all the children had a blast together.

As a mother, you may feel a tremendous amount of guilt spending even a half-an-hour away from your children. But that half-an-hour should be used to take the time for renewing your energy and your total well-being.

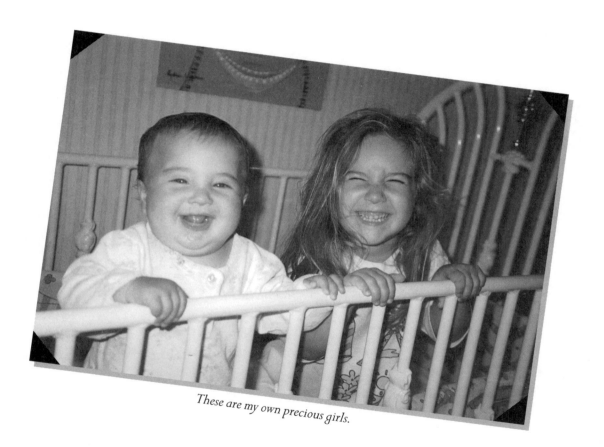

These are my own precious girls.

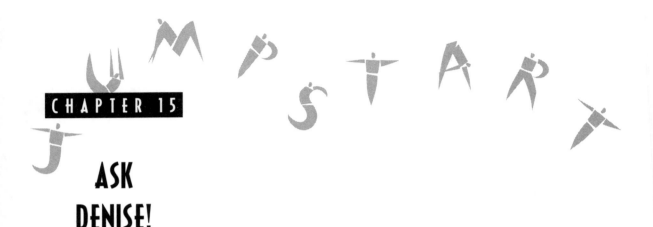

CHAPTER 15

ASK DENISE!

ere are the answers to the top twenty questions I get asked most frequently, either by letter or on the road! Some of them may be a little repetitive, after you've just recently work through the 21 Day JumpStart Plan. But I thought this might be a great way to provide a handy method of recap and review. Maybe you can use these questions to test your own fitness savvy.

What Is the Best Time of Day to Exercise?

Whatever time best suits your schedule, stick with that same time daily so that it's part of your day. But it is my opinion, and studies support this, that the best time to exercise is first thing in the morning. It seems the sooner we all get it over with, the less chance there is that we will find an excuse not to do it!

How Many Days per Week Should I Exercise Aerobically?

Three to four days per week is ideal for burning fat, increasing your aerobic capacity, and really reshaping your body. That is not to say that if you can only fit it in twice a week you will not get anything out of it. . . . You will! But there is no doubt that the more you exercise aerobically, the faster you will lose fat and achieve the results you are looking for.

What if I Have No Time to Exercise?

One of the most basic principles of my philosophy of fitness is that everyone can find time to exercise, even if they have to squeeze it in among their regular activities; that is why I wrote the chapter "A Day With Denise."

Some of my favorite recommendations to someone with a hectic schedule are: walk or bike to work or to the train station instead of driving; keep a set of light hand weights at the office for quick upper-body toning; or, park in the last spot in the parking lot and walk the rest of the way! All exercise adds up. Look for ways to exercise creatively as a part of your busy day.

What Is the Best Way to Flatten My Stomach After a Baby?

Achieving a tight tummy after a baby is no different than tightening that tummy any other time—it just seems to take a lot longer! As with everything else, consistency is the key. Once your doctor okays exercise, begin doing crunches every day. Within this book, I have shown you several different exercises for your tummy. Pick the one or two you like best and do them religiously.

What Is the Best Way to Get Rid of Cellulite?

Losing cellulite is no more mysterious than losing fat because that is what it is—fat! The most effective way to rid yourself of this unattractive fat that seems to collect in the buns and thighs is with aerobic exercise, toning up, and a sensible low-fat diet.

Shouldn't I Lose Weight Before I Start to Lift Weights?

No. This is a common misconception. A lot of people think that if they have fat on their body and they start to lift weights, their fat will turn into muscle. This is impossible. Fat is fat and muscle is muscle! They are not interchangeable or components of each other. In fact, lifting weights actually contributes to fat loss, since the added muscle increases your metabolism. And speeding up that metabolism helps you to lose weight even more quickly.

I Am Doing My Aerobics, but I Am Not Losing Any Weight. Why?

Check the intensity of your workouts. My guess is that you are working out at too high an intensity to burn fat. The most efficient level of activity for fat burning is slow to moderate. Your body needs to have the time and freedom to zero in on fat stores as energy. High-intensity workouts need fast energy, which comes in the form of glycogen found in the muscles, not fat. So slow it down. After all, exercise should be fun—and something you can maintain for at least 15 to 20 minutes. Take the talk test or monitor your heart rate to check if you are working out in a slow-to-moderate range.

How Much Fat Is Good to Eat?

We need some fat in our diets to be healthy, but the average American overshoots the healthy level by leaps and bounds every day. My recommendation is to strive for a diet that is around 20 percent fat, realizing that you will exceed that target on occasion.

How Do I Know What Percentage of Fat Is in the Food I Eat?

The new label laws have really helped here. Every food product now comes with a detailed nutritional information label that clearly states the percentage of fat in a food, as well as grams per serving. If you want to figure it out yourself, the formula is easy. Each gram of fat has 9 calories. Multiply the number of grams of fat by 9 (use 10 if that is easier for you to calculate). Divide the total number of calories by the number of fat calories. The number you get is the total percentage of fat in the food.

If I Skip Meals Will I Lose Weight More Quickly?

The answer to this is a great big NO. When you skip meals, you actually slow your progress! Going hungry decreases your metabolic rate and the amount of calories that you are able to burn. It is better to eat small, healthy meals frequently throughout the day. And, of course, eat a healthy snack if you get hungry in between.

What Is the Training Zone?

The *training zone* is a measure of the intensity of an exercise using your heartbeat. See chapter 6 for a more in-depth explanation. But, in a nutshell, the body most effectively burns fat at no more than 65 percent of your maximum heart rate. Your target zone is approximately 65 to 85 percent of the maximum times your heart can beat per minute.

What Percentage of Body Fat Is Good?

The average body fat recommendation for women is 22 to 24 percent. But every woman and physique is different, so I recommend that you remain where you feel and look your best. Some women look better with a little extra fat; others need to carry less.

What Exercises Burn the Most Fat?

Aerobic exercise done at low intensity for at least 20 minutes.

Is It Possible to Lose Weight Just in Certain Areas?

Spot reducing is a myth. Fat loss occurs throughout the entire body. Think of it this way: If you could lose weight in your thighs by doing leg lifts, then chewing gum would make your face skinny!

Is It Okay to Drink Alcohol?

The latest research shows that alcohol reduces the rate at which your body burns fat. Also, alcohol contains calories that are virtually empty of any nutritional value. And, finally, alcohol consumption tends to make us want to snack on high-fat foods like chips and peanuts, or at the very least softens our resolve to eat healthy foods. Anything is okay in moderation, but think of alcohol as one of your more fattening food choices.

What Is the Best Exercise for a Bad Back?

Increasing your abdominal and lower-back strength, combined with improving your hamstrings (the long muscle that runs from ankle to the top of your rear) is the best way to prevent back pain and future back trouble! Of course, consult your doctor if you experience serious back pain.

At What Age Should My Kids Start to Exercise?

I suggest that you encourage your children to exercise and be active as a normal course of life from a very early age. Family walks and games with movement help them develop coordination and flexibility, and are fun! Passing on healthy habits is a lifelong gift to your children.

What Do I Do if I Injure Myself While Exercising

First, stop exercising! Apply R.I.C.E: *R*est, *I*ce, *C*ompression, and *E*levation. Consult your physician if pain persists more than a day or two. And do not return to physical activity without your doctor's okay.

How Much Time Should I Spend Exercising?

An ideal, and effective, program is 30 minutes a day. It should include aerobic exercise, muscle toning, and stretching.

What Is the Best Way to Speed Up My Metabolism?

The top three components of speeding your metabolism are:

1. Eat several times a day. Don't give your metabolism a chance to rest!
2. Add toning exercises to your routine. Remember, increased muscle burns increased fat!
3. Exercise aerobically. Done at a low intensity for a 20-minute period of time does wonders for fat loss!

What Time of Day Is Best for Aerobic Exercise?

Anytime it fits your schedule, because studies have shown that people who set a designated time of the day to exercise and keep that time each day are more likely to stick to a fitness schedule. I like to get up half an hour early to get my exercise routine in before the pressures of the day distract me.

How Many Days a Week Should I Exercise Aerobically?

I recommend that you invest 20 to 30 minutes at least three days a week engaging in some form of aerobic exercise. Please remember, however, that this number is a minimum. The more you do, the more results you will see, and the better you will feel! I personally do an aerobic activity 4 days a week.

What Is the Best Form of Aerobic Exercise?

It is impossible to isolate a best aerobic exercise. In my opinion, the best aerobic exercise is one that you personally enjoy, and are most likely to continue to participate in consistently.

Is Walking Aerobic?

Yes! Aerobic walking is a bit more intensive than a stroll through the park, though. To be aerobic, by definition, you must elevate your heart rate. I use 120 steps per 15 to 18 minutes as a rule of thumb. One of the reasons that my TrimWalk tape has been so successful is that I keep pace for you! So, put some spring in that step and let your arms move with you—enjoy nature's bounty as you walk your way to a better body!

What Is the Recommended Time to Spend Doing Aerobic Exercise?

Twenty minutes is generally recommended as the minimum time you can devote to aerobic exercise and still see great results. The more time you spend, however, the more dramatic the changes will be. Since exercise increases the metabolic rate, the longer you move, the more you burn!

Is It Okay to Eat in the Evening?

Yes. As with everything else, apply your good common sense. If you are really hungry in the evening, eat! It is never a good idea to starve your body. Just try to avoid an overload of complex carbohydrates late in the evening. These are primarily energy calories. As a result, they are more difficult for the body to break down at night, because the metabolism has slowed for sleep. Proteins and fibrous vegetables are the best choices for a late night meal.

If I Get Really Hungry in the Middle of the Day, What Should I Eat?

Contrary to popular belief, snacking between meals is okay! Just take the time to think about it and make the wisest choice possible. Snacks such as chips, cookies, and crackers are high in fat, so try to avoid those if you can. A better bet is vegetables like carrot and celery sticks. They travel well, so you can keep a supply with you. Grab an apple instead of a candy bar: It is much more nutritious and will be just as effective in getting you through the remainder of your day!

If I Change the Way I Eat, Will I Lose Weight?

Yes! As long as you are not eating more calories than you burn. Remember, the basic principle of weight loss is that calories burned must *exceed* calories consumed. That is why you must keep moving in order to lose those excess pounds.

What About the Holidays?

I believe in the importance of holidays, family gatherings, and festive feasts. I use moderation as my best defense against holiday weight gain. I eat whatever I want, and try not to overeat. If your mother makes some of your favorite dishes only once a year, then indulge! You deserve a holiday, too. No one ever gained a significant amount of weight because they chose to eat high-fat foods for one day. If you take good care of your body throughout the year, a break now and then is well deserved. So enjoy the holidays!

How Much Water Should I Drink?

There is no doubt that your body needs lots of water, and that the average American does not get enough! Water is even more important when you are exercising. I suggest a minimum of eight 8-ounce glasses per day. Water is essential to flush the body of toxins. It also does great things for the complexion and has the added benefit of curbing the appetite. Toting a water bottle is the fashion now, so take water wherever you go!

JUMPSTART

RECIPES YOU CAN COUNT ON— IN-A-HURRY RECIPES FOR HEALTHY COOKING

Here is a wide variety of my favorite personal recipes, ones I can always count on . . . even when I'm "In a Hurry." You'll make fabulous dinners that are delicious, healthy, and easy . . . because if it isn't easy, I won't do it. And most of these dinners can be on the table in less than 30 minutes. I have also included some great breakfast and healthy sandwich ideas; low-fat sauces, dressings, and appetizers; and scrumptious nonfat desserts.

Enjoy! Food is fabulous.

GRANDMA KATNICH'S PEAS

My grandma was a wonderful cook. These slavic peas is one of my favorite dishes she would make us. Grandma was from the old country, born in a small Austrian village close to Italy on the Adriatic Sea. The recipe is so simple that it's basically just assembly. The bay leaves add a distinct flavor that makes the dish special.

Prep and cooking time:
12 minutes

2   cans of Del Monte Sweet Peas
1   small can of Hunt's Tomato Sauce
1   medium onion, chopped fine
1-2 tablespoon flour
3   bay leaves
    Cooking spray
    Pepper to taste

Lightly spray a nonstick pan with cooking spray. Sauté chopped onion over medium heat until transparent and slightly soft. Add peas and liquid from cans. Pour in tomato sauce and stir. Sprinkle flour into mixture and continue stirring until mixture is thickened. Add pepper and bay leaves.

Simmer on low heat for 10 minutes.

Makes six servings
Calories: 80
Fat: Less than 1g

CHICKEN DENISE OVER BROWN RICE

This favorite dish of mine has some of the flavorings and spices I have tasted so often in the Caribbean. I know you'll learn to appreciate the flavors of allspice, bay leaves, and citrus . . . they work so well together, without calories.

Prep and cooking time:
35 minutes

4   boneless, skinless chicken breasts
1   cup whole-wheat flour
1   tablespoon olive oil

$\frac{1}{3}$ cup red wine vinegar
$\frac{1}{2}$ teaspoon allspice
2   bay leaves
    Salt and pepper to taste
4   cups cooked brown rice
$\frac{1}{2}$ cup orange juice
    Orange slices and parsley (for garnish)

Rinse chicken breasts and dip in flour, turning to cover all sides. Set aside.

Pour olive oil in large nonstick pan and turn heat to high. Place chicken in pan and sauté 5 minutes on each side until golden brown. Remove from heat and drain excess oil.

Add orange juice, vinegar, allspice, and bay leaves and return pan to low heat. Cover and simmer chicken for 15 to 20 minutes.

Divide cooked, warm rice onto 4 plates. Ladle chicken breasts with sauce over rice. Garnish with orange slices and parsley.

Makes four servings
Calories: 350
Fat: 6g

DENISE'S TUNA SALAD

I've given my tuna fish a tangy twist and it's just great. If you have any balsamic vinegar in your pantry, try that, too. It's very fruity, even slightly sweet, and gives everything a whole different character.

Prep and cooking time:
5 minutes

1   10-ounce can white-meat tuna, packed in water
$\frac{1}{2}$ onion, chopped fine
2   stalks celery, chopped fine
2   teaspoons red wine vinegar
    Dash of salt and pepper to taste

Drain tuna and rinse well. Combine tuna and other ingredients in bowl and mix thoroughly. Serve with crackers.

Makes four servings
Calories: 100
Fat: 2g

SPICY BROWN RICE AND BEANS

I absolutely love beans for their taste and nutritional content, and try to eat them often. You can try this recipe with different kinds of beans. A dash of hot sauce and a squeeze of lime can give this simple recipe some pizazz!

Prep and cooking time: 12 minutes

1	cup brown rice, cooked
½	can of black beans
	Salsa to taste

Mix all ingredients together and microwave on high for 1 minute.

**Makes one serving
Calories: 250
Fat: 2g**

CHICKEN MADEIRA

Madeira is a fortified wine from Portugal. It gives this dish its intensity. The rich sweetness of the wine makes this chicken very luxurious.

Prep and cooking time: 50 minutes

6	boneless, skinless chicken breasts
	Flour for dusting, seasoned with a dash of salt and pepper
1	bunch of green onions, chopped
12	mushrooms, sliced
1	cup water mixed with ½ teaspoon instant chicken bouillon
¼	cup Madeira wine
1	tablespoon cornstarch

Preheat oven to 300°.

Dust chicken breasts lightly with seasoned flour, shaking off the excess. In a large skillet, spray a little olive oil or light cooking spray. Place chicken in to brown on both sides. Remove chicken from pan and place in baking dish.

Add mushrooms and onions to pan. Cook down a little and add chicken broth and Madeira. Add cornstarch to thicken, and pour over chicken. (This may be prepared earlier in the day.) Bake for 45 minutes.

Makes six servings
Calories: 514
Fat: 6g

LEMON HERB CHICKEN

Nothing is as irresistible as a big dose of fresh lemon juice with a blend of herbs. Fortunately, there are some great herb mixtures on the market that make recipes like this easy. Sometimes the simplest recipes are the best!

Prep and cooking time:
35 minutes

1   *fryer, cut into pieces*
    Juice of 2 lemons
A dash of each of the following:
    Onion powder
    Garlic salt
    Freshly ground black pepper
    Italian seasonings
    Paprika

Preheat broiler.

Place chicken on a cookie sheet skin side down. Sprinkle heavily with lemon juice, onion powder, garlic salt, Italian seasoning and paprika.

Broil chicken for 15–20 minutes on one side. Turn and season other side. Broil 15–20 minutes. (This may be prepared earlier in the day and kept in the refrigerator to marinate. Broil at dinnertime.)

Remember to remove the skin before eating.

Makes 2 servings
Calories: 190
Fat: 4g

HONEY MUSTARD CHICKEN

The perfect balance of flavor in so many recipes comes from just enough sweetness to offset the tangy, savory ingredients. This dish does just that!

Note: This dish is best prepared the day before.

**Prep and cooking time:
75 minutes**

4	skinless, boneless chicken breast halves
½	cup honey
½	cup dijon mustard
1	tablespoon curry powder
2	tablespoons soy sauce

Place chicken breasts snugly in flat baking dish in one layer. Mix other ingredients and pour over chicken. Refrigerate overnight.

Preheat oven to 350°.

When ready to bake, turn chicken, cover dish with foil and bake 1 hour. Remove foil, baste well, and bake uncovered an additional 15 minutes.

**Makes four servings
Calories: 150
Fat: 3.6g**

SWEET AND SPICY PORK CHOPS

Did you know that preserves can flavor many meat dishes? It's a great secret and does the trick in a lot of speedy sauces. In this recipe, the sweet preserves are nicely balanced with the salty soy sauce and tangy white wine.

**Prep and cooking time:
45 minutes**

4	pork chops, about ¾-inch thick
½	cup apricot-pineapple preserves
¼	cup soy sauce
¼	cup white wine
	Cooking spray

Trim fat from pork chops. Spray large skillet with cooking spray. Brown chops on both sides over medium-high heat. Spray shallow baking dish with cooking spray. Place chops in baking dish. Combine preserves, soy sauce and wine; pour over chops. Cover and bake for 45 minutes or until chops are tender.

Makes four servings
Calories: 150
Fat: 3.6g

FRESH SCALLOP SAUTÉ

Scallops are great as long as you can get them really, really fresh. There is no waste and almost always no prep involved. They take so little time to cook that they're truly a convenience food. Here's a trick to remember the size of sea scallops compared to bay scallops: Sea scallops are larger because they come from a larger body of water—the sea or ocean. Bay scallops are tiny because they come from a smaller body of water—a bay.

Prep and cooking time:
10 minutes

15	sea scallops
½	lemon
1½	teaspoons dill
	Cooking spray
½	tablespoon garlic, minced
½	cup white wine
¼	cup water

Wash and pat dry scallops.

Spray skillet with cooking spray. Sauté garlic for 2 minutes in pan. Add scallops to pan and stir to coat with garlic. Cook for 5 minutes on medium heat. Add wine and water. Sprinkle with lemon juice and dill. Stir to combine. Cook until done, about 5 more minutes

Makes four servings
Calories: 150
Fat: Less than 1g

BROILED FISH FILLETS

This is as quick and easy and healthy as can be! To get your children to eat fish, add extra cracker meal and slice the fillets to make healthy fish sticks—my kids love them.

Prep and cooking time:
12 minutes

4   white fish fillets (flounder or sole)
    Olive oil cooking spray
    Cracker meal
    Paprika

Preheat broiler.

Spray olive oil cooking spray on fillets. Lay fillets on a cookie sheet sprayed with olive oil spray. Sprinkle lightly with cracker meal and paprika.

Place fish under broiler and cook about 10 minutes, or until light golden brown and flaky.

Note: Don't salt before cooking, as salt toughens fish.

Makes four servings
Calories: 120
Fat: 1.5g

PORK CHOP BARBECUE

You'll love this barbecue! Pork is much leaner than it used to be because of modern breeding—pork is 30 percent lower in fat than it was 10 years ago. The loin is one of the leanest cuts of pork—just trim all visible fat from the edges before cooking your chops. Substitute beef, veal, or lamb for another delicious dinner.

Prep and cooking time:
1 hour

4   loin pork chops
½   cup catsup
¼   cup lemon juice
2   teaspoons brown sugar
2   teaspoons Lea & Perrins (Worcestershire or steak sauce)
½   cup water
¾   cup chutney (I like mango or peach chutney)

Preheat oven to 350 degrees.

Spray skillet with cooking spray. Brown chops over medium-high heat. Place in a baking dish. Combine rest of ingredients. Cook in small pot over medium heat for a few minutes. Pour over chops and bake, covered, one hour.

Makes four servings
Calories: 260
Fat: 9g

PITA PIZZAS

This recipe is so simple, I'll bet you almost always have these ingredients on hand. What a bonus that they're delicious and very low in fat! The whole family will love them.

Prep and cooking time:
5 minutes

2   *large whole-wheat pita breads*
¼   *teaspoon salt*
1   *medium green pepper, diced*
1   *medium onion, diced*
1   *medium tomato, diced*
1   *cup grated mozzarella cheese*
2   *tablespoons chopped scallions*
      Dash of oregano

Preheat oven to 500 degrees.

Spray each half of pita with cooking spray. Place in toaster oven. Toast.

Spray a skillet with cooking spray. Sauté onion and green pepper in skillet until tender. Add tomato. Stir often.

Sprinkle about one-third cheese over each half pita. Arrange a layer of the onion/tomato mixture on pita. Sprinkle with remaining cheese, scallions, and oregano. Cook pizzas in oven until cheese is bubbly and slightly browned.

Makes two servings
Calories: 150
Fat: 3g

PIZZA CHICKEN

Pizza is one of the healthiest dinners you can eat. It's high in protein from the cheese and meat. If you're careful with the products you use when making pizza, it can be low fat, nutritious, and delicious!

**Prep and cooking time:
45 minutes**

4   *boneless, skinless chicken breasts*
1   *jar of pizza sauce*
4   *slices of skim milk mozzarella cheese*
1   *teaspoon Italian seasoning*
4   *teaspoons Parmesan cheese*

Preheat oven to 350°.

Place chicken in baking dish. Cover with sauce, sprinkle Italian seasoning and Parmesan cheese. Bake for 45 minutes. Remove, add more sauce if chicken looks dry, and top with mozzarella. Return to oven until cheese melts.

**Makes four servings
Calories: 250
Fat: 6g**

CARIBBEAN BAKED BEANS WITH HAM

Beans are one of the best foods going when we consider their nutritional value and low fat. Try to eat beans frequently, because they fill you up and give loads of energy. This recipe is a dish with an "island" feeling.

**Prep and cooking time:
30 minutes**

2   *cans (about 15 ounces each) butter beans or large limas*
1   *can (8 ounces) juice-packed crushed pineapple*
½   *cup tomato-based barbecue sauce*
1   *small onion, chopped fine*
¼   *cup light brown sugar, firmly packed*
4   *ounces diced cooked ham*
2   *tablespoons fresh lime juice*
1½ *teaspoons powdered ginger*
1   *tablespoon dijon mustard*

Preheat oven to 400 degrees.

Spray a 1½ quart shallow baking dish with cooking spray. Rinse and drain beans; drain pineapple. Mix all ingredients in the casserole until well blended. Bake casserole, uncovered, for 25 minutes, stirring occasionally. Serve immediately. (Casserole may also be cooled at this point and then frozen for future use.)

Makes four servings
Calories: 273
Fat: 2.98g

MEXICAN PASTA CASSEROLE

This recipe is really speedy, and is great for a group. The kids will love it! Believe it or not, you don't have to precook the ground beef, which saves a lot of time. The recipe can be cut in half or it can be frozen once it has been baked.

Prep and cooking time:
30 minutes

½   *onion, chopped fine*
1   *28-ounce can chopped tomatoes with juice*
1   *1¼-ounce package taco mix*
1   *15–16 ounce can black beans, rinsed and drained*
8   *ounces very lean ground round, crumbled*
3   *cups cooked ziti or penne pasta (about 6 ounces dried)*
1   *cup nonfat ricotta*
½   *cup nonfat shredded cheddar cheese*

Heat the oven to 425°.

Spray a 7-by-11-inch baking dish with cooking spray. In a medium bowl or food processor, blend onion, tomatoes, taco mix, and black beans.

Spread 1 cup of the tomato sauce on the bottom of the baking dish. Add the cooked pasta. Dot with the ricotta and then spread cheese with a knife.

Stir the ground beef pieces into the remaining tomato sauce and spoon over the ricotta. Sprinkle with the shredded cheese. Bake 25-30 minutes. Serve immediately.

Makes four servings
Calories: 336
Fat: 5.97g

PORK-GRAPEFRUIT STIR-FRY

1-1/2   pounds lean boneless pork
3/4   cup frozen Florida grapefruit juice concentrate, thawed
3/4   cup cold water
3   tablespoons reduced-sodium or regular soy sauce
2   tablespoons cornstarch
1   tablespoon honey
1/2   teaspoon ground ginger
1   tablespoon cooking oil
3   cups sliced zucchini
1   medium red or green sweet pepper, cut into bite-size strips
1   tablespoon sesame seeds, toasted
3   cups hot cooked rice

Trim fat from pork. Put pork in freezer until partially frozen, just until firm. Thinly slice pork across across the grain into bite-sized strips; set aside.

For sauce, in a bowl stir together thawed concentrate, water, soy sauce, cornstarch, honey, and ginger; set aside.

Pour oil into a wok or 12-inch skillet. Preheat over medium-high heat. Add zucchini and pepper strips; stir-fry for 2 to 3 minutes or until vegetables are crisp tender. Remove vegetables and set aside.

Add half of the pork to wok. Stir-fry for 2 to 3 minutes or until no pink remains. (If necessary, add more oil, 1 teaspoon at a time, to prevent sticking during cooking.) Remove pork and repeat with remaining meat. Return all pork and vegetables to the wok. Push from center of wok. Stir sauce and add to center of wok. Cook and stir until thickened and bubbly. Stir all ingredients together to coat with sauce. Sprinkle with sesame seeds. Serve over rice.

Makes 6 servings
Calories: 344
Fat: 31 g

ENERGY-BOOST LINGUINE

This pasta dish is so full of flavor that you'll be amazed that it's packed with such nutrition, too! Did you know that one red bell pepper has more vitamin C than an orange? This is the speediest of dishes, taking less than thirty minutes to prep and cook. My favorite trick is to cook extra boneless, skinless chicken breasts for a recipe so that I'll have enough left over to make this dish the next night.

Prep and cooking time:
Less than 30 minutes

8	ounces dried linguine
1	cup frozen bell pepper slices
½	cup nonfat ricotta
1	cup chicken broth
2	scallions, finely sliced
2	cloves garlic, minced
1	tablespoon freshly chopped basil (or 1 teaspoon dried)
1	6-ounce jar marinated artichoke hearts, drained and coarsely chopped
2	cups cooked diced chicken (white meat preferred)

Cook linguine according to package directions. After the linguine has cooked for five minutes, add the bell pepper slices and cook in the water with the pasta for another 2 to 3 minutes.

Meanwhile, in a medium bowl, mix together ricotta, chicken broth, scallions, garlic, basil and artichoke hearts.

Drain pasta and bell pepper strips in a colander and then return to the warm pot. Add the ricotta mixture and the chicken and toss quickly until all is mixed and heated through. Serve immediately.

Makes four servings
Calories: 401
Fat: 5.79g

GUILT-FREE FRITTATA

In this recipe it's really best to work with a heavy nonstick skillet that has an oven-safe handle. Then you can pop it right into the oven.

Prep and cooking time:
25 minutes

1	teaspoon canola oil
1	medium onion, chopped fine
1	medium zucchini (about 6 inches long), sliced thin
1	medium crookneck squash (about 6 inches long), sliced thin
2	cloves garlic, minced
6	egg whites, lightly beaten (or equivalent egg substitute)
1	cup fresh bread crumbs (from about 1 large slice bread)
2	teaspoons dijon mustard
½	teaspoon salt
½	cup shredded nonfat mozzarella cheese (or cheese of your choice)

Preheat oven to 400°.

Heat a medium nonstick skillet (with an oven-proof handle) over medium-high heat. Add oil. Add onion and squashes and sauté for 8 minutes. Add garlic, eggs, bread crumbs, mustard, and salt. Reduce heat to medium and continue cooking while stirring egg mixture until it begins to set.

Sprinkle the cheese evenly over the top and place in hot oven. Bake for about 15 minutes or until frittata is firm, but not hard, and just beginning to puff. Cut into wedges and serve from the skillet.

Makes six servings
Calories: 81
Fat: 1.3g

CHUTNEY CHICKEN BREASTS

This is one of the tastiest chicken breasts recipes that I know. It's also so quick, you'll want to make it all the time, diet or not!

**Prep and cooking time:
15 minutes**

4	boneless, skinless chicken breast halves (3–4 ounces each)
	Salt and pepper
	Flour for dusting
¼	cup lemon juice
½	teaspoon Worcestershire sauce
⅓	cup white wine (or chicken broth)
⅓	cup mango chutney (such as Major Grey's)
3	thinly sliced scallions, white separated from the green
¼	cup raisins
1	tablespoon toasted chopped almonds

Sprinkle chicken breasts with salt and pepper and then dust lightly with flour. Heat a large nonstick skillet over medium high heat. Spray with cooking spray and, when hot, add chicken breasts and cook for 2 minutes per side. To the same pan, add the lemon juice, Worcestershire sauce, wine, chutney, white part of the scallions, and raisins. Stir to mix and then cover. Reduce heat to medium and simmer chicken breasts in the sauce for 15 minutes or until firm to the touch. Serve chicken breasts along side or over noodles, spooning extra sauce over the top. Sprinkle with scallion greens and toasted almonds.

**Makes four servings
Calories: 282
Fat: 3.6g**

TUNA ST. TROPEZ

This dish sparkles with the fresh taste of lots of vegetables encircling the tuna fillet. Sometimes just a different arrangement of food on a plate can make a great meal even more exciting.

**Prep and cooking time:
25 minutes**

4   (3–4 ounces) fresh tuna fillets, ½-inch thick, blotted dry (grouper or halibut may also be used)
1   small crookneck squash, cut into ½-inch cubes
1   small zucchini, cut into ½-inch cubes
1   medium red bell pepper, cut into ½-inch cubes
1   small eggplant, cut into ½-inch cubes
2   tablespoons fresh thyme or ¾ teaspoon dried
2   tablespoons fresh lemon juice

Spray a large skillet with cooking spray and heat on medium-high until hot. Add fish and sear to brown. Cook for 4 to 5 minutes per side. Remove and keep warm. Spray the pan with additional cooking spray. Add vegetables and sauté, stirring a few times, for 8–10 minutes or until vegetables are cooked but still slightly crunchy. Stir in thyme and return fish to pan, being careful not to break. Cook until fish is hot.

Serve on a platter or individual plates with vegetables surrounding fish. Drizzle fish and vegetables with lemon juice, salt, and pepper to taste.

**Makes four servings
Calories: 167
Fat: 1.47g**

SPEEDY GONZALES SOUTHWESTERN CHICKEN

Most of us can never get enough recipes for boneless, skinless chicken breasts, so here is another great one that's bound to become a favorite. This recipe can also be made with a mild fish fillet like grouper, halibut, or red snapper. You don't need to change a thing in the recipe.

**Prep and cooking time:
Less than 30 minutes**

4 boneless, skinless chicken breast halves, lightly flattened to $\frac{1}{2}$-inch thick
$\frac{1}{2}$ cup fat-free Italian salad dressing
$1\frac{1}{2}$ cups crumbs from corn creakfast cereal (such as corn flakes or Crispix), placed in a medium plastic bag or shallow bowl and crushed in the bag with a rolling pin
$1\frac{1}{2}$ cup salsa (medium hot)
1 15–16 ounce can black beans, rinsed and drained

Blot the chicken breasts with paper towels to dry. Place chicken in a shallow bowl and cover with dressing, tossing to coat. Cover and refrigerate 1 to 4 hours to marinate, if possible.

Preheat oven to 400°.

Remove each chicken breast half from the dressing and toss in corn cereal crumbs until well coated (you may have to press them to adhere).

Place coated chicken on a flat greased baking sheet. Bake for 16 to 18 minutes in hot oven. While chicken is baking, mix salsa and black beans. If chilled, heat to room temperature by microwaving. To serve, spoon salsa generously over each chicken breast half.

**Makes four servings
Calories: 395
Fat: 2.56g**

PASTA PUTTANESCA WITH EGGPLANT

Pasta dishes are always a sure bet for convenience and taste. This is a fabulous dish that supplies plenty of protein without any meat. It is a classic meal that combines lots of great vegetables in a robust red sauce.

**Prep and cooking time:
Less than 30 minutes**

8   ounces dried linguine or spaghetti
2   cups Healthy Choice Red Pasta Sauce with mushrooms
1   onion, peeled and sliced thin
1   small eggplant, sliced into ⅜-inch rounds, then into ½-inch strips
1   teaspoon olive oil
2   cloves fresh garlic, minced
1   16-ounce can chickpeas, rinsed and drained

Cook the pasta according to package directions.

In a large nonstick skillet, heat olive oil until hot. Add eggplant and sauté for 3 minutes. Add oil and green pepper and sauté 5 more minutes. Add garlic, chick peas, and sauce, lower heat slightly and heat through.

Drain pasta, place in a large bowl, pour sauce over and toss. Place most of the veggies on top of the pasta. Serve immediately. (This dish is also great served cold as a salad.)

**Makes four servings
Calories: 454
Fat: 5g**

QUICK CIOPPINO

San Franciscans have long had a love affair with this full-bodied seafood stew that is not unlike the bouillabaisse of France. Shellfish and white fish swimming in a garlicky tomato-and-white-wine base are the standard ingredients. Fennel bulb adds a delicate sweetness, and works well with fish. This entree is deceptively simple and very low in fat.

**Prep and cooking time:
Less than 30 minutes**

1	teaspoon olive oil
1	cup coarsely chopped fennel bulb
1	large onion, diced
4	cloves garlic, minced
1	16-ounce can tomatoes with juice, broken into pieces
1	6-ounce can tomato paste
¾	cup dry white wine or vermouth
¾	cup vegetable or clam stock
¼	teaspoon red pepper flakes
1	teaspoon thyme
2	tablespoons chopped fresh basil
8	littleneck clams
6	ounces white fish fillet, cut into 1-inch cubes
4	ounces sea scallops
4	ounces medium shrimp, peeled

In a large nonstick dutch oven or soup pot, add olive oil and heat over medium high until oil is hot. Add fennel, onion, and garlic and cook, stirring occasionally, for 6 to 8 minutes. Add the tomatoes, tomato paste, wine, stock, thyme, and basil.

Keep heat on medium high and cook for 5 minutes more. Add fish cubes, scallops, and shrimp and cook 5 to 7 minutes. Clams should be open and fish firm but not rubbery. Serve in large shallow soup bowls or over pasta or rice.

**Makes four servings
Calories: 277
Fat: 7.7g**

CHICKEN SALAD VINAIGRETTE

You won't miss the mayonnaise in this chicken salad. It's light, fresh, and delicious!

**Prep and cooking time:
25 minutes**

1	tablespoon dijon mustard
2	tablespoons lemon juice
2	tablespoon basil
8	ounces chicken (cooked, boned, skin removed)
1	tablespoon scallions, cut into 1/4-inch slices
1	tablespoon red wine vinegar
1/2	teaspoon mustard
1	small head boston lettuce

Preheat oven to 350°.

Slice chicken into 1-inch strips. Combine mustard, lemon juice, and basil; toss chicken in mixture. Place in baking pan which has been sprayed with cooking spray. Cover with foil. Bake for 20 minutes.

Meanwhile, combine vinegar and mustard. Arrange cooked chicken on lettuce leaves. Pour vinaigrette over chicken. Sprinkle cut scallions over chicken. Serve.

**Makes four servings
Calories: 200
Fat: 4g**

GREAT GOULASH

Just the right addition to a fabulous buffet. Also, a quick and easy dinner. I make this for my kids. They get protein and great taste.

**Prep and cooking time:
15 minutes**

1	pound extra lean hamburger or ground turkey
1	large jar Ragu spaghetti sauce
1	large package elbow macaroni

Fry hamburger meat, then drain. Add spaghetti sauce to hamburger meat in frying pan and simmer for 10 minutes while you boil the macaroni. Add sauce just before serving. Sprinkle with cheese. For dinner, serve with green salad and garlic bread.

Makes six servings
Calories: 300
Fat: 8g

SPICY PORK TENDERLOIN

I love spicy foods, and this is one of my favorites. Make sure before cooking that you trim all visible fat from the tenderloin. Also, try this with other meats such as veal or chicken.

Prep and cooking time:
50 minutes

1	tablespoon oregano
1	tablespoon garlic powder
1	tablespoon paprika
1	tablespoon thyme
1	tablespoon extra-virgin olive oil
1/2	teaspoon black pepper
1/2	teaspoon cumin
1/2	teaspoon light salt
1/2	teaspoon nutmeg
1/2	teaspoon cayenne pepper
2	pounds pork tenderloin

Preheat oven to 350 degrees.

Blend the spices in a plastic bag. Rub the tenderloin with olive oil, and then roll the tenderloin in the spices on a piece of wax paper. Bake for 40 minutes or until no longer pink inside.

Makes eight servings
Calories: 302
Fat: 14g

HEALTHY SPINACH PIE

Spinach quiche is a favorite of mine, but I hate all the fat and calories it contains. This recipe, because of the cheese and pie crust, gives me the feeling of eating quiche without the fat and calories.

**Prep and cooking time:
40 minutes**

4	ounces Second Nature egg product
¾	cup nonfat cottage cheese
¾	cup shredded low-fat mozzarella
1	teaspoon olive oil
2	tablespoons Italian parsley
6	ounces mushrooms, sliced
1	tablespoon lemon juice
1	teaspoon black ground pepper
12	ounces fresh spinach, chopped
	Dash of nutmeg and salt
2	tablespoons chopped fresh chives
	9-inch pie crust

Preheat oven to 350°.

In a large bowl, mix together the egg product, cottage cheeese, mozzarella, and parsley.

In a large skillet, heat oil over medium heat. Add the mushrooms, lemon juice, pepper and salt, and sauté until tender. Add the spinach and nutmeg, cover for 2 minutes. Remove cover and sauté for 1 more minute. Spinach should be cooked. Remove from heat and stir in chives. Cool for 3 minutes.

Combine all mixtures and pour into 9-inch pie crust. Bake for 30 minutes or until the top is lightly browned.

Cool for 10 to 15 minutes before serving.

**Makes eight servings
Calories: 85
Fat: 4g**

CHICKEN NORMANDY

This is delicious served with white and wild rice mix. You can use a packaged rice mix and discard the spice packet.

	Butter-flavored vegetable spray
4	boneless, skinless chicken breast halves (about 4 ounces each)
2	medium Granny Smith apples, unpeeled, cored, sliced
6	green onions and tops, sliced
2/3	cup apple cider or unsweetened apple juice
2	teaspoons chicken bouillon crystals
1-1/2	teaspoons dried sage leaves
2/3	cup 2% milk
2	teaspoons flour
1-3/4	teaspoons Equal for Recipes or 6 packets Equal sweetener or 1/4 cup Equal Spoonful
	Sage or parsley sprigs, for garnish

Spray large skillet with cooking spray; heat over medium heat until hot. Sauté chicken breasts until browned, 3 to 5 minutes on each side. Season to taste with salt and pepper.

Add apples, onions, apple cider, bouillon, and sage to skillet; heat to boiling. Reduce heat and simmer, covered, until chicken is tender, 10 to 12 minutes. Remove chicken and apples to serving platter. Continue simmering cider mixture until almost gone.

Mix milk, flour, and Equal, in glass measuring cup; pour into skillet. Heat to boiling; boil, stirring constantly, until thickened, about 1 minute. Season to taste with salt and pepper; pour over chicken and apples. Garnish with sage.

Makes 4 servings
Calories per serving: 240
Fat: 2g

GRAPEFRUIT AND BLACK BEAN SALAD

	Lettuce leaves
2	Florida grapefruit, peeled and thinly sliced and seeded
1	15-ounce can black beans, rinsed and drained
1	medium cucumber, halved lengthwise and sliced
1	cup cubed papaya, drained
2	ounces reduced-fat Monterey Jack cheese, cut into 1/4-inch cubes
1/3	cup frozen Florida grapefruit juice concentrate, thawed
1/4	cup water
2	tablespoons snipped fresh cilantro
2	teaspoons honey
1/4	teaspoon ground cumin

Line 4 salad plates with lettuce. Arrange grapefruit slices on plates. Arrange beans, cucumber, and papaya in mounds on lettuce. Sprinkle with cheese.

For dressing, in a screw-top jar combine thawed grapefruit juice concentrate, water, cilantro, honey, and cumin. Cover and shake well. Drizzle some of the dressing over the salads. Pass remaining dressing.

Makes 4 servings
Calories: 219
Fat: 4 g

GINGER AND LIME CHICKEN

What a tangy delight! Lime juice is used to moisten chicken and then accented with ginger! This recipe is quick and easy and can add life to that boring chicken breast.

**Prep and cooking time:
28 minutes**

6	boneless chicken breasts
1/4	cup Rose's lime juice
3/4	cup red currant jelly
2	tablespoons light soy sauce
2 1/2	tablespoons dry sherry
	Pinch each cayenne pepper, chili powder, paprika, and garlic powder
1/2	teaspoon ground black pepper
1	tablespoon minced fresh ginger
2	tablespoons orange juice
1	tablespoon I Can't Believe It's Not Butter Light

Preheat oven to 375°.

Place chicken in a glass baking dish.

Blend remaining ingredients in a small saucepan, cook over medium heat until jelly is dissolved. Pour sauce over chicken and cook for 20 minutes or until done.

**Makes six servings
Calories: 200
Fat: 6g**

TOMATO MELT WITH
LOW-FAT MOZZARELLA CHEESE SANDWICH

Tomatoes are superb in the summertime, and make for great quick and easy sandwiches.

**Prep and cooking time:
5 minutes**

4   large tomato slices
2   pieces oat bran bread
4   slices part-skim mozzarella cheese

Preheat toaster oven to broil.

Put 2 tomato slices on each slice of bread and then top each with a mozzarella slice. Broil open faced in the toaster oven until the cheese is melted.

**Makes 2 servings
Calories: 175
Fat: 7.5g**

QUICK QUESADILLAS

A quesadilla is a take on a grilled cheese sandwich but Tex-Mex style. As easy to do for the whole family as for one; just double or triple the recipe. I love this for a quick snack!

**Prep and cooking time:
2 minutes**

1   flour tortilla
1   ounce low-fat Jack cheese
1   tablespoon salsa

Place thin slices of cheese in the center of the tortilla. Add the salsa, fold in the sides and roll up.

Place on a paper plate or microwavable dish, cover with wax paper, and microwave on high for 1 minute.

**Makes one serving
Calories: 165
Fat: 4g**

TORTELLINI WITH CHICKEN AND CHERRY TOMATOES

This wonderful Italian dish will make your mouth water. The mixture of tomatoes and chicken broth will make you think twice before eating a cream sauce.

Prep and cooking time: 30 minutes

9	ounce package of cheese or vegetable tortellini
4	boneless, skinless, chicken breasts
8	cherry tomatoes, halved
1	can low-fat chicken broth
3	tablespoons olive oil
1½	tablespoons white wine vinegar
2	tablespoons balsamic vinegar
1	tablespoon ground black pepper
	Dash salt

Preheat oven to 350°.

Cook pasta 5 minutes in boiling water, drain, place in bowl.

Place chicken in a glass baking dish and pour chicken broth over chicken. Bake chicken for 20–25 minutes.

Cool for 10 minutes, then slice chicken into bite-size strips. In a bowl, add pasta, chicken, and cherry tomato halves. Pour dressing over. Serve immediately.

**Makes four servings
Calories: 253
Fat: 6.4g**

EASY SALSA CHICKEN

I'm always looking for a new way to bake chicken and this one is so delicious and so easy you'll love it. It's light and spicy.

Prep and cooking time:
30 minutes

4   boneless skinless chicken breasts
1   jar of medium-hot salsa verde (green salsa)

Preheat oven to 400°.

Place each piece of chicken in a piece of foil and top with a generous amount of salsa. Fold foil and place on cookie sheet. Bake for 30 minutes.

Makes four servings
Calories: 160
Fat: 4g

PENNE WITH FRESH ROMA TOMATOES

Pasta is a great source of carbohydrates. It gives you the stamina to make it through a busy day. I love this pasta dish because anything with goat cheese tastes so good! I like to serve this dish at lunch when a couple of my girlfriends come over. It's good hot or cold. Goat cheese is soft and only mildly tart.

Prep and cooking time:
20 minutes

3   tablespoons olive oil
2   tablespoons lemon juice
1   tablespoon white wine vinegar
½   teaspoon crushed black pepper
¼   teaspoon light salt
16   ounces cooked penne pasta
5   fresh roma tomatoes, chopped into pieces
5   small slices fresh low-fat goat cheese (optional)

Mix olive oil, lemon juice, white wine vinegar, crushed black pepper, and salt in small bowl. Pour over pasta, and add the roma tomatoes and low-fat goat cheese.

Makes six servings
Calories: 280
Fat: 7g

STEAMED VEGETABLE MEDLEY

To me, there's nothing as fulfilling as a mix of fresh vegetables, steamed just right. You don't need butter or a thick, fatty sauce. A squeeze of lemon will enhance the flavor. If you don't have a vegetable steamer, just bring ½ inch water to a boil in a pan with a tight-fitting lid. Steam right in the pan according to directions. That's all there is to it.

Prep and cooking time:
8 minutes

4   medium carrots, pared, cut into 1½-inch sticks
10 ounces green beans, trimmed
1   small onion, slivered
1   red pepper, stemmed, seeded, slivered
    Salt
    Pepper
    Lemon juice from ½ lemon

Place carrots, beans, and onion in steamer set over boiling water. Steam, tightly covered, until not quite tender (5 to 6 minutes). Add peppers and toss.

Makes two servings
Calories: 150
Fat: 1g

ALL-RED FRUIT SALAD

What a delicious treat on a hot summer day!

Prep time: 10 minutes

1	cup red grapes
1	cup strawberries, sliced
1	cup red apples, diced
1	cup red plums, sliced
1	cup red raspberries
½	cup golden raisins
¼	cup vanilla low-fat yogurt
¼	cup nonfat cottage cheese
1	tablespoon honey
1	tablespoon lemon juice
1	tablespoon orange juice

Combine all fruit in a bowl. Blend all other ingredients in a blender until smooth. Pour over fruit. Let chill for 1 hour before serving.

Makes eight servings
Calories: 180
Fat: 2g

COOL GAZPACHO

If you're unusually hungry and nothing seems to whet your appetite, this soup is a tasty way to fill you up. It contains only 50 calories and it's great to keep frozen and pop in the microwave for a quick lunch or snack.

Prep time: 20 minutes

2	red tomatoes, peeled, seeded, diced
2	red peppers, diced
1	cucumber, sliced
3	cloves garlic, chopped fine
½	cup red onion, chopped fine
1	tablespoon lime juice
1	cup tomato juice
⅛	cup olive oil

1   hot pepper, deseeded and chopped
$\frac{1}{2}$ cup cilantro, chopped
$\frac{1}{4}$ teaspoon white pepper
     Pinch salt
     Pinch Tabasco
$\frac{1}{4}$ cup cold water

Blend all together in a food processor until smooth. Chill for 2 to 3 hours.

**Makes eight servings
Calories: 50
Fat: 3g**

ENERGIZING BREAKFASTS

BUTTERMILK PANCAKES

Pancakes are always a hit, and this recipe gives you a rich, fluffy cake. You can also add fresh fruit to the batter to make them extra special. I some times add blueberries, banana slices, diced or grated apple, sliced f strawberries, or even red raspberries.

**Prep and cooking time:
10 minutes**

1   cup reduced-fat Bisquick
2   egg whites or $\frac{1}{4}$ cup egg substitute
$\frac{1}{2}$ cup skim milk or nonfat buttermilk
1   teaspoon fat-free sour cream

Mix all ingredients and beat until well blended. P
hot griddle sprayed with cooking spray. Cook u
cook until golden. Makes 8 pancakes.

**Makes two servings
Calories: 200
Fat: 2.5g**

SCRAMBLED MEXICAN EGG WHITE

No fat, hardly any calories, and lots of protein! There is no better way to begin your morning—with zest!

**Prep and cooking time:
5 minutes**

3   egg whites
2   tablespoons thick, chunky salsa

In bowl whisk egg whites and add salsa. Heat frying pan and spray with cooking spray. Scramble eggs in pan until done to your taste.

**Makes one serving
Calories: 58
Fat: 0g**

BANANA-TOASTED ENGLISH MUFFIN

This fabulous recipe gives you two taste treats in one. First you have a crunchy toasted muffin and, then, a topping that tastes like flambéed bananas! I have tried it with raisin and other English muffins and they're all great.

ling time:

English muffins
honey

roiler and remove.

with cooking spray. Arrange banana slices on
and sprinkle with cinnamon. Spray tops of
g spray.

ntil tops are browned.

NUTTY CRUNCH CINNAMON MUFFINS

Nothing is better on a cold winter morning than a hot muffin with a cup of hot tea or coffee and these are great because you can make them ahead of time and freeze them. All you have to do is pop them in the oven or microwave and enjoy. A great quick breakfast for your children.

**Prep and cooking time:
30 minutes**

2½   cups all-purpose flour, sifted
1¼   cups brown sugar, firmly packed
½   teaspoon salt
1   teaspoon ginger
1   tablespoon cinnamon
½   cup canola oil
¼   cup chopped walnuts
2   teaspoons baking powder
½   teaspoon baking soda
4   ounces Second Nature egg product
¾   cup skim milk

Preheat oven to 350°.

Spray muffin tins with cooking spray. In a large bowl, stir in the flour, sugar, salt, ginger, and one-half the cinnamon. Add the canola oil and mix well. Mixture will be somewhat dry.

Remove one-half the mixture to a small bowl, and add the nuts and remaining cinnamon. Set aside.

To the remaining flour mixture, add baking powder and baking soda. Stir well. Add the egg product and skim milk until well blended.

Spoon the batter into the muffin tins, filling each cup two-thirds full. Sprinkle one-half tablespoon of the dry topping over each muffin.

Bake for 15 to 20 minutes or until a toothpick comes out clean. Cool f[or ?] minutes, then remove from tins.

**Makes sixteen muffins
Calories: 160
Fat: 5g**

HONEY AND CINNAMON BAKED APPLES

This is the simplest of recipes, and turns a healthy apple into an indulgence. Honey is much better for you than refined sugar. So, if you like it, use it instead of sugar whenever possible.

**Prep and cooking time:
25 minutes**

2	golden delicious apples, cored and quartered
¼	teaspoon cinnamon
2	tablespoons honey

Preheat oven to 350°.

Spray bottom of baking dish with cooking spray. Arrange apple slices on bottom. Spray top of apples with cooking spray, drizzle honey over top. Sprinkle cinnamon over apples.

Bake for 20 minutes.

**Makes two servings
Calories: 70
Fat: 0g**

ENERGY SHAKE

Don't have time for breakfast? Then make my shake for your drive to work. It's fast, easy, and much better for you than that doughnut at the office.

Prep time: 3 minutes

1	cup skim milk
½	cup strawberries (fresh or frozen, full size, about 5)
½	banana
¼	cup nonfat plain yogurt
	cubes

...nder for about 1 minute. Ready to eat!

363

PEACHY ORANGE YOGURT WHIP

Prep time: 5 minutes

1	8-ounce carton plain nonfat yogurt
1/4	cup frozen orange juice concentrate
1/4	cup skim milk
3 or 4	packets Equal sweetener or 1 to 1-1/4 teaspoons Equal for Recipes
2	cups frozen sliced peaches
1	cup ice cubes

In a blender container, combine yogurt, juice concentrate, milk, and Equal. With the blender running, add peaches a few at a time through opening in lid. Blend till smooth, then add ice cubes one at a time through opening in lid, blending until slushy. Pour into glasses.

**Makes 4 7-ounce
servings
Calories: 99
Fat: 0 g**

SPEEDY NONFAT DESSERTS

RUBY POACHED PEARS WITH GINGER CRUNCH

You get all the nutrients from fruit here, with a special twist that really satisfies for dessert.

**Prep and cooking time:
10 minutes**

2   ripe pears, cut lengthwise into 4 halves and cored
2   cups low-calorie cran-raspberry juice
2   tablespoons reduced-sugar raspberry jam or preserves
6   gingersnap cookies, coarsely crumbled

In a medium saucepan or a skillet, bring pear halves and their juice to a boil. Reduce heat and simmer 5 to 8 minutes or until pears are tender when pierced with a knife.

Just before serving, mix raspberry preserves and gingersnap cookie crumbs. (Don't do this too early because the cookies will get soggy.)

Place each pear half on a serving plate with the well side up. Fill each well with an equal portion of raspberry-gingersnap mixture. Serve immediately.

**Makes 4 servings
Calories: 134
Fat: 1.4g**

SWEET-AND-WARM LEMON YOGURT SAUCE

There are some great low-fat baked goods on the market now, so it's easy to whip up a quick sauce like this, and have an instant dessert.

**Prep and cooking time:
7 minutes**

1   6-ounce container frozen lemonade concentrate, thawed
1   tablespoon cornstarch
2   tablespoons sugar
1   cup nonfat plain yogurt
4   1-inch thick slices low-fat pound cake (such as Entenmann's)
1   tablespoon sliced almonds, toasted

For the sauce, mix all of the ingredients together in a medium microwavable bowl. Microwave on 100% for 3 to 5 minutes, stirring after 2 minutes. Sauce should be thickened and smooth.

Serve warm over pound cake slices. Sprinkle each dessert with equal portions of toasted almonds.

Makes four servings
Calories: 272
Fat: .9g

WHOLE-WHEAT CHOCOLATE CHIP COOKIES

If you're craving chocolate, try these. They're a chocolate lover's dream. They're so easy to make that even my children enjoy making them.

Prep and cooking time:
25 minutes

½	cup canola oil
½	cup brown sugar, packed firmly
½	cup white sugar
1	teaspoon vanilla extract
1	tablespoon water
4	ounces Second Nature egg product
1¼	cup whole-wheat flour
1	cup all-purpose flour
1	teaspoon baking soda
½	teaspoon salt
8	ounces semi-sweet chocolate chips
¾	cup chopped walnuts

Preheat oven to 375°.

Combine oil, sugars, vanilla, and water in a large bowl. Beat in the egg product.

In separate bowl combine flours, baking soda, and salt. Gradually add this to the wet mixture, blending well. Stir in chips and nuts.

Drop, by tablespoons, onto ungreased cookie sheet. Bake 8 to 10 minutes.

Makes 3 dozen cookies
Calories: 80
Fat: 3g

FATLESS CHOCOLATE CAPPUCCINO CUPS

If you thought marshmallow treats were just for kids, think again. These delicious darlings are fat free! Sometimes, you deserve a real special treat. Remember, sugar does have calories, so you shouldn't eat the whole batch yourself. It's best to use nonstick muffin tins if you have them. Aside from saving a few calories, you save clean-up time.

**Prep and cooking time:
5 minutes**

5   ounces (about 20) regular marshmallows
2   tablespoons unsweetened cocoa powder
1   teaspoon vanilla extract
3   cups Rice Krispies breakfast cereal
8   tablespoons frozen nonfat yogurt (cappuccino or coffee flavor)
8   large fresh strawberries

If using regular muffin tins, spray 8 of the cups with cooking spray.

Place marshmallows in a medium microwave-safe bowl and microwave on 100% power for one minute. Stir in cocoa and microwave 30 seconds longer if marshmallows have not melted. Stir in cereal and vanilla.

Divide the marshmallow-cereal mixture into eight of the muffin cups and, with greased fingers, press into the cups and around the edges to create a well or pocket in each center. Let firm at room temperature or, for faster firming, place in the freezer for about 4 minutes.

Just before serving, gently lift the chocolate mixture out of the muffin tin and place 1 tablespoon of nonfat frozen yogurt in the well of each. Top each tablespoon of nonfat yogurt with 1 sliced strawberry. Serve immediately.

**Makes six servings
Calories: 127
Fat: .43g**

CHOCOLATE MOUSSE PIE

YUM! You will never miss the fat and calories in this chocolate mousse pie. Whip this up a few hours before having a dinner party—freeze and it's ready to serve! See if any of your guests realize how light this pie is! I guarantee you will have your guests feeling guilty. Don't tell!

Prep time: 5 minutes
Freeze: 4-5 hrs

4	ounces Bakers sweet chocolate
½	cup skim milk
8	ounce package light cream cheese, softened
8	ounce container light Cool Whip
8-inch	Oreo cookie crust
2	tablespoons sugar

Melt chocolate with 2 tablespoons skim milk over low heat.

Beat cream cheese and sugar. Add remaining milk and blend in chocolate well. Gradually add light Cool Whip until all ingredients are blended.

Pour into Oreo cookie crust. Freeze 4 to 5 hours before serving.

Makes eight servings
Calories: 220
Fat: 5.5g

FROZEN WATERMELON BALLS

Great for the summertime, and for the kids!

Prep time: 10 minutes

1	whole watermelon, seedless
10–15	Popsicle sticks

Cut the watermelon in half. Using an ice cream scooper, scoop out rounds of watermelon and place in a bowl. Push a Popsicle stick into the middle of each watermelon ball, freeze overnight.

Makes twenty servings
Calories: 40
Fat: 0g

SAUCES AND DRESSINGS

DENISE'S CREAMY SALAD DRESSING

Salad dressings are one of the biggest challenges when it comes to eliminating all the fat from the oil while keeping a full flavor that will coat well. Yogurt is a fabulous solution to this problem . . . plus it gives you calcium. This dressing is rich, creamy, and loaded with taste from the onion, garlic and herbs. Fat-free dressings may look tempting in the supermarket, but read the ingredients and nutritional breakdown. Usually sugar and sodium have been greatly increased and, of course, these dressings contain additives and thickeners to replace the oil. But not this homemade salad dressing!

Prep time: 5 minutes

- 1¼ cup plain nonfat yogurt
- ¼ cup water
- 3 tablespoons minced onion
- 3 teaspoons chopped fresh dill
- 1 clove garlic, minced
- ¼ teaspoon basil
- ¼ teaspoon oregano
- ¼ teaspoon pepper

Blend all ingredients in bowl. Cover and refrigerate until ready to serve.

**Makes eight servings
Calories per serving: 25
Fat: 0g**

GRAPEFRUIT-MINT DRESSING

Serve this fruity, tangy dressing over fruit salad or meat or poultry salad.

Prep time: 2 minutes

- 1/2 cup Florida grapefruit juice
- 1/2 cup salad oil
- 2 tablespoons light corn syrup
- 1 tablespoon snipped fresh mint or 1/2 teaspoon dried mint, crushed

**Makes about 1 cup
Calories per 1 tablespoon
serving: 40
Fat: 3 g**

In a screw-top jar, combine grapefruit juice, oil, corn syrup, and mint. Cover and shake well to mix. Chill in the refrigerator at least 1 hour before using. Shake well before serving.

SASSY SWEET AND SOUR DRESSING

Prep time: 5 minutes

Use 1 tablespoon poppy seeds instead of celery seed for a different taste!

1	cup plain lowfat yogurt
1/3	cup cider vinegar
2	tablespoons finely chopped onion
1-3/4	teaspoons Equal for Recipes or 6 packets Equal sweetener or 1/4 cup Equal Spoonful
1	teaspoon dry mustard
1	teaspoon celery seed
1/2	teaspoon salt

Process all ingredients in food processor or blender until smooth and well mixed. Refrigerate until ready to serve.

**Makes 12 servings
Calories per 2 tablespoon
serving: 19
Fat 0 g**

TERIYAKI MARINADE

Prep time: 2 minutes

This marinade is ideal for well-trimmed pork chops or skinless chicken pieces. Allow them to marinate for 4 hours for maximum flavor!

1/3	cup sodium-reduced soy sauce
2	tablespoons Equal Spoonful
2	tablespoons white vinegar
1	teaspoon ground ginger
1/2	teaspoon garlic powder

In small bowl, whisk together soy sauce, Equal Spoonful, vinegar, ginger, and garlic powder. Use to marinate meat or chicken. Reserve small amount of marinade for basting during broiling or grilling.

**Makes about 1/2 cup
Fat: 0 g**

371

LOW-FAT GUACAMOLE

Do you love guacamole with your favorite Mexican recipes, but hate all the fat? Then you'll love this low-fat, quick recipe. Remember, avocados have lots of fat so pick the smallest avocados you can find.

Prep time: 5 minutes

½   cup nonfat sour cream
4   avocados
1   small red onion
1   jalapeño pepper, seeded
3   cloves garlic, minced
1   tablespoon lime juice
   Dash Tabasco
¼   cup cilantro
2   cups diced tomatoes

Combine all the ingredients, except tomatoes, in a food processor. Blend well. Add diced tomatoes.

Refrigerate for at least 1 hour.

Makes three cups
Calories per
3 tablespoons: 15
Fat: 2g

SALSA ON THE GO

Prep time: 3 minutes

1   16-ounce jar of your favorite salsa
1   15-ounce can black beans, drained
1   4-ounce package sweet corn, thawed
2   tablespoons fresh cilantro

Mix all together. Chill before serving.

Makes four cups
Calories per ¼ cup: 35
Fat: .6g

PESTO WITH CILANTRO

Prep time: 5 minutes

$\frac{1}{2}$ cup unsalted pecans
$\frac{1}{2}$ cup parsley
$\frac{1}{2}$ cup cilantro
3   cloves garlic, chopped
$2\frac{1}{2}$ tablespoons light olive oil
Pinch salt

Blend ingredients in food processor.

**Makes about one cup.
Calories per
$1\frac{1}{2}$ tablespoons: 40
Fat: 4g**

SKINNY "CREAM" SAUCE

To use just about anywhere—soups, sauces, and stews. Add a squeeze of lemon to make a fat-free sour cream for baked potatoes.

Prep time: 3 minutes

1   cup part-skim ricotta cheese
2   tablespoons flour
1   tablespoon skim milk

Mix all the ingredients in a food processor or blender until smooth.

**Makes about one cup
Calories per
tablespoon: 20
Fat: 2g**

HUMMUS DIP AND SPREAD

Great to serve with pita wedges or to dip with raw vegetables. Also, you can spread it on a sandwich instead of mustard or mayo.

Prep time: 3 minutes

1   can chickpeas (garbanzos)
1   tablespoon lemon juice
2   tablespoons tahini* (sesame seed paste)
1   clove garlic, chopped or pressed
2   tablespoons water

Drain and rinse chickpeas. Blend all ingredients in a food processor or blender until smooth.

*Tahini is available in health-food stores, Middle Eastern markets, and some supermarkets

Makes eight servings
Calories per
2 tablespoons: 74
Fat: 2 g

STRAWBERRY JAM

2   quarts fresh or frozen strawberries (do not use strawberries frozen in syrup)
1   package (1-3/4 ounces) no-sugar-needed pectin
4   tablespoons Equal for Recipes or 40 packets Equal sweetener or
    1-2/3 cup Equal Spoonful

Mash strawberries to make 4 cups pulp. Combine strawberries and pectin in large saucepan. Let stand 10 minutes, stirring frequently. Cook and stir over medium heat until mixture comes to a boil. Cook and stir 1 minute more. Remove from heat; stir in Equal. Skim off foam if necessary.

Immediately fill containers, leaving 1/2 inch head space. Seal and let stand at room temperature several hours or until set. Store up to 2 weeks in refrigerator or 6 months in freezer.

Makes 4 (1/2 pint) jars
Calories per
tablespoon: 8
Fat: 0 g

374

HEALTHY SANDWICHES

- 1 slice of roast beef and tomato with a little horseradish.

- Sliced chicken with tomato, lettuce, and mustard.

- Tunafish made with light mayonnaise, chopped celery, and onion.

- Junior club—Sliced chicken or turkey, crisp turkey bacon, lettuce, tomato, and light mayonnaise

- Sliced cold meatloaf (made with white turkey meat) with cocktail sauce or catsup.

- Corned beef with chives, cucumbers, and sliced tomato.

- Sliced ham, chicken, crisp turkey bacon, lettuce, and tomato, topped with fat-free Thousand Island dressing.

- Turkey burger, mustard, thinly sliced red onion, and dill pickle.

- Ham with mustard-dill sauce.

- Open-faced mushroom sandwich. Cook mushrooms and onions in microwave for 4 minutes. Toast an English muffin. Pile mushrooms and little onion on top (you can add any type of light cheese; I like skim milk mozzarella). Place under broiler until cheese melts.

- Open-faced smoked salmon with capers, lemon juice, and cracked pepper on rye.

- Denise's vegetarian special—Hummus, sprouts, and tomato on whole-wheat pita bread.

APPETIZERS

ASPARAGUS HAM ROLL UPS

Boiled low-fat ham, sliced very thin
Asparagus
Mustard-dill sauce (p. 371)

Blanch asparagus for a few minutes and plunge in ice water to retain crispness. Spread ham with mustard-dill sauce. Place an asparagus spear at one end and roll up.

SMOKED FISH SPREAD

Use any good smoked white fish. Flake fish in a bowl. Squeeze lime juice over fish. Add a little horseradish and a little light mayonnaise to bind. Serve with crackers or toast.

MEXICAN QUICKIE

Mix fat-free cottage cheese with salsa, and serve with fat-free tortilla chips

FOR ASPARAGUS LOVERS

When asparagus are in season, clean and trim asparagus to the same length. Blanch for a few minutes until they are fork-tender but still crisp. Plunge into ice water to stop cooking. Serve with mustard-dill sauce or horseradish sauce. Place on a platter and arrange in a sunburst pattern. Very pretty and very low in calories.

CHEESY GARLIC TOAST

I love garlic toast with my pasta or as an appetizer, but I hate all the fat and calories. To make it low fat and yummy, take a piece of French bread, spread ricotta cheese over it, and sprinkle with garlic and onion powder. Place it in oven on broil or toast it in toaster oven until crispy.

OVEN-FRIED POTATOES

My children love french fries (as do I), but I hate feeding them extremely high-fat foods, so I make these. Just take a potato and slice it thin. Dip in 1 beaten egg white mixed with onion powder and pepper. Bake on 450 degrees for 30 minutes on a nonstick cookie sheet.

STUFFED BELGIAN ENDIVE

**Prep and chill time:
20 minutes**

Easy as 1-2-3. Low fat and quick, for a delicious appetizer. You can vary this recipe by adding chopped tomatoes or chopped red peppers.

4   Belgian endives, washed and leaves separated
8   ounce package light cream cheese, softened
5   chives, chopped

Mix the cream cheese and chives and spread onto the endive. Refrigerate for 15 minutes. Serve.

**Makes twenty servings
Calories: 23
Fat: 2g**

HELPFUL TIPS

Low-Fat Substitutions

- Use evaporated skim milk in place of cream, especially in soups and casseroles.
- Use plain yogurt to replace sour cream in all recipes. You might need to add a table-spoon of flour to keep it from getting runny.
- Use plain yogurt to replace mayonnaise in some of your recipes, or just try light or fat-free mayonnaise.
- Use low-fat cottage cheese in casserole recipes that call for cheddar cheese

More Great Tips

- To thicken any sauce, use cornstarch.
- To thin a sauce, use wine.
- Do not wash berries until just before eating them.
- Soak eggplant in salt water for 20 minutes to remove bitterness.
- A dash of Lea & Perrins Worcestershire Sauce brings out the flavor of turkey meat—makes it taste like a hamburger.
- Squeeze a little lemon juice over avocados and fruit to prevent discoloring.
- If your fingers get smelly from chopping garlic, squeeze a little lemon on them. Sometimes I squish my fingers in a lemon half—it takes the smell right out.
- Add a pinch of baking soda to greens to remove any bitterness.
- Add a dash of sugar in boiling water to cook broccoli to help it retain its bright green color.
- To keep snow peas crisp, plunge in boiling water until they turn bright green. Remove and pour ice-cold water over them immediately.

JUMPSTART

LOW-FAT HEALTHY CHOICES

have compiled a list of some of my favorite product choices. I hope this will save you time at the grocery store. Of course, this is not a complete list; if I have left out your favorite brand, just check the labels and compare fat content and calories.

BREADS

Choose whole-grain breads over refined whites, because those highest in fiber keep your intestinal tract in working order, just like a scrub brush. Here are a few tips for buying breads.
- Make sure the first ingredient is whole-wheat or another whole-grain flour, like rye flour.
- Make sure that there are no more than two grams of fat per slice.
- Make sure that there are no more than 200 milligrams of sodium per slice.

Product	Serving Size	Calories	Fat
Wheat			
Country Hearth:			
Honey Wheat Berry	1 slice	80	.5 gm
Oat Bran n' Fiber	1 slice	75	.2 gm
7 Whole Grain	1 slice	80	.2 gm
Honey Nut n' Oat Bran	1 slice	85	1 gm
100% Whole Wheat	1 slice	60	.5 gm
Pepperidge Farm:			
100% Whole Wheat	1 slice	90	1 gm
Nine Grain	1 slice	90	1 gm
Crunchy Grains	1 slice	90	1 gm
Very Thin Sliced Wheat	1 slice	36	.5 gm
Soft 100% Whole Wheat	1 slice	60	.5 gm
Whole Wheat Thin Sliced	1 slice	60	1 gm
Wonder Soft:			
100% Whole Wheat	1 slice	55	1 gm
Roman Meal:			
100% Whole Wheat	1 slice	60	1 gm
French			
Francisco	1 slice	55	1 gm
Pioneer	1 slice	60	.5 gm
Webbers:			
Plain	1 slice	60	1 gm
Sourdough	1 slice	60	.5 gm
Rye			
Jewish Rye	1 slice	70	1 gm
Extra Sour Rye	1 slice	70	1 gm
Dark Rye	1 slice	70	1 gm

Product	Serving Size	Calories	Fat
Pita			
Thomas':			
White Pita Plain	1 whole	150	1 gm
Sourdough Pita	1 whole	140	1 gm
Mr. Pita:			
Plain	1 whole	130	.5 gm
100% Whole Wheat	1 whole	130	1 gm
Bagels			
Fresh (any flavor except egg)	1 whole	210	2 gm
English Muffins			
Thomas':			
Raisin	1 whole	140	1 gm
Oat Bran	1 whole	120	1 gm
Sourdough	1 whole	120	1 gm
Plain	1 whole	120	1 gm
Tortillas			
Light Flour	1 whole	70	1 gm
Corn	1 whole	60	.5 gm
French Rolls			
Plain	1 roll	210	2.5 gm
With Sesame	1 roll	220	3.5 gm
Hamburger Buns			
Country Hearth:			
Oat Bran	1 bun	100	.5 gm
Sesame	1 bun	100	1 gm
Roman Meal:			
Plain	1 bun	110	2 gm

Most of these brands of products are sold nationally or will be soon. If you can't find them in your grocery store, look for brands with comparable calories and fat.

DAIRY

Product	Serving Size	Calories	Fat
Yogurt			
Dannon:			
Light Fat Free	8 oz.	100	0 gm
Blended	6 oz.	150	0 gm
Light 'n Crunchy	8 oz.	140-150	0 gm
Yoplait:			
Light Fat Free	6 oz.	90	0 gm
Original	6 oz.	180	1.5 gm
Custard Style	6 oz.	170	2.5 gm
Weight Watchers:			
Fat Free	8 oz.	90	0 gm
Colombo:			
Fat Free	8 oz.	200	0 gm
Lucerne:			
Nonfat	6 oz.	90	0 gm
Low-fat	8 oz.	250	2.5 gm
Jello:			
Bits & Yogurt	6 oz.	220	1.5 gm
Lowfat	4.4 oz.	130	1 gm
Cheese			
Alpine Lace:			
Mozzarella	¼ cup	45	0 gm
Cheddar	¼ cup	45	0 gm
Healthy Choice:			
Mozzarella	¼ cup	45	0 gm
Cheddar	¼ cup	45	0 gm
Philadelphia Free Cream Cheese	2 tbsp.	30	0 gm
Weight Watchers Fat Free:			
Parmesan	1 tbsp.	15	0 gm
Milk			
Skim	1 cup	80	0 gm

TOMATO SAUCES AND BEANS

Product	Serving Size	Calories	Fat
Pasta Sauce			
Prego:			
Zesta Basil Extra Chunky	½ cup	130	3 gm
Zesta Oregano Extra Chunky	½ cup	140	3 gm
Garden Combo Extra Chunky	½ cup	90	1 gm
Newman's Own:			
Spaghetti Sauce	½ cup	60	2 gm
Ragu:			
Traditional	½ cup	80	3.5 gm
Pizza Sauce			
Prego:			
Traditional Pizza Sauce	3 tbsp.	35	1 gm
Ragu:			
Pizza Sauce	¼ cup	30	1 gm
Pizza Quick Sauce	¼ cup	40	1.5 gm
Beans			
Refried, Vegetarian	½ cup	120	2.5 gm
Refried, Zesty Fat Free	½ cup	100	0 gm
Refried, Traditional Fat Free	½ cup	120	0 gm
S&W:			
Black Beans	½ cup	70	0 gm
Progresso:			
Black Beans	½ cup	100	1 gm
Canned Tomatoes	½ cup	25	0 gm

PIZZA

Product	Serving Size	Calories	Fat
Stouffer's:			
Lean Cuisine Deluxe	1 pizza	330	6 gm
Lean Cuisine Pepperoni	1 pizza	330	7 gm
Healthy Choice:			
Cheese French Bread	1 pizza	310	4 gm
Supreme French Bread	1 pizza	340	6 gm
Tombstone:			
Light Vegetable	⅕ pizza	240	7 gm
Weight Watchers:			
Deluxe Combo	1 pizza	380	11 gm
Lean Pockets:			
Pepperoni	1 pocket	270	8 gm
Ellio's:			
Cheese	1 pizza	320	5 gm
Just Help Yourself:			
Cheese French Bread	1 pizza	280	4.5 gm
Pizza Grande	1 pizza	310	7 gm
Pepperoni French Bread	1 pizza	310	7 gm
Vegetarian French Bread	1 pizza	300	5 gm

CONDIMENTS

Product	Serving Size	Calories	Fat
Pace Thick & Chunky Salsa (mild or medium)	2 tbsp.	10	0 gm
Guiltless Gourmet:			
Black Bean Dip	2 tbsp.	30	0 gm
Pinto Bean Dip	2 tbsp.	35	0 gm
Land O Lakes:			
No Fat Salsa Dip	2 tbsp.	25	0 gm
Ranch Dip	2 tbsp.	30	0 gm
French Onion Dip	2 tbsp.	30	0 gm

Product	Serving Size	Calories	Fat
French's Mustard	1 tsp.	0	0 gm
Grey Poupon Dijon	1 tsp.	5	0 gm
Bullseye Barbecue Sauce	1 tbsp.	30	0 gm
Vinegar (any brand)	1 tsp.	5	0 gm
Hunts Catsup	1 tsp.	15	0 gm
Heinz Catsup	1 tsp.	15	0 gm

Light Mayonnaise

Product	Serving Size	Calories	Fat
Kraft Light	1 tbsp.	40	3 gm
Miracle Whip Light	1 tbsp.	40	3 gm
Hellman's/Best Foods			
Low Fat	1 tbsp.	25	1 gm
Light	1 tbsp.	50	5 gm

SALAD DRESSING

Product	Serving Size	Calories	Fat
Kraft Free:			
Peppercorn Ranch	2 tbsp.	50	0 gm
Thousand Island	2 tbsp.	45	0 gm
Blue Cheese	2 tbsp.	45	0 gm
Honey Dijon	2 tbsp.	50	0 gm
Pritikin:			
Dijon Balsamic	1 tbsp.	6	0 gm
Honey Dijon	1 tbsp.	6	0 gm
Ranch	1 tbsp.	18	0 gm
Naturally Fresh Fat Free:			
Raspberry Vinaigrette	2 tbsp.	12	0 gm
Thousand Island	2 tbsp.	20	0 gm
Ranch	2 tbsp.	25	0 gm
Honey French	2 tbsp.	25	0 gm
Wishbone:			
Lite French Style	2 tbsp.	25	1 gm
Lite Creamy Italian	2 tbsp.	25	1 gm

SYRUPS

Product	Serving Size	Calories	Fat
Aunt Jemima Light	½ cup	100	0 gm
Mrs. Butterworth's Light	¼ cup	100	0 gm
Log Cabin Light	¼ cup	100	0 gm
Fruit Syrup	¼ cup	100	0 gm

JAMS AND PRESERVES

Product	Serving Size	Calories	Fat
Knott's Preserves:			
All Berry Flavors	1 tbsp.	20	0 gm
Smucker's:			
Low Sugar Preserves All Berry Flavors	1 tbsp.	25	0 gm
Simply Fruit (Strawberry, Boysenberry, Raspberry, Apricot) (full size)	1 tbsp.	50	0 gm

LUNCH MEATS AND TUNA

Product	Serving Size	Calories	Fat
Lunch Meats			
Oscar Mayer 96% Fat Free:			
Ham	3 slices	60	2.5 gm
Smoked Ham	3 slices	60	2.5 gm
Turkey Breast	3 slices	70	2.5 gm
Foster Farms:			
Turkey Pastrami	1 slice	35	1 gm
Turkey Ham	1 slice	30	1 gm
Smoked Turkey	1 slice	30	.5 gm

Product	Serving Size	Calories	Fat
Healthy Choice:			
Ham	6 slices	60	1.5 gm
Oven Roasted Turkey	6 slices	60	1.5 gm
Louis Rich:			
Turkey Ham	3 slices	80	2.5 gm
Smoked Turkey	3 slices	70	2 gm
Empire Kosher:			
Turkey Pastrami	3 slices	60	2 gm

Tuna Fish

Star Kist Solid White in Spring Water	3 oz. can	100	1 gm
Bumble Bee White in Spring Water	3 oz. can	100	1 gm

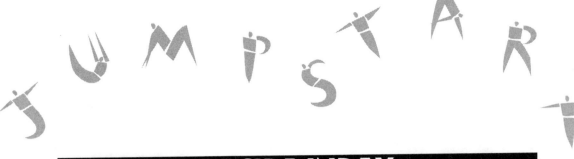

RECIPE INDEX

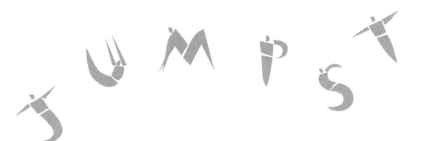

EXERCISE INDEX

ONCE AGAIN, DENISE AUSTIN DEFINES "SURVIVAL OF THE FITTEST."

"I get so many letters from people saying they just can't find the time to exercise. That's why I created Hit The Spot, a series of short, no-nonsense, 30-minute videos that everyone can afford . . . that every woman can find the time to use . . . and that zero in on the four areas my viewers are concerned about most—their arms, hips, thighs, and butts."   —**Denise Austin**

Now, after selling over five million videos, Denise Austin hits the spot with exactly what her fans want now—target spot workouts for hips, thighs, arms, and abs, all at a very affordable price.

IT'S A FACT . . .

Denise Austin is the **most watched and most listened to exercise expert in the world.** Her ESPN show, *Getting Fit with Denise Austin,* is seen by over one million people a day in the U.S. and countless more millions in 25 countries throughout the world.

To order call: 1-800-272-4214
PPI Entertainment Group, 88 St. Francis St., Newark, NJ 07105
Copyright © 1995 Parade Video/Peter Pan Industries, Inc.

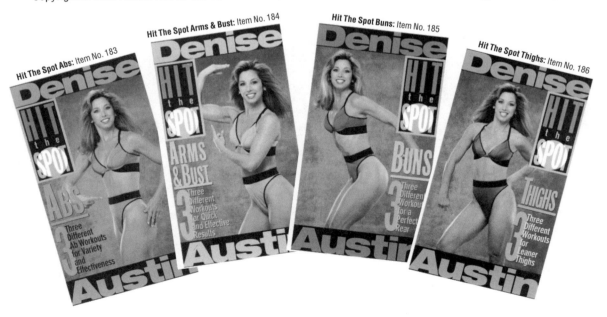

Hit The Spot Abs: Item No. 183
Hit The Spot Arms & Bust: Item No. 184
Hit The Spot Buns: Item No. 185
Hit The Spot Thighs: Item No. 186

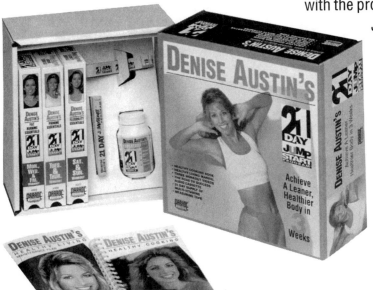

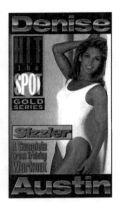
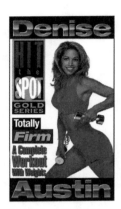
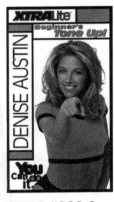
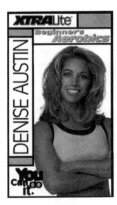

At 5'4" and 112 pounds, Denise Austin has been dubbed "America's favorite fitness expert." Born on February 13, 1957, Denise grew up in San Pedro, California. She started gymnastics at the age of twelve and earned an athletic scholarship to the University of Arizona. She transferred to California State University, Long Beach, where she earned her degree in 1979. She began teaching aerobic exercise classes in the Los Angeles area, earning her own local television program two years later. In 1983, Denise married Jeff Austin, a sports attorney and brother of tennis champ Tracy Austin. They moved to Washington, D.C., when Jeff accepted a job with a sports marketing firm.

From 1984–1988, Denise was the resident fitness expert on NBC's *Today* show. She also wrote a column for the *Washington Post* and received a prestigious award from the President's Council on Physical Fitness and Sports.

In 1987 Denise created her ESPN television show, *Getting Fit*. Today she is seen on Lifetime TV's *Denise Austin's Daily Workout* and she spends four months a year taping her popular program at the most beautiful resorts in the world, traveling with her family as often as possible. Her television show, which has aired for ten years, is rated #1 and is seen in eighty-two countries.

Denise has created twenty-two exercise videos, has her own line of workout equipment, and appears monthly on QVC. She can be seen motivating people on talk shows and is often used as a fitness expert for magazine articles. Her sensible, realistic, and enthusiastic approach to fitness (she works out only 30 minutes a day) and eating (she never skips a meal) has won fans throughout the United States, from whom she receives over 700 letters a week. Making a difference in the lives of people and her strong belief that she can inspire people to feel better about themselves are what gives Denise the energy to tackle challenges and achieve her success.

She was honored with the distinguished Alumna of 1997 by her alma mater and gave the commencement address to the graduates. She was appointed by Governor George Allen of Virginia as chairman of the Governor's Commission on Physical Fitness and Sports.

A dynamo of energy in a size 5, Denise Austin is a true motivator and has become a veritable fitness empire. But Denise believes her greatest achievement yet is being a mom to her two daughters, Kelly and Katie.